MEDICAL LASER ENDOSCOPY

Developments in Gastroenterology

VOLUME 10

The titles published in this series are listed at the end of this volume.

Medical
Laser Endoscopy

edited by

DENNIS M. JENSEN, M.D.
UCLA School of Medicine
Los Angeles, California, U.S.A.

and

JEAN-MARC BRUNETAUD, M.D.
Lille Medical School
Lille, France

Kluwer Academic Publishers
Dordrecht / Boston / London

Library of Congress Cataloging-in-Publication Data

Medical laser endoscopy / edited by Dennis M. Jensen, Jean Marc
Brunetaud.
          p.   cm. -- (Developments in gastroenterology ; v. 10)

      1. Laser endoscopy. 2. Gastrointestinal system--Diseases-
  -Treatment. 3. Gastrointestinal hemorrhage--Treatment. 4. Laser
  coagulation.   I. Jensen, Dennis.   II. Brunetaud, Jean Marc.
  III. Series: Developments in gastroenterology ; 10.
    [DNLM: 1. Endoscopy. 2. Lasers--therapeutic use.   W1 DE997VYB v.
  10 / WB480 M489]
  RD73.L3M43 1990
  617'.05--dc20
  DNLM/DLC
  for Library of Congress   89-26800

ISBN-13: 978-94-010-6714-0   e-ISBN-13: 978-94-009-0507-8
DOI:10.1007/ 978-94-009-0507-8

Published by Kluwer Academic Publishers,
P.O. Box 17, 3300 AA Dordrecht, The Netherlands.

Kluwer Academic Publishers incorporates
the publishing programmes of
D. Reidel, Martinus Nijhoff, Dr. W. Junk and MTP Press.

Sold and distributed in the U.S.A. and Canada
by Kluwer Academic Publishers,
101 Philip Drive, Norwell, MA 02061, U.S.A.

In all other countries, sold and distributed
by Kluwer Academic Publishers Group,
P.O. Box 322, 3300 AH Dordrecht, The Netherlands.

Printed on acid-free paper

TABLE OF CONTENTS

Atlas of color plates between pages 134 and 135

PREFACE

There has been incredible progress over the last decade in therapeutic endoscopy. Such therapies are either easier now than ten years ago or are possible when previously they were inconceivable. These advances have depended upon major improvements in diagnostic endoscopy for different subspecialties. Simultaneously, a major innovation for therapeutics through endoscopes is the application of medical lasers.

This book is written by renowned biophysicists and laser endoscopists of different subspecialties where the application of lasers has revolutionized medical care. In some cases treatments which were not previously possible are now routine. Laser palliation of obstructing tumors in different subspecialties is an example of this. In other cases, resective surgery is obviated by the application of lasers via endoscopy such as for the control of gastrointestinal bleeding. The authors of different medical or surgical subspecialties which use endoscopic lasers write about the pathology and clinical problems, their personal experience and results. However, they also emphasize their techniques of laser endoscopy through case examples, technical discussions, and colored illustrations. Their discussions will give the reader a better understanding about the role of laser treatment of different conditions compared to routine medical or surgical therapy. In several instances, randomized controlled trials involving medical lasers were discussed in this book because they fundamentally changed our understanding of common problems such as upper gastrointestinal bleeding.

We predict continued progress in therapeutic endoscopy. Because medical lasers were the first to open new frontiers of treatment and many patients have benefited, lasers will be the standard for comparison of newer endoscopic techniques.

We wish to express our appreciation to the authors of this book, to Mary Carroll the word-processor and editorial assistant, and to our families who gave us the moral support to complete this work. To them we dedicate this book.

Dennis M. Jensen, M.D.
UCLA School of Medicine
Los Angeles, California

Jean-Marc Brunetaud, M.D.
Lille Medical School
Lille, France

LIST OF CONTRIBUTORS

DAVID C. AUTH, Ph.D., Professor of Electrical Engineering and Biophysics, University of Washington. Director of Biophysics International, Bellevue, Washington.

JACQUES BISERTE, Professor of Urology, Lille Medical School, Lille, France.
Co-author: Jean Marc Brunetaud, M.D.

STEVEN G. BOWN, M.D., Director, National Medical Laser Center, Faculty of Clinical Sciences, University College, The Rayne Institute, London.

JEAN-MARC BRUNETAUD, M.D., Laser Unit of Lille Regional Hospital, Associate Professor of Medicine, Lille Medical School, Lille, France. Co-authors: Serge Mordon, Ph.D., V. Maunoury, D. Colchelard, A. Cortot, J.C. Paris, Alain Cornil, Joseph Scopelliti, M.D.

KENNETH R. CASEY, M.D., Pulmonary Disease Division, University of Utah School of Medicine, Salt Lake City, Utah.

JOHN A. DIXON, M.D., Professor of Surgery, University of Utah, Laser Institute, Salt Lake City, Utah.

DAVID E. FLEISCHER, M.D., Associate Professor of Medicine, Georgetown University, Washington, D.C.

JEFFREY J. GILBERTSON, M.D., Research Fellow, Department of Surgery, University of Utah School of Medicine, Salt Lake City, Utah. Co-author: John A. Dixon, M.D.

YOSHIHIRO HAYATA, M.D., Professor and Chairman, Department of Surgery, Tokyo Medical College, Tokyo, Japan.
Co-author: Jutaro Ono, M.D. Department of Surgery

A.G. HOFSTETTER, M.D., Professor, Doctor of Medicine, Director Urology Clinic, Medizinesche Hochschule Lubeck, Lubeck, Germany.
Co-author: E. Keiditsch, M.D.

DENNIS M. JENSEN, M.D., Professor of Medicine, Director, GI Procedures Unit, UCLA Center for the Health Sciences, Los Angeles, California.

JAMES H. JOHNSTON, III, M.D., Associate Clinical Professor, University of Mississippi, Jackson, Mississippi.

PETER KIEFHABER, M.D., Doctor of Medicine, Chief of Medicine and Gastroenterology, Stadtkrankenhaus Traunstein, Traunstein, Germany. Co-authors: Drs. K. Kiefhaber, F. Huber and G. Nath.

RENE LAMBERT, M.D., Professor of Gastroenterology, Director, GI and Laser Endoscopy Unit, Hopital E. Herriot, Lyon, France.

GUSTAVO MACHICADO, M.D., Associate Clinical Professor, UCLA, Los Angeles; Chief of GI, Valley Hospital Medical Center, Van Nuys.

CLAUDE PERSONNE, Director of Pulmonary Laser Unit.
Co-authors: Drs. A. Colchen, G. Vourc'h, J.F. Dumon, A. Meric.

JEAN-LUC POULY, M.D., Department of Obstetrics and Gynecology, Polyclinique Ph. Marcombes, Clermont Ferrand, France.
Co-authors: Drs. Gerard Mage and Maurice A. Bruhat.

JOSEPH A. SMITH, JR., M.D., Professor of Urology, Urologic Oncology, University of Utah, Salt Lake City, Utah.

C. PAUL SWAIN, M.D., Consultant, Department of Gastroenterolgy, St. James and University College Hospitals, London.

1. FUNDAMENTALS OF LASERS FOR ENDOSCOPY AND LASER TISSUE INTERACTIONS

DAVID C. AUTH

Introduction

For the past 60 years, surgeons have used high frequency electrical current for cutting and coagulating tissue. With Bovie's monumental work of the 1920's (1), the field of electrosurgery was to become yet another achievement of the electrical age. In 1960, Theodore Maiman (2) demonstrated the first optical 'maser', later to be dubbed the 'laser'. Scarcely months later, surgeons were coagulating the retina of the eye and blasting cancerous tumor cells around the laboratory. Each form of energy carries a set of physical properties that need to be understood in order to best develop devices and methods of treatment for medical and surgical practice. Actually, high frequency electrical energy is precisely the same form of energy as that emitted by the laser. Physicists refer to it as electromagnetic (EM) energy or electromagnetic waves. Figure 1.1 is a schematic diagram of the electromagnetic spectrum extending from 0 Hz to 10^{21}Hz.

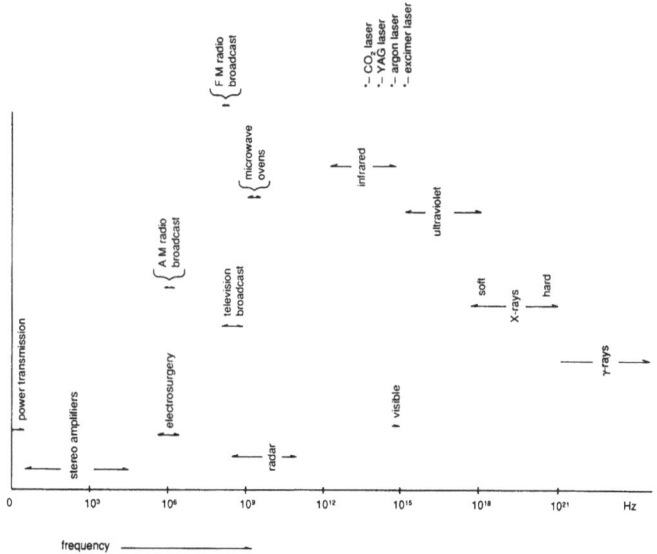

Fig. 1.1. The electro-magnetic spectrum.

D.M. Jensen and J.M. Brunetaud (eds), Medical Laser Endoscopy. 1-15.
© 1990 Kluwer Academic Publishers, Dordrecht

The cluster of laser frequencies representing the CO_2, YAG, argon, and excimer laser, although spanning the range for the middle infrared to the near ultraviolet, take up a very small space of the spectrum used by man for a variety of applications. The ubiquitous X-ray machine uses 60 Hz electricity (i.e., electromagnetic energy) for its primary source of power. It then converts this low frequency energy to X-ray energy at a frequency of approximately 10^{19} Hz. Although the form of energy is the same, the frequency is different by about seventeen orders of magnitude. This vast difference in frequency is responsible for a vastly different tissue response. 60 Hz EM energy shocks the human nervous system, can cause fibrillation, and at high currents, will burn tissue. X-ray frequencies (10^{18}-10^{20} Hz) penetrate tissue handily, photochemically activate silver compounds in photographic plate, and can cause genetic transformation. The Bovie or electrosurgical scalpel/coagulator operates at a frequency of 500,000–3,000,000 cycles per second or .5–3 Hz. In this frequency range, the neuromuscular response of the human body is non-existent and therefore very high currents can be delivered to the tissue without any perceptible shock. In fact, the currents are so high that tissue can be rapidly vaporized or coagulated because of the dissipation of the electrical energy in the tissue. When the tissue is subjected to a voltage, electrons within the tissue matrix are forced to move, thereby constituting an electrical current. As these electrons travel through the tissue latticework, they collide with the atomic structure and give up a portion of their energy to the lattice in the form of molecular vibration or heat.

Thus, electrical current causes heat which, in turn, leads to coagulation or evaporation. Laser radiation or optical radiation can also cause the electrons to move within the tissue and secondarily to impart molecular agitation to the latticework. Again, this agitation is thermal energy or heat which can lead to coagulation, cutting, or evaporation of tissue. Lasers which operate in the visible or near-infrared region of the electromagnetic spectrum have a frequency of 2×10^{14}–6×10^{14} Hz, or 200 to 600 trillion cycles per second. Although the frequency is different, the physical action is the same whether one is using the Bovie or a laser.

Laser physics

Terminology

The word 'l a s e r' is an acronym signifying '*l*ight *a*mplification by *s*timulated *e*mission of *r*adiation'. The device which historically preceded the laser was known as the 'm a s e r' which signified *m*icrowave *a*mplification by *s*timulated *e*mission of *r*adiation. Microwave radiation refers to electromagnetic energy in the frequency range of 1–100 billion cycles per second.

The discovery in the early 1950's of the maser was heralded largely because a new form of atomic interaction made possible the amplification of microwave radiation. This interaction referred to as 'stimulated emission' involved the extraction of energy from atoms 'upon command'.

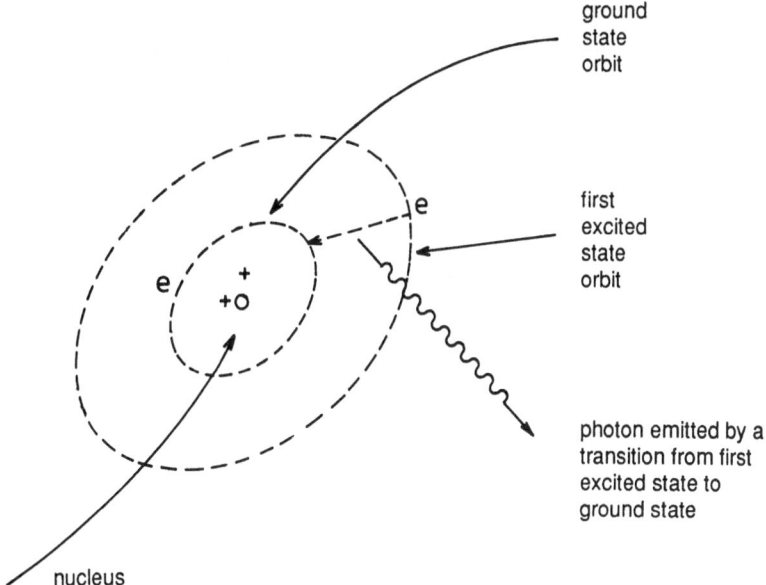

Fig. 1.2. Spontaneous photon emission resulting from electron decaying from first excited state to ground state.

In Fig. 1.2, an excited atom is shown emitting a photon. For the sake of this discussion, a photon is a particle of light or quantitized bundle of electromagnetic radiation. An atom exchanges its energy with the ambient environment by absorbing or emitting photons. Thus, when color pigment absorbs light, it is capturing photons. When the hot wire of the light bulb emits light, it is emitting photons. Individual atoms emit photons when their electrons, orbiting about the nucleus, undergo a downward energy transition. Nature conserves energy by allowing the energy which is lost by the downward energy transfer of the electron to go off as a photon of equivalent energy. Conversely, when a photon is absorbed, the electron makes an upward energy transition exactly equal to the energy of the absorbed photon. Since atoms can only exist in certain energy states, not all photons can be absorbed. Thus, for a photon to be absorbed, it must first of all have an energy which 'agrees' with the available energy states of the atom. This process of absorption and emission of radiation or photons is a reciprocal process; i.e., the atom which is capable of emitting a certain energy photon is also capable of absorbing the same energy photon. In fact, most systems in nature are constantly exchanging

3

energy in just this way. What characterizes the process of natural absorption and emission of radiation is spontaneity and probability. A photon may be emitted at any time by an excited atom. One can say statistically that there will be a 50% probability of emission within some 'lifetime' such as 10^{-8} seconds, but the actual moment is not currently predictable by physics. In 1917 (3), Einstein correctly identified the phenomena of 'stimulated emission.' An excited atom can be encouraged to emit its radiation at some particular time by the presence of radiation at the same frequency as the light which would be given up if the atom were to spontaneously emit. This process is analogous

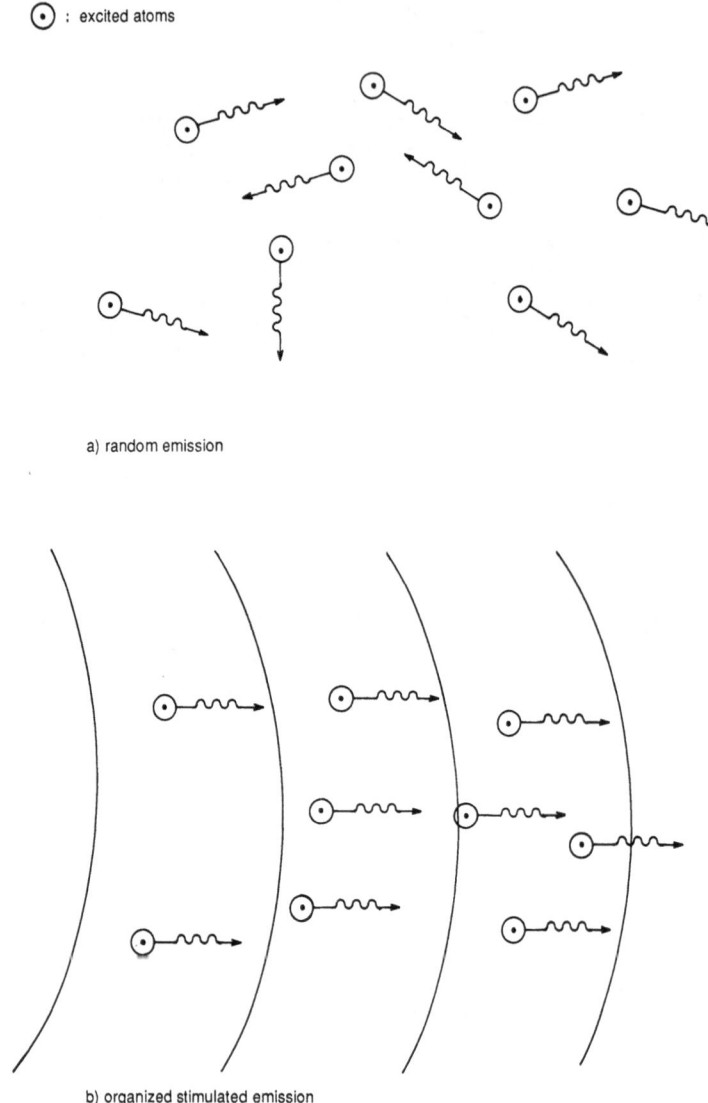

⊙ : excited atoms

a) random emission

b) organized stimulated emission

Fig. 1.3. a) random emission; b) organized stimulated emission.

to resonance excitation of two tuning forks. It is known that a tuning fork which is vibrating at its characteristic frequency will excite another tuning fork into vibration provided it has the same natural frequency as the original tuning fork. Thus, what Einstein observed was that atoms always improve their emission rate when they are stimulated at the proper frequency. Furthermore, Einstein pointed out that the improvement in emission rate was directly proportional to the intensity of the stimulus. Again, this is analogous to the tuning fork case. Although nature has always been exchanging energy between radiation and atoms with proper regard for both spontaneous and stimulated emission, it was not until the 1950's that man was able to engineer a device that could harness this stimulation property to amplify an electromagnetic wave. The maser was the first demonstration of such a device. Although the maser was of itself an important device, physicists longed for an 'optical maser' or laser which could provide amplification of visible light in a controllable way. This quest for a laser was particularly acute since no coherent light source existed up to that point in time. In contrast, microwave sources were routinely available that produced coherent signals. A coherent signal is one in which the wave looks like a single sinusoidal 'wiggle' instead of a jumble of 'wigglets'. Figure 1.3 depicts this distinction.

Engineers view this jumble of wigglets as a noisy source and one that is impossible to tightly focus. In contrast, the coherent source is one that orchestrates the vibrations of all of the atoms into one cohesive symphony of vibration which may be focused to a tiny spot of the dimensions of a single

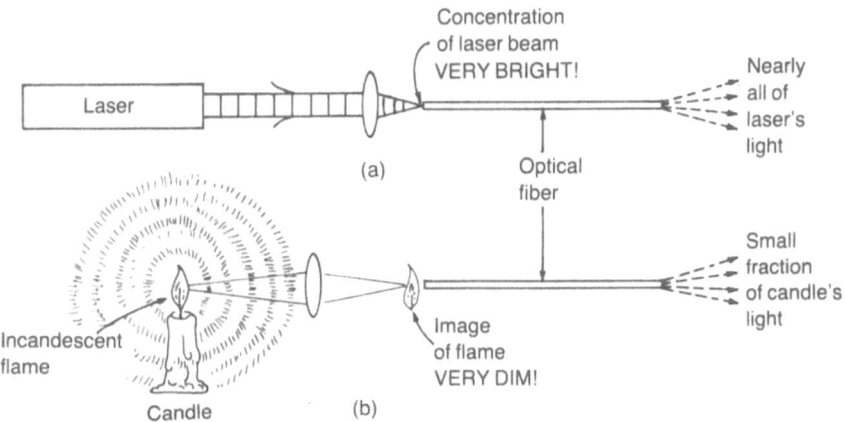

Fig. 1.4. Coupling of light into an optical fiber waveguide. (a) Efficient coupling of laser light having high directivity into fiber; (b) inefficient coupling of light from an incandescent source having poor directivity. Optical coherence is depicted in example (a). Optical incoherence is depicted in example (b). (Reprinted with permission from Auth, D.C.: Laser Photocoagulation Principles. In Papp, J.P. (Ed): Endoscopic Control of Gastrointestinal Hemorrhage. Copyright 1981, CRC Press, Inc.).

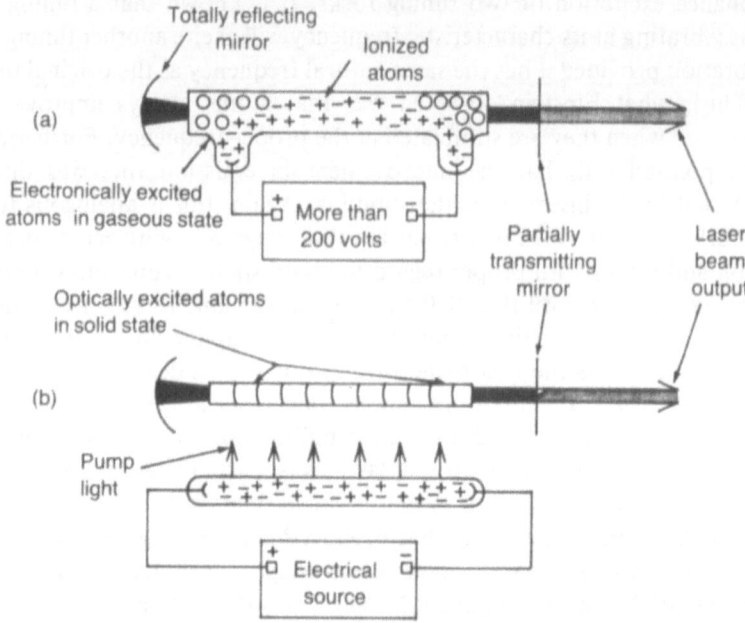

Totally reflecting
mirror

Ionized
atoms

(a)

Electronically excited
atoms in gaseous state

More than
200 volts

Partially
transmitting
mirror

Laser
beam
output

Optically excited atoms
in solid state

(b)

Pump
light

Electrical
source

Fig. 1.5. Two common laser systems. (a) Electrical discharge pumped gas laser representative of the argon and CO_2 lasers; (b) optically pumped solid-state laser representative of the Nd:YAG and ruby lasers. Each system typifies the parallel mirror laser cavity or resonator. (Reprinted with permission from Auth, D.C.: Laser Photocoagulation Principles. In Papp, J.P. (Ed): Endoscopic Control of Gastrointestinal Hemorrhage. Copyright 1981, CRC Press, Inc).

wavelength of light. It is this focusability which made the laser so attractive for medicine and surgery. It means that microscopic precision of surgical procedures is facilitated, for example, production of micron-size coagulation spots on the retina. Furthermore, this focusability enables injection of the light into a single filament of glass fiber for flexible conveyance of the light through endoscopic instruments. Figure 1.4 illustrates this principle.

The Laser Cavity

Figure 1.5 depicts the optical structure which is used to provide the 'orchestrating' function for the laser. Light is confined by two mirrors which force the optical wave to bounce back and forth. When excited atoms are placed in the space between the two mirrors, they are subjected to the vibrational motion of the electromagnetic wave which is bouncing back and forth. Thus, the stage has been set for stimulated emission of radiation by the atoms when they are excited. If it is possible to excite atoms, then as soon as a spontaneous photon is emitted in the direction perpendicular to the mirrored surface, an electromagnetic wave will vibrate within the two mirror structure.

6

But, notice that this vibration is the right frequency for exciting atoms of the same species since it arose from one of the flock. Other excited atoms will then be induced to emit their energy as a result of stimulated emission. They do so and the strength of the wave grows exponentially which further increases the stimulation and so forth and so on. Very quickly, a single electromagnetic signal is sloshing back and forth between the mirrors in beautiful synchrony. If all of the energy is confined totally between the mirrors, how do we put it to work? Answer: We let a little bit leak out without damaging the orchestra. This leakage may be in the form of a tiny hole in one of the mirrors or more conveniently by designing the coating on one of the mirrors so that instead of reflecting 100% of the light it reflects a little less, such as 98%, thereby permitting the other 2% to exit the mirrored cavity to do useful work. Typically, this will be of the order of 0.1% of the light which is used up because of inefficiency in the mirror. The technology of laser mirrors has grown enormously in the twenty-five years since the first demonstration of laser action. The optical engineer can now specify an arbitrary reflection coefficient for a mirror which varies from 0.1% to 99.9% with only 0.1% inefficiency. This means of organizing the optical vibration between two mirrors was the subject of a famous patent issued to Townes and Schawlow in 1958 (4).

The Population Inversion

Because of the reciprocal nature of absorption and stimulated emission, an excited atom in the vicinity of a proper frequency electromagnetic wave will emit a photon with the same probability as it would absorb it if it were not excited. Thus, a stream of photons passing through a sea of non-excited atoms of the proper energy structure will be absorbed by those atoms and thus experience attenuation or negative gain. Conversely, a stream of photons passing through a sea of excited atoms of proper energy structure will encourage more photon emission (by stimulation) and thus the stream will increase in size and positive gain will be realized. When the population of excited and non-excited atoms is the same, the *net* gain is zero. Thus, for positive gain, as is desirable in a laser, there needs to be more excited than non-excited atoms. Since nature normally prefers to lie in its lowest energy state, having more atoms in an upper energy state is referred to as a population inversion. Choosing atomic species whose populations are relatively easily inverted is one of the primary goals in laser engineering.

The Energy Pump

In order to supply the energy necessary for a population inversion, some means must be found for coupling energy into the atoms. As mentioned

7

before, light may be absorbed and indeed optical production of the population inversion is possible. In the original laser of Maiman, the ruby crystal (2) was subjected to the intense flash of light produced by a photographic flash lamp which surrounded the ruby rod. Ruby consists of sapphire crystal (Al_2O_3) which is doped with an impurity of chromium. The chromium atom is the actual lasing element in the ruby laser.

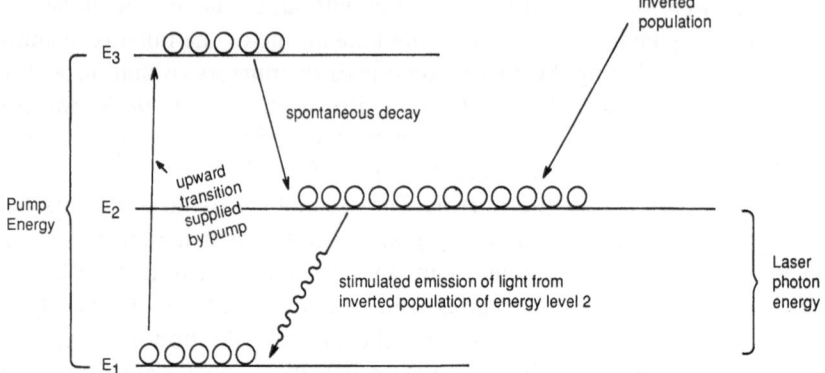

Fig. 1.6. Energy level schematic for a 3-level laser such as a ruby laser depicting population inversion.

Figure 1.6 depicts the optical pumping scheme employed in the ruby laser. The pump light forces electrons from the lowest energy state (or ground state) up to the third energy level. As the third level becomes heavily populated, the rate of net absorption of pump radiation is reduced because some of the electrons are being stimulated by the pump to re-emit photons at the pump energy. However, electrons in the third level undergo rapid transition to the second or middle level as shown in Figure 1.6. Here they can be stored without fear of stimulation by the pump light because the energy associated with decay to the ground state is different from that used for pumping. In time, a large population inversion can be produced between levels 1 and 2. The stage is then set for laser action when a spontaneous photon is emitted by an atom in energy level 2. If that spontaneous photon is trapped in a cavity, then, it can stimulate other atoms within the cavity to emit and add to its own energy. They in turn stimulate others, until the cavity contains an intense level of radiation at one precise photon energy.

Another form of pumping is electron discharge or, in other words, a sustained weak spark. Electrons colliding with atoms can cause them to jump to higher energy states, thereby preparing a population inversion. Since crystals are damaged by spark discharges, they are better pumped with optical radiation. Gases are readily pumped by spark or arc discharge and thus gas discharge lasers are commonplace. The familiar neon sign is an example of atomic re-emission of light after arc excitation in the gas of the tube. The fluorescent light is another example.

Laser tissue interactions

Penetration Depth

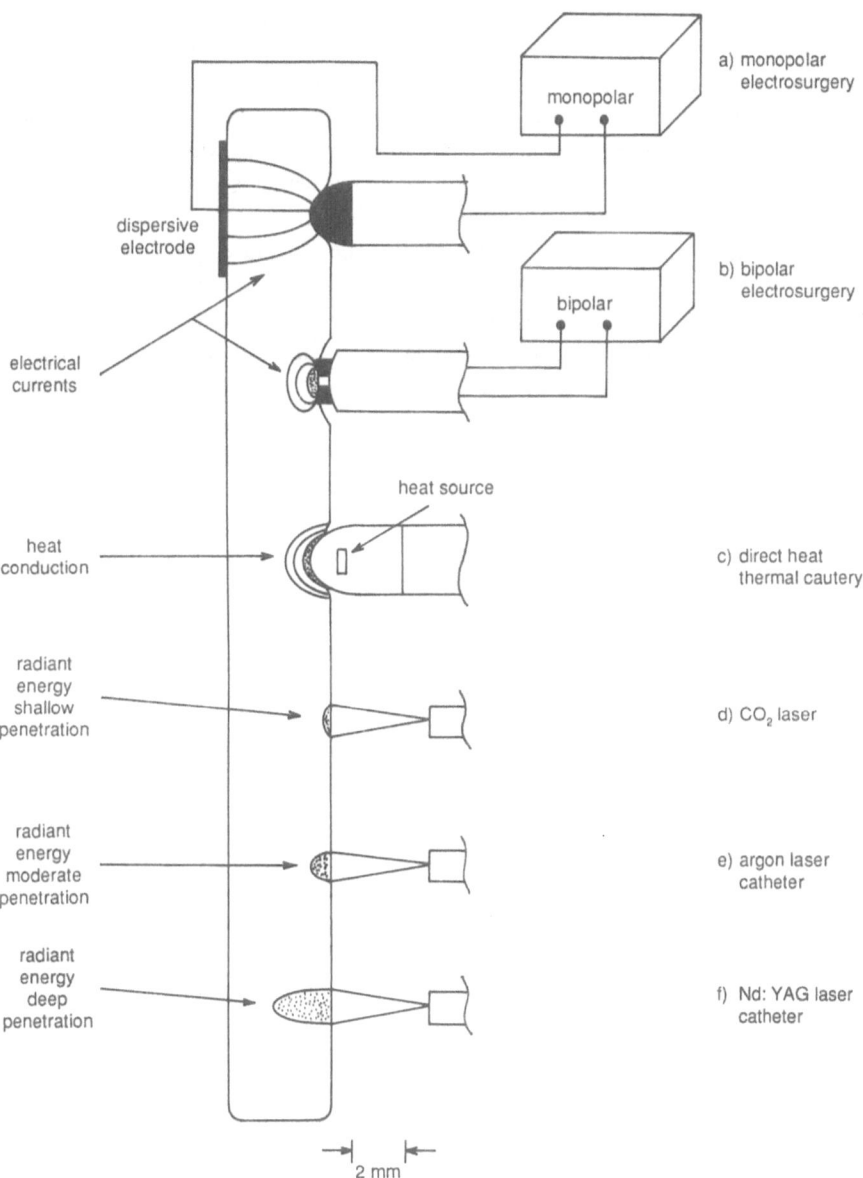

Fig. 1.7. Energy release in tissue. Six different endoscopic modalities.

Figure 1.7 depicts a 6-way comparison of the relative penetration of laser and non-laser energy into tissue. The familiar monopolar Bovie-type electrosurgery electrode is shown with its electrical currents and hence heat formation descending into tissue as it completes the circuit to the external and distal patients plate. The bipolar electrosurgical probe is shown with its highly confined electrical currents and resultant heat flux. Figure 1.7c depicts the hot cautery probe where heating is external to the tissue and transferred into the tissue by thermal conduction, similar to normal cooking. Figures 1.7d, 1.7e, and 1.7f depict respectively the CO_2 (carbon dioxide), argon, and neodymium: YAG (Nd:YAG) laser beams as they impinge on tissue. YAG is an acronym signifying Yttrium Aluminum Garnet which is a gem quality solid crystal. When doped with neodymium, its color changes from clear to light blue. In normal, moderately vascular tissue, the CO_2 laser penetrates about 0.1 mm, the argon laser penetrates about 0.5 mm and the YAG laser about 2.5 mm. Penetration in this sense refers to the actual propagation at the speed of light of the laser's electromagnetic beam into the tissue depth. Of course, thermal conduction will carry the heat energy deeper and more lateral than the actual contour of the beam energy. Therefore, the depth of tissue coagulation cannot be equated with penetration as used here. In a general sense, deeper penetrating radiation is capable of depositing heat deeper which, when it builds up with time, will exceed the limit for cell viability (about 43°C). As further time passes, protein denaturation (coagulation) occurs when the deposited heat raises the temperature to about 57°C. The actual time interval for coagulation may be less than 0.1 second if the rate of radiant energy deposition and transformation to heat is high enough. During the deposition of heat, some heat energy will be conducted away by thermal conduction or by vascular convection. This can cause a local spreading of the thermal effect beyond the strict boundaries of the radiant energy profile. The depth of radiant energy penetration is not perfectly delineated since the energy falls off exponentially due to the absorption of the light during its passage in the tissue. Figure 1.8 depicts a margin of tissue necrosis below the coagulation zone. This is a result of the exponential fall-off of the radiant energy in the tissue and to thermal conduction. Thus, in the space adjacent to the 57°C isothermal contour line, there will be a zone above 43°C but below 57°C such that necrosis without coagulation can occur. The CO_2 laser operates at 10.6 microns in the middle-infrared region of the spectrum. It is heavily absorbed by the water molecule and this accounts for its very shallow penetration depth. The argon laser operates in the blue-green region (.488 and .514 microns) of the visible spectrum. The hemoglobin molecule absorbs heavily in the green and blue (hence the red appearance of blood) and this accounts for the relatively shallow penetration depth of the argon laser. The Nd:YAG laser operates at 1.06 microns in the near-infrared region of spectrum where its energy is moderately absorbed by hemoglobin. With reduced hemoglobin absorption, the YAG laser is able to penetrate more deeply into the tissue.

For a given amount of laser energy, a shallow penetrating laser beam will impart a greater volumetric energy density to the tissue. This can lead to rapid boiling of entrained water within the tissue matrix. If this boiling is very rapid, the steam produced in the depth of tissue will not have time to escape by normal diffusion. When this happens, a microexplosion of the steam vesicle occurs, leading to rupture of the tissue and expulsion of small fragments of the tissue in some cases. This microrupture of the tissue can be used to good advantage for surgical ablation or cutting of the tissue. With deeper penetrating lasers, more energy is required to bring the tissue water up to the boiling point. Frequently, sufficient energy is imparted to raise the temperature to 60–100° centigrade which is sufficient to denature the protein molecule and cause thermal coagulation. Thus, a laser can achieve coagulation without surgical cutting and ablation when the energy is released sufficiently slowly within the tissue. Since the 'wake' of thermal heating is rather narrow in the vicinity of a CO_2 laser beam within tissue, the corresponding margin of coagulation adjacent to the beam is narrow. This narrow margin is capable of sealing only small vessels of capillary size or slightly larger. With the argon laser, vessels of the order of .25 mm can be sealed due to its somewhat larger margin of denaturation and thermal coagulation. The Nd:YAG laser can seal vessels approaching 1 mm in diameter because of its still larger margin of coagulation. Unfortunately, larger vessels have rapidly flowing blood which can easily drain away heat faster than it is produced, and thus the Nd:YAG laser and the argon laser frequently are unable to stop bleeding vessels of larger than 0.5 mm diameter. The velocity of blood in a 0.5 mm artery is typically about 30 cm per second. Thus, for a laser beam spot size of 3 mm, the moving hemoglobin molecule is only illuminated for 1/100th of a second. In most cases, the coagulation is very inefficient in larger arteries since a lot of energy is wasted heating the blood which is carried off to the distal circulation.

Coagulation proceeds in a complicated fashion by inducing swelling of the surrounding tissue and partial stagnation of the flowing blood which in turn permits a larger rise in temperature in the intraluminal blood. In turn, the vessel walls eventually rise in temperature leading to shrinkage (5). In some cases, the process of swelling, shrinkage, and intraluminal coagulation of blood leads to total hemostasis for larger vessels. Compression of the vessel before application of heat is a well established technique (6, 7) to improve hemostasis.

In addition to tissue rupture secondary to steam vesicle formation, the laser can actually evaporate tissue directly. More energy is required since the tissue must reach much higher temperatures. As the tissue temperature approaches 300-400 degrees Celsius, oxidation and hence combustion occurs, which in effect incinerates the tissue, leaving only ash. This is similar to the action in a self-cleaning oven. The ash can be evaporated if the laser energy is sufficiently intense to raise the temperature to 3000-4000 degrees Celsius. These higher temperatures are not usually observed in medical procedures, but the laser is capable of producing them when confined to a small spot size.

Laser Tissue Energetics

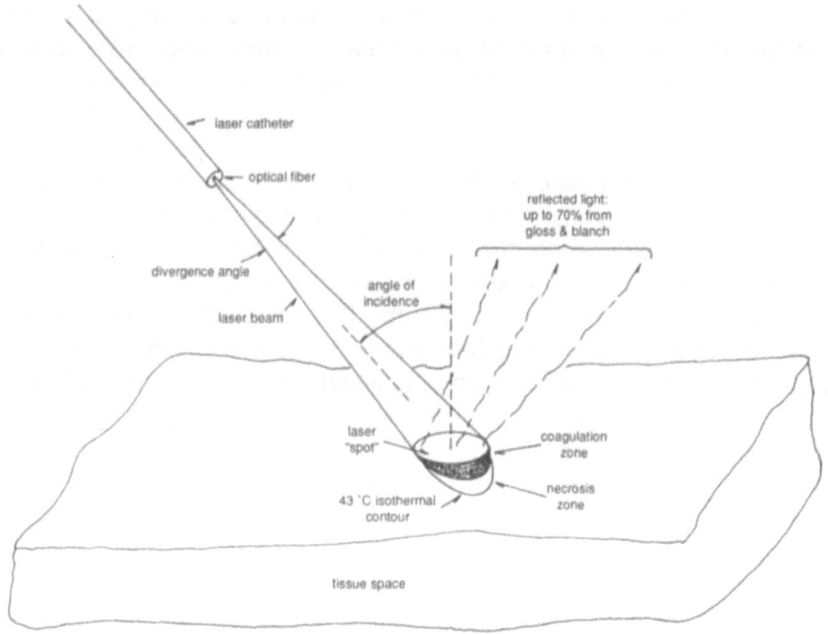

Fig. 1.8. Dynamics of laser beam impingement on tissue.

Table 1.1. Glossary of terminology used in laser surgery and electrosurgery.

---

absorption coefficient – the amount of radiant energy absorbed per unit path length

angstrom unit – a unit of length measurement for wavelength of light, equal to one ten billionth of a meter or one ten thousandth of a micron

ablation – removal of tissue by vaporization

beam diameter – the diameter of that portion of the laser beam which contains 86 percent of the power

brightness – the visual sensation of the luminous power of a light beam, as opposed to scientifically measured power of the beam

calorimeter – an instrument which measures the power or energy of a light beam

C.I.E. – abbreviation for Commission International de L'Eclairage, the French translation for International Commission on Illumination

carbonization – thermal expulsion of hydrogen, oxygen, and nitrogen from tissue leaving black carbonaceous residue; occurs at temperatures in excess of 200°C

combustion – burning of tissue usually resulting from application of heat in an oxidizing atmosphere such as air *denaturation* – reconfiguring the natural shape of a molecule usually referring to the hardening of liquid protein due to spiral conformation after application of heat

desiccation – drying of tissue by evaporation of water usually accelerated by application of heat

desiccative electrosurgery – spark-free contact of tissue for coagulation by electroresistive heating

diffusion – propagation of heat or vapor through tissue

CO_2 *laser* – a gas laser operating in the middle infrared region of the spectrum characterized by high operating efficiency and high absorbance in tissue

coaxial gas – shield of gas flowing around and over an optical fiber to blow away blood and debris, protect the output end of the fiber, and partially back-pressurize the circulation

collimation – the process by which divergent rays of light are converted into parallel rays

CW – abbreviation for continuous wavefront; the continuous emission of a laser as opposed to pulsed operation

depth of field – the working range of a laser beam; particularly important for use in microsurgery

divergence angle – the angle at which the laser beam spreads as it propagates away from the fiber tip

erosion – undesirable removal of tissue by vaporization

fluorescence – the glow induced in a material when bombarded by light of higher energy

flux – the radiant, or luminous power of a light beam; the time rate of flow of radiant energy across a given surface area

focus – the point where rays of light meet upon convergence by a lens or mirror

frequency – the number of complete vibrations or cycles per unit time

fulguration – sparking from an electrosurgery machine directed at tissue to perform ablation or coagulation

gas discharge laser – a laser containing a gaseous lasing medium in a glass or ceramic tube in which an electric arc is sustained for the purpose of pumping the lasing atoms

heat sink – an adjunctive medium which drains away heat

Hertz – unit of frequency in the International System of Units (SI) abbreviated Hz; replaces cps for cycles per second

incident light – a ray of light that falls on the surface of tissue; the angle of incidence is the angle made by the ray with a perpendicular to the tissue surface

ion laser – a type of laser employing a very high discharge current passing down a small bore tube to ionize a noble gas such as argon or krypton; the ionized atom becomes the lasing element

intensity – the magnitude of radiant energy, such as heat or light per unit surface area per unit time

Joule – a measurement of energy equal to 1 watt-second

incandescence – emission of visible light resulting from tissue temperature in excess of 500°C

energy density – Joules per unit area

micron – unit of measurement equal to 1 millionth of a meter, frequently used to denote wavelength of laser light

monochromatic light – light consisting purely of one wavelength; a characteristic of many lasers

nanometer – unit of measurement of wavelength equal to 1 billionth of a meter

optical fiber – a thin cylinder of quartz or glass for propagation of laser light or conventional light; ranges in diameter from 100 microns to 1000 microns

output power – the energy per second (in watts) emitted by a laser or electrosurgery generator

power density – the number of watts of radiant energy per unit surface area exposed

power meter – an accessory used to monitor laser beam power

pulse energy – the energy of a single brief emission from a laser operating in pulsed (not CW) mode

reflectance – the ratio of the reflected flux to the incident flux or the ratio of the reflected light to the light falling on an object

resonator – the mirror or reflectors making up the laser cavity

RMS – root mean square – a mathematically correct average for the power of modulated electromagnetic waves

temperature clamping – holding temperature at some fixed level because of an energy intensive phase transformation, usually arising from boiling of water at 100°C

spot size – the diameter of the laser beam at the point of impingement upon tissue

white spot – a white colored zone signifying denaturation of protein which leads to broad spectrum (white) scattering and reflection of light

working distance – distance from optical fiber tip to tissue

TEM – abbreviation for transverse electric and magnetic mode: TEM_{oo} refers to lowest order, hence purest and most coherent mode of operation of a laser; it permits focusing to the smallest possible spot

transmission – in optics the passage of radiant energy (light) through a medium

wave – an undulation or vibration; a form of local movement as energy is transmitted through the media

wavelength – the length of the light wave; usually measured from crest to crest; common units of measurement are microns; nanometers, or angstroms.

Table 1.1 presents a glossary of terminology which is widely used in electrosurgery and laser surgery and coagulation. Many of the terms used in this section are addressed in Table 1.1. The laser beam used in endoscopy is frequently conveyed via a flexible glass fiber. It emerges from the fiber with a certain divergence angle. This angle is typically about 10–15°. By varying the distance from the tip of the optical fiber to the tissue, the endoscopist in effect varies the spot size of the laser beam on the tissue. Figure 1.8 illustrates the fall-off in laser beam energy density as the beam propagates from the optical fiber to the tissue. The energy density on the tissue is also a function of the angle of incidence (see Fig. 1.8) since the beam spreads out along the surface as the angle of incidence is increased (becomes more oblique). Beam spreading on the surface reduces the energy density since the surface area is increased. Additionally, with increasing angles of incidence, the actual amount of radiation entering the tissue is reduced still further because more of the light is reflected at oblique angles. With YAG laser operating at 80 Watts of power, a power intensity of 8000 Watts per square centimeter is readily possible since this would imply a spot size of 1/100th of a square centimeter or about 1.1 mm diameter. Such power density can be used to incise tissue for endoscopic surgical procedures. Such a density would not be desirable for coagulation since it would be more apt to induce bleeding rather than stop it. Such induced bleeding would be more moderate than a frank, cold knife incision since there would be some margin of radiant heating and subsequent thermal coagulation and necrosis. Tissue has a heat capacity approximately equal to water, which is 1 calorie per cubic centimeter per degree Celsius. A calorie is equal to 4.18 joules or 4.18 Watt-seconds. Thus, an 80 Watt laser operating for 1 second produces 80 Watt-sec of energy or 80 joules. 80 joules equals about 20 calories. 20 calories can raise the temperature of 1 cubic centimeter of tissue approximately 20° Celsius which would be sufficient to cause irreversible thermal damage and bring the tissue to the coagulation point. Of course, this is ignoring the heat which may be lost due to circulation. The amount lost due to circulation can be highly variable depending upon the local vascular anatomy. The same 20 calorie pulse of energy would, if confined to a 100 cubic millimeters of tissue bring its temperature quickly to 100°C., having used only 6.3 calories in doing so. This follows because of the 63 C temperature differential between body temperature and the boiling point of water, and the fact that 100 cubic millimeters is equal to 1/10th of a cubic centimeter. Thus, of the 20 calories, 14 can be used to offset the heat of vaporization of water which is equal to 535 calories per cubic centimeter (or gram) or 0.535 calories per cubic millimeter. In this example, the remaining 14 calories can be used to evaporate 14/.535 or approximately 26 mm^3 of water. This would cause appreciable desiccation of the original 100 cubic millimeters of tissue. In some cases, evaporation of this much water might lead to steam vesicle eruption when vascular cooling is not present.

Summary and conclusion

Laser energy can be useful for the endoscopist as a means of coagulation, ablation, controlled necrosis, or surgical cutting of tissue. It can be used to highlight fluorescent dyes, activate photochemical dyes or break molecular bonds within the tissue. It is significant for the endoscopist because it can (for some laser wavelengths) be conveyed through flexible fibers. Rigid endoscopy can also benefit from laser technology since the light can be focused to very tiny spots and provide surgical precision. Choice of laser wavelength can be made to enhance depth of penetration for tumor destruction, or activation of tumor specific drugs. Although there are thousands of different atoms which can be used for lasers, only a few are available which produce several Watts of CW (see glossary) power in a price range suitable for the medical market. We have discussed the big three: CO_2, argon, and the Nd:YAG. Other lasers of growing importance such as the dye laser, the excimer laser, and the frequency doubled YAG will undoubtedly play a larger medical- surgical role as they are further developed. The optimal choice of energy, whether laser or non-laser, is frequently the result of protracted research in animals and careful clinical trials.

References

1. Cushing WT, Bovie WT. Electrosurgery as an aid to the removal of intracranial tumors. Surg Gynecol Obstet 1928;47:751-784.
2. Maiman TH. Nature 1960;187:493-494.
3. Einstein A. Zur quantentheorie der strahlung. Phys Z 1917;18:121.
4. Schawlow AL, Townes CH. Phys Rev 1958;112:1940-1949.
5. Gorisch W, Boergen KP. Heat-induced contraction of blood vessels. Lasers in Surg and Med 1982;2:1-13.
6. Sigel B, Dunn MR. The mechanism of blood vessel closure by high frequency electrocoagulation. Surg Gynec Obstet 1965;121:8230-831.
7. Siegel B, Hatke FL. Physical factors in electrocoaptation of blood vessels. Arch Surg 1967;95:54-58.

2. OPTIC FIBERS FOR LASER THERAPEUTIC ENDOSCOPY

JEAN-MARC BRUNETAUD, SERGE MORDON,
ALAIN CORNIL AND JOSEPH SCOPELLITI

History of endoscopic laser fibers

The recent proliferation of laser use in medicine was the direct result of advances in the technology of laser light transmission. The first methods of laser light transmission used direct transmission or articulated mirrors. However, these systems are bulky and are now used only for CO_2 lasers. The reasons are 1) optic fibers transmitting the 10.6 um wavelength of CO_2 are still under development, and 2) optic fiber transmission would not allow the sharply focused point necessary for surgical incision. The development of optic fibers in the seventies facilitated the adaptation of lasers to endoscopy. The principle of transmission is based upon total internal reflection. The waveguide is made up of two components, an inner core which transmits the light and an outer cladding which continuously reflects the light internally. The first work in the development of laser light transmission by fiber-optics was carried out between 1973 and 1975 by two groups in Germany. Fruhmorgen, Boden et al. (1) for argon laser and Nath, Kiefhaber et al. (2) for Nd:YAG laser. Boden et al. (1) used a plastic fiber with a polymethyl methacrylate core (i.e. plexiglass). However, power loss through the fiber was a major problem, and this particular fiber produced a 50% loss per meter of fiber length. Also, the divergence angle at the fiber tip was over 12 degrees making its application clinically quite difficult. Nath, et al. (2) developed the 'Triconic fiber' which is still used clinically by Kiefhaber. This fiber allows the transmission of Argon and Nd:YAG light with little power loss (less than 20% for 4 meters) and a narrow beam divergence (2 to 4 degrees). But this fiber is very fragile; it has to be fixed in a specially modified endoscope. Protection from contamination is made by a quartz window screwed in the tip of the endoscope.

In 1977, the first commercial fibers with a silicon quartz core were developed for medical use (3). Originally developed for industrial and telecommunications uses, their characteristics adapted perfectly for medical needs. Based on a 200 to 1000 micron quartz core and a silicone rubber optical cladding, the first generation of these fibers, denoted QSF, yielded 85 to 90% power transmission from a 5 meter long fiber for Argon or Nd:YAG light. The divergence angle ranged from 6 to 12 degrees.

The next generation of optical fibers, denoted QSF-AS, was developed and applied in 1980 (4). The quartz core remained unchanged but the silicone

D.M. Jensen and J.M. Brunetaud (eds), Medical Laser Endoscopy. 17-26.

cladding was doped with fluoride and the whole fiber was covered with a silicone rubber coating for mechanical protection. QSF-AS fibers were available in 200 and 400 um core diameter. The main advantage over the QSF was a lower beam divergence: 8 degrees for a 200 um fiber (QSF:12) and 6 degrees for a 400 um fiber (QSF:8). QSF and QSF-AS were manufactured by a French company, Quartz and Silice and were available in long lengths at a low cost.

These two fibers (QSF and QSF-AS) can be utilized in endoscopy in several ways: 1) Some endoscopists like Lambert (5) have a raw fiber in direct contact with the tissue. The fiber tip burns like a candle. This system does not need gas insufflation or maintenance. However, the reproducibility of the effects mainly depends on the endoscopist's experience. The lack of neutral gas circulation does not protect against explosion in the colon or rectum where special care is required. 2) Joffe (6) has developed another type of contact system which is manufactured by Surgical Laser Technologies (Keyghley, England). The fiber is inserted into a teflon sheath and an 'universal connector' is fixed at the tip of the fiber.

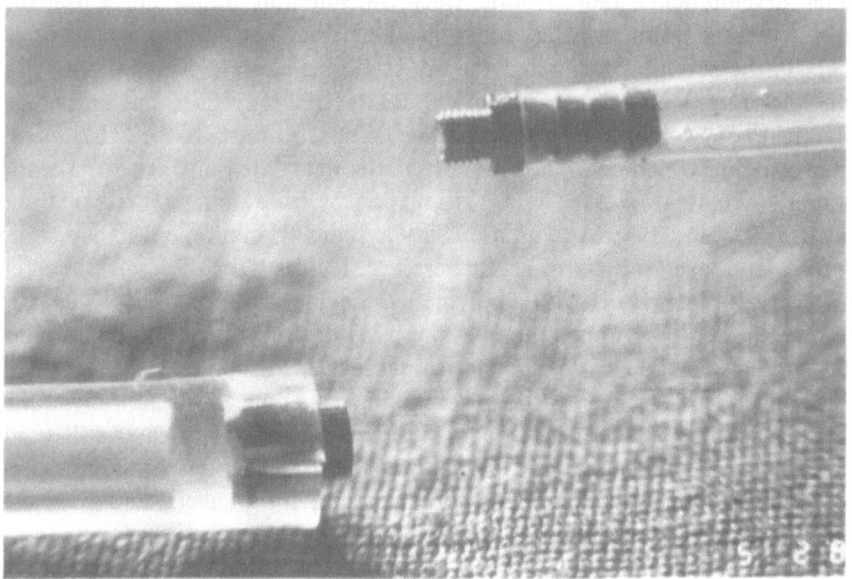

Fig. 2.1. Universal connector fixed at the tip of the fiber.

Different sapphire tips can be screwed on the universal connector: flat for hemostasis (Fig. 2.2) or round for vaporization (Fig. 2.3).

Gas insufflation is still required, but at a low flow rate, less than one liter per minute. The optic power with Nd:YAG laser is limited to 20 W. This system is presently under evaluation in our laser center. 3) Emphasis will be placed on the third system, the endoscopic laser probe, which is the most commonly used in endoscopy.

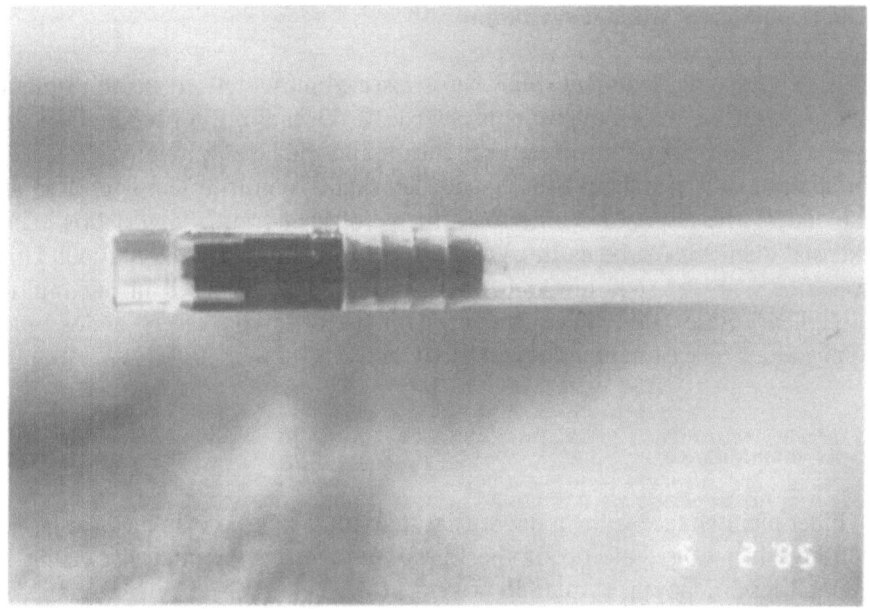

Fig. 2.2. Flat sapphire tip for hemostasis is screwed on the universal connector.

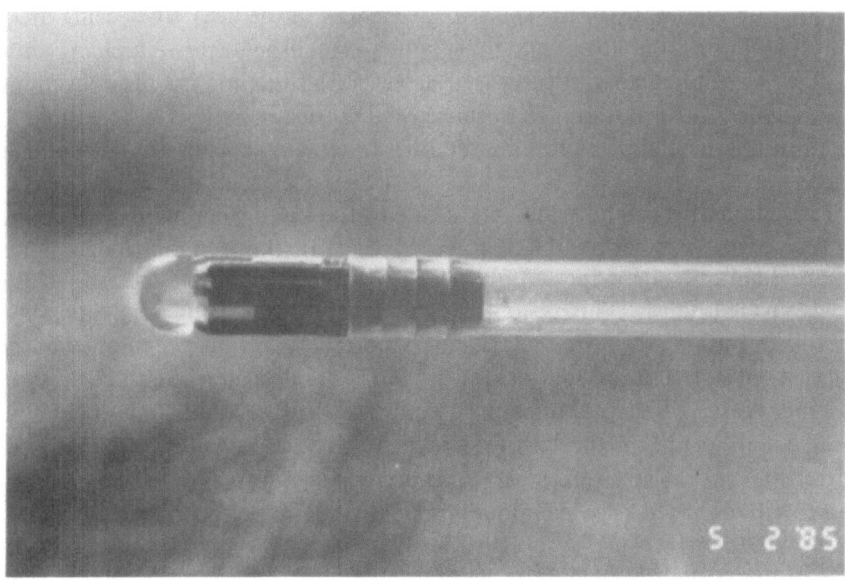

Fig. 2.3. Round sapphire tip for vaporization is screwed on the universal connector.

Endoscopic laser probe constitution

For endoscopic treatment, the fiber is inserted into a teflon sheath through which a protective coaxial gas jet is passed. At the end of the fiber a metal tip is attached to hold both the catheter sheath and the laser waveguide in place. In addition, the metal tip is designed such that a Venturi effect is created at the end of the laser waveguide to further protect it from flying debris. The external diameter of the entire system ranges from 1.6 mm (200 and 400 Um core fibers) to 2.2 (600 um core fibers). Such fibers are used in our multi-disciplinary laser unit for different Nd:YAG or argon lasers endoscopic applications in gastroenterology, urology and ENT.

Fiber maintenance

Fiber maintenance is the most crucial step in the upkeep of a medical laser. Through heavy use, the tip of the fiber is progressively damaged causing a gradual loss of power output. Replacement of the old fiber by a new one is expensive so it is worthwhile to repair rather than replace laser probes. There are two systems for cutting the quartz fiber tip for optimum working order. Both methods have the same end-point: a flat surface which is exactly perpendicular to the path of the laser light and completely free of surface irregularities.

One system requires the tip of the optical fiber to be polished to a high level of smoothness. This is carried out using specially designed polishing stones with a progressively smaller grit. The surface irregularities must be removed to an order of magnitude of the specific wavelength of the laser fiber being used. This method has the advantage that the newly polished tip is extremely close to exact perpendicular with every try. However, this method is time consuming and requires specific training. Because of these features, it is not feasible to perform this technique in the middle of a treatment session should the need arise.

The alternative method involves cleaving the laser fiber with a diamond cutting edge. A superficial defect is created with the diamond edge. Then longitudinal pressure is exerted on the fiber until it separates at the site of the newly created defect. This system has the advantage of being very quick and easy. The equipment is simple as well as portable, and the technique can be done in the laser unit or anywhere necessary. The surface of the fiber tip after cleaving is free of irregularities and requires no further polishing. The main disadvantage of this method is that a perpendicular axis cannot be guaranteed. Distortion of 0 to 10 degrees can be expected.

We will describe the technique used at Lille for repairing a damaged endoscope fiber:

Step 1: When the fiber has been damaged, the first step in maintenance is to extend the fiber tip from its teflon sheath. The metal tip is then removed from the distal end of the optic fiber. The fiber is then put back into the sheath and the terminal part of the teflon sheath is cut with a scalpel (Fig. 2.4).

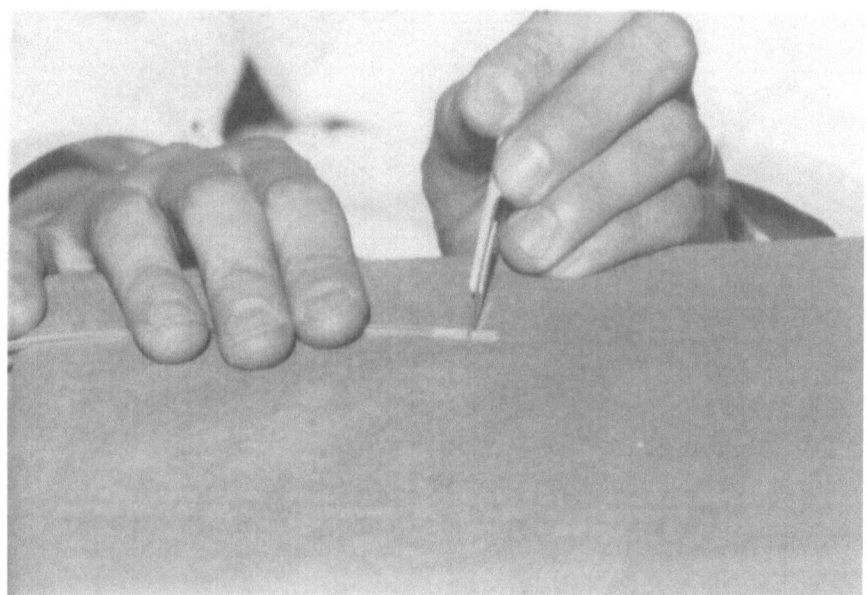

Fig. 2.4. Cutting the terminal part of the teflon sheath.

Step 2: The optical fiber is advanced beyond the teflon sheath and the fiber is clamped in the cutting tool. (Infocut by A.T.I., France). The upper part of the mechanical protection of the fiber is removed with a scalpel (Fig. 2.5).

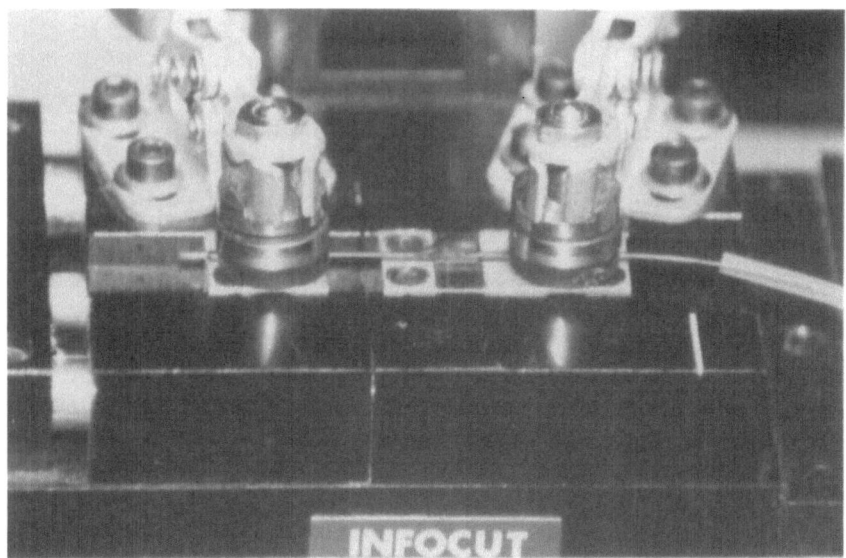

Fig. 2.5. Removal of the upper part of the cladding that protects the fiber.

Step 3: A superficial defect is created on the fiber core using a sawing motion with the diamond cutting edge (Fig. 2.6).

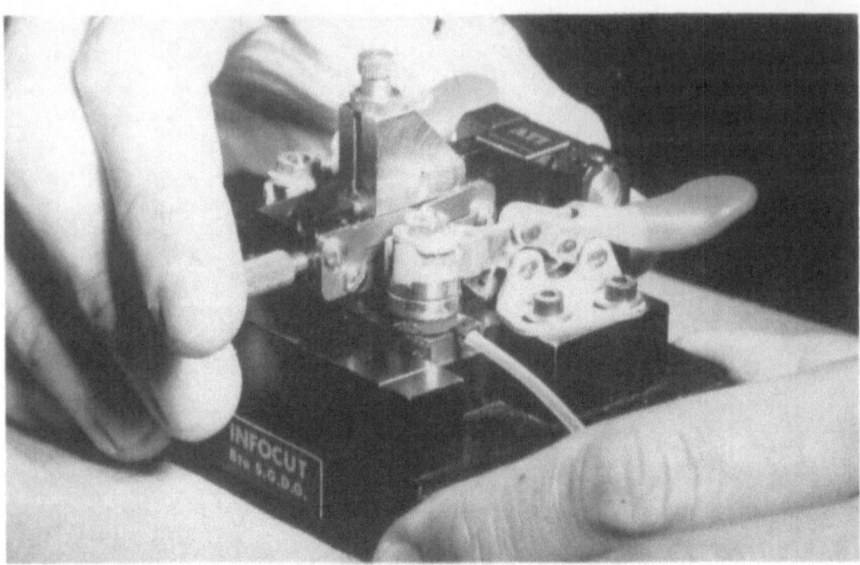

Fig. 2.6. Creation of a superficial defect by moving the diamond.

Step 4: Distilled water is placed on the newly created defect. With the clamping mechanism of the diamond cutter, longitudinal pressure is exerted on the optic fiber. This results in the separation of the distal portion of the optic fiber and results in a clean fiber tip (Fig. 2.7).

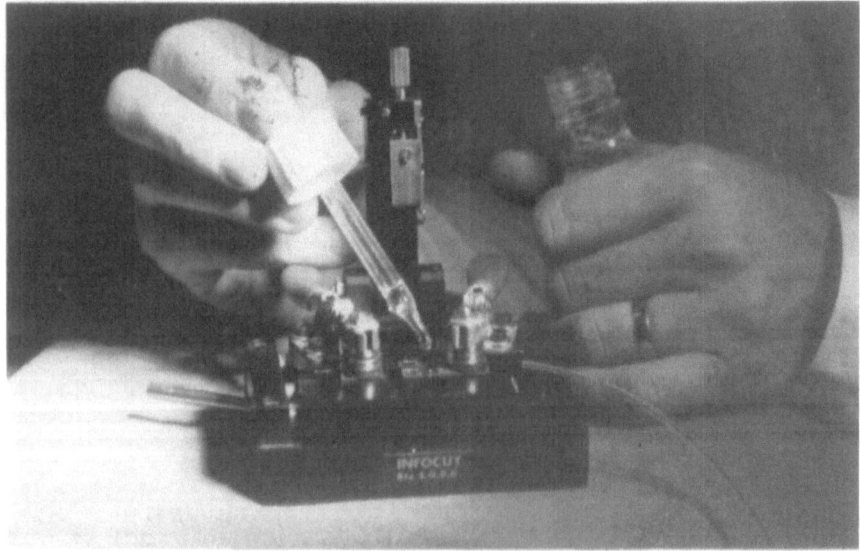

Fig. 2.7. Distilled water is placed on the newly created defect to improve the cutting efficacy.

Step 5: The optical fiber is removed from the clamping mechanism and the silicone rubber is stripped off the distal tip for a distance of approximately 3 mm (Fig. 2.8).

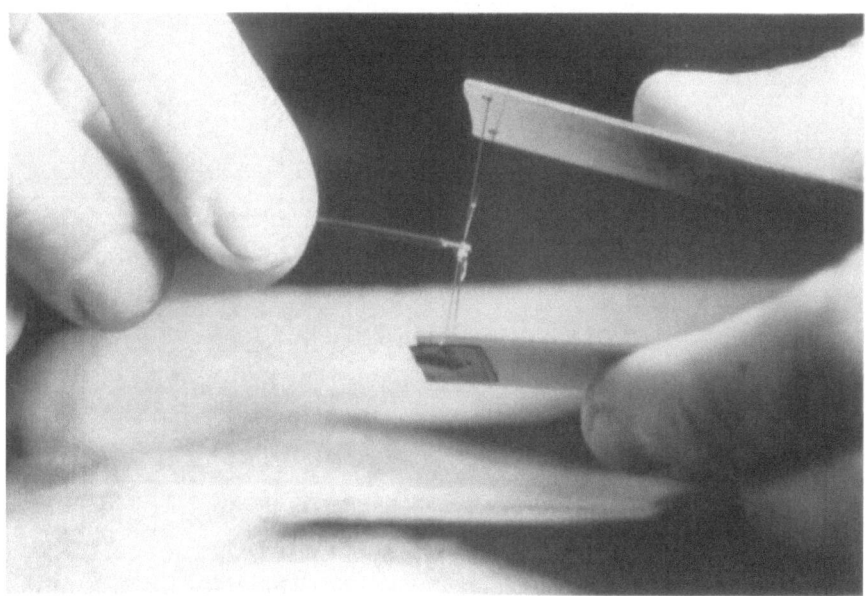

Fig. 2.8. Stripping the silicone rubber from the distal part of the fiber.

Step 6: The new fiber tip is inspected using a magnifying lens (Fig. 2.9) and further cleaned with acetone. Any residual silicone rubber is scrubbed away using acetone (Fig. 2.10).

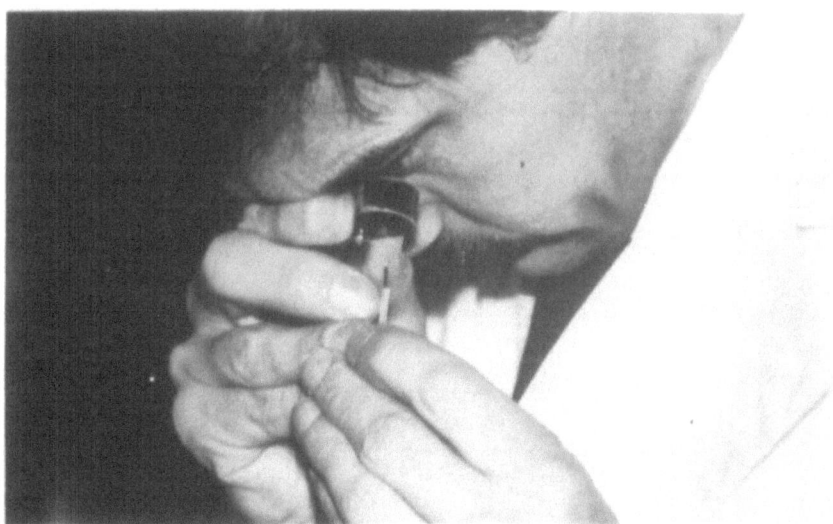

Fig. 2.9. Inspection of the fiber tip with a magnifying lens.

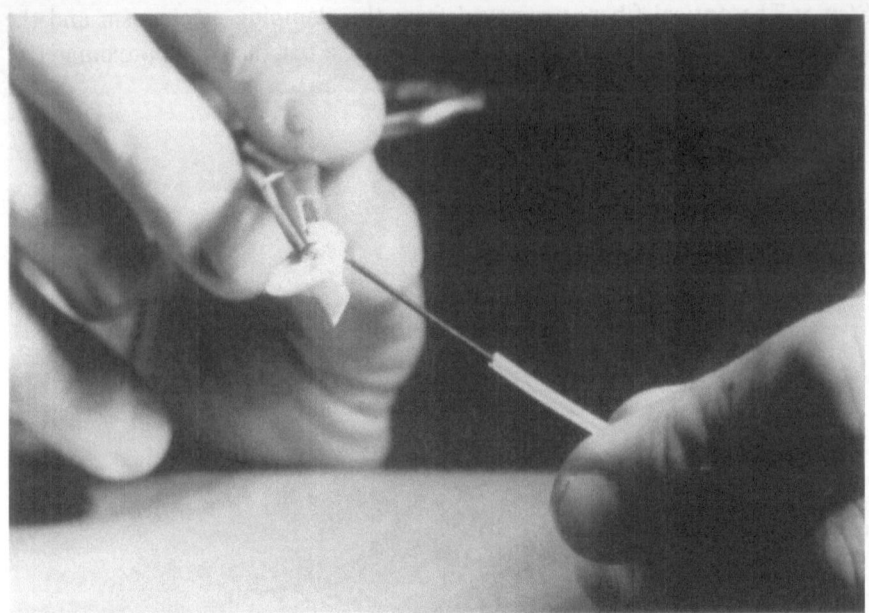

Fig. 2.10. Cleaning the fiber tip with lens paper and acetone.

Step 7: The metal tip is then reapplied to the distal fiber. It is important that the fiber tip be properly threaded onto the distal fiber (Fig. 2.11).

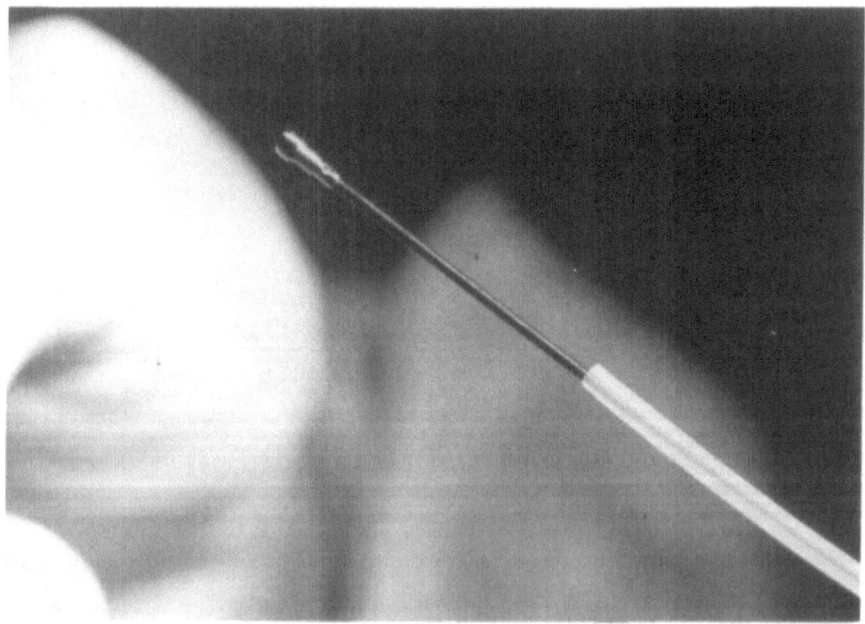

Fig. 2.11. The metal tip is threaded onto the distal fiber.

Step 8: The fiber tip is then reinserted within the teflon sheath and the laser fiber tested (Fig. 2.12).

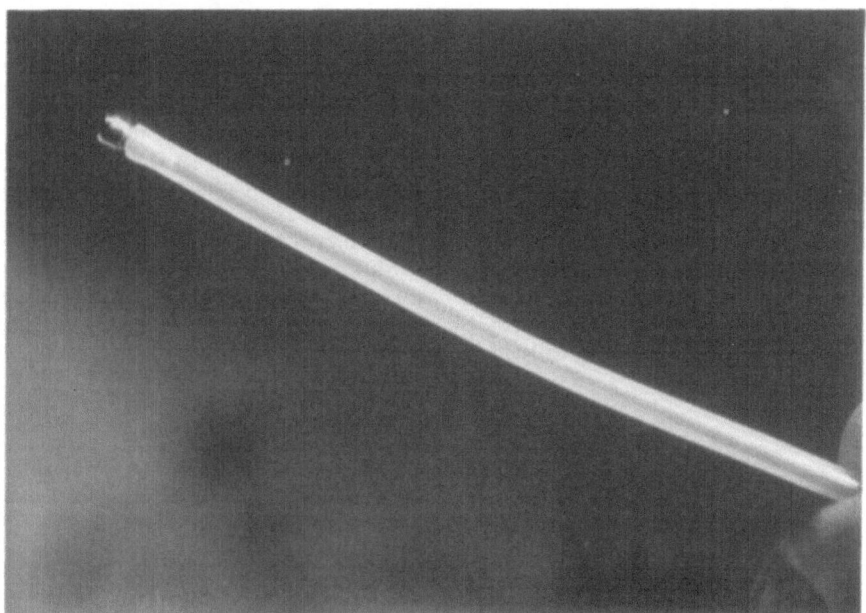

Fig. 2.12. The fiber is reinserted within the teflon sheath.

Three specific evaluations should be made at this time. The first is that adequate gas flow has been maintained after reassembly of the optic fiber. The second is a test firing of the laser to be certain that the fiber tip does not glow indicating a misalignment in the reassembly of the optic fiber. Finally, the power output should be tested using an optic power meter.

The metal tips have been designed in our Biomedical Engineering Department (INSERM, Unit 279). They can be reused after a cleaning in hydrogen peroxide. A 5 meter long fiber may be cut several times before becoming too short. Our center is also equipped for the manufacture of new fibers. A unique system has been adapted to all our treatment and research lasers which makes the fibers exchangeable.

Maintenance is a real problem. We have described our solution which gives good results. At the time of laser purchase, one must ask the representative of the laser company what his solution is for fiber maintenance. Training for one of the staff (nurse, technician or medical doctor) is strongly recommended to avoid interruption in the treatment.

References

1. Fruhmorgen P, Reidenback MD, Boden F et al. Experimental examination on laser endoscopy. Endoscopy 1974;6:116-122.
2. Nath G, Gorisch W, Kiefhaber P. First laser endoscopy via a fiberoptic transmission system. Endoscopy 1973;5:208-213.
3. Brunetaud JM, Maffioli C, Enger A et al. Endoscopic laser coagulation in the digestive tract: Development of a photocoagulation and experimental study. Laser 77, IPC Science and Technology, Guilford 1977;355-360.
4. Brunetaud JM, Moschetto Y, Lenoir P et al. Les applications thérapeutiques des lasers: une nouvelle génération de fibres. Photon 1980. Proceedings 285-291.
5. Lenz P, Sabben G, Lambert R et al. Quartz fibers laser therapy in tissue contact. Photon 1983, May 16-19, 1983, Paris. SPIE Proceedings, 405, 97-104.
6. Joffe SN, Sankar MY, Slazer D et al. Preliminary clinical application of the contact surgical rod and endoscopic microprobes with the Nd:YAG laser. American Society for Laser Medicine and Surgery, May 27-29, 1985, Orlando.

3. MULTIDISCIPLINARY APPROACH TO MEDICAL LASER USE

JEAN-MARC BRUNETAUD AND SERGE MORDON

Wide spread application of laser therapeutics has been developing in many different fields of medicine. But a universal laser source does not exist. One specialty may need two lasers, like Gastroenterology (Argon and Nd:YAG) or Dermatology (Argon and CO_2), without having the budget to buy two different laser sources. When a specialty starts to explore the possibilities of laser treatment, it may require several laser sources for one particular indication. This has facilitated the sharing of laser facilities among different specialists. After three years of informal multidisciplinary work (1978-1982) in the laser room of the gastroenterology department, a Multidisciplinary Laser Center was created at the Lille University Hospital (May 1982). This chapter will describe the Center and its activity.

1. Description of the Laser Center

1.1. The Laser Rooms

The laser center has four rooms specialized for laser treatment: one operative theater for use of the CO_2 laser (Fig. 3.1), one room containing the argon and Nd:YAG systems (Fig. 3.2), one room for oncology with an argon-dye laser (Fig. 3.3), and one room containing all the equipment for dental treatment (Fig. 3.4).
The Laser Center also has a waiting room, recovery room, physicians' office and rooms for the secretary and assistants. All rooms are located on the same floor of the hospital building. In addition, the Laser Center has a room at the Lille Medical School specially equipped for experimental surgery on animals (Fig. 3.5).
An easy connection by elevators allows transportation of laser sources between the hospital and the medical school.

1.2. Laser Sources

This center has six laser systems for treatment. The Ercelas 40 CO_2 laser (Biophysic Medical, Clermont Ferrand, France) has a TEM 00 emission with

D.M. Jensen and J.M. Brunetaud (eds), Medical Laser Endoscopy. 27-36.

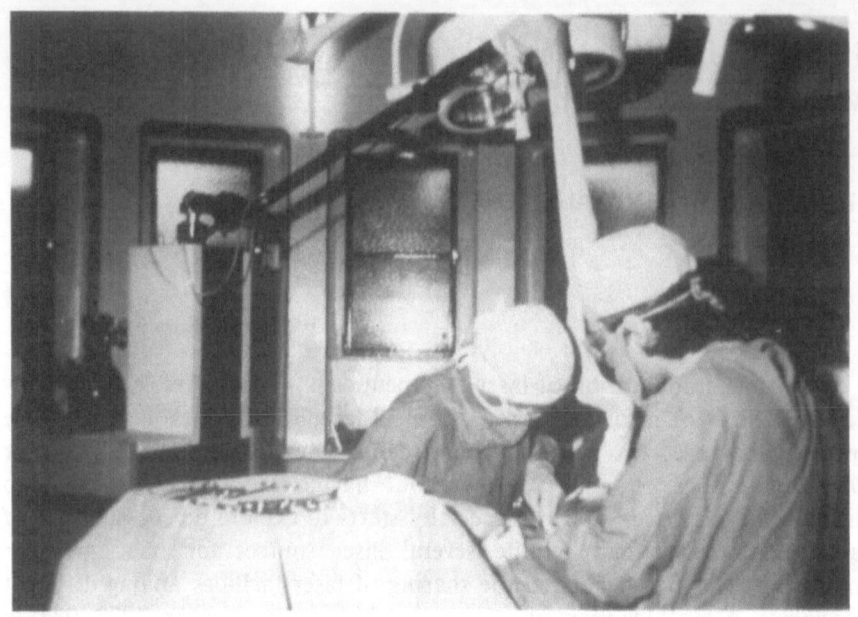

Fig. 3.1. Operative theater with a CO_2 laser.

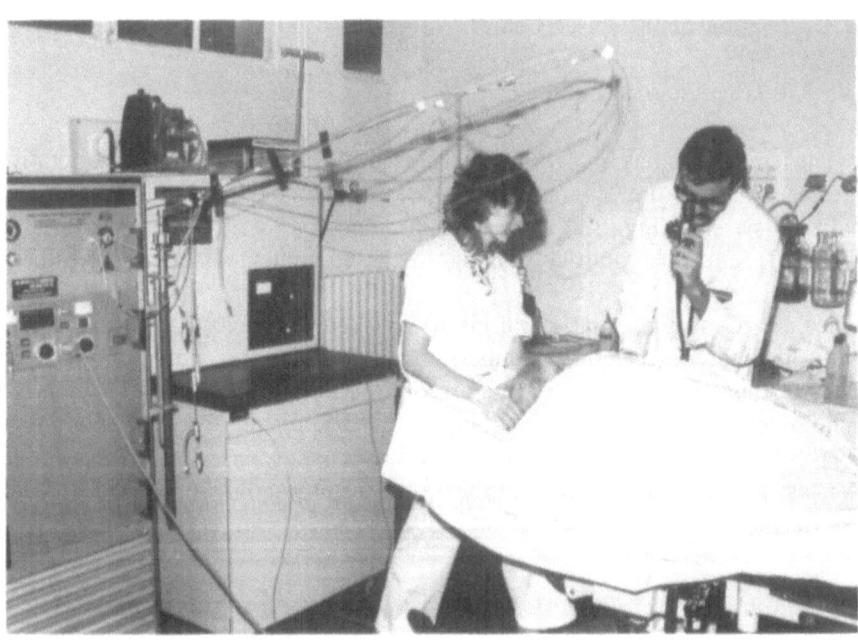

Fig. 3.2. Endoscopic laser room with the Nd:YAG (left) and the Argon (right). Treatment of an esophageal cancer.

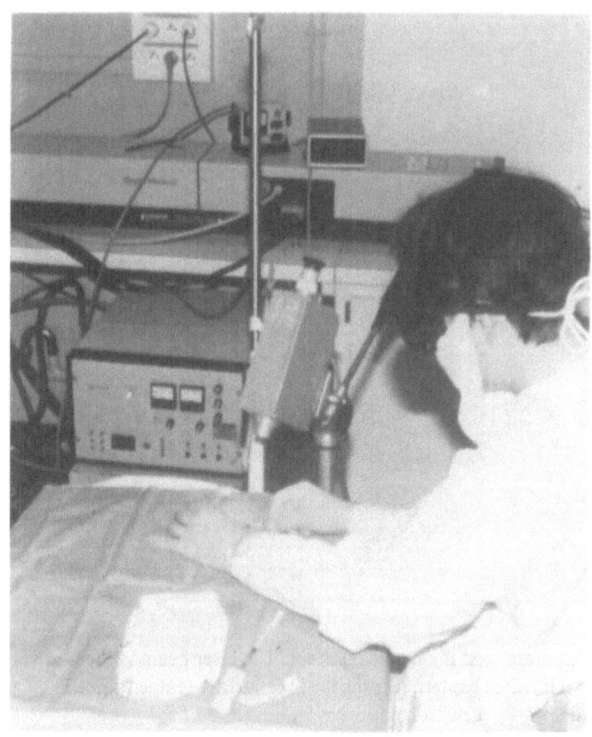

Fig. 3.3. Dye laser room. Treatment of an experimental cancer on a mouse. The camera is a pyrometer which records the surface temperature of the skin during treatment. In the back, the argon-dye laser and optic power meter.

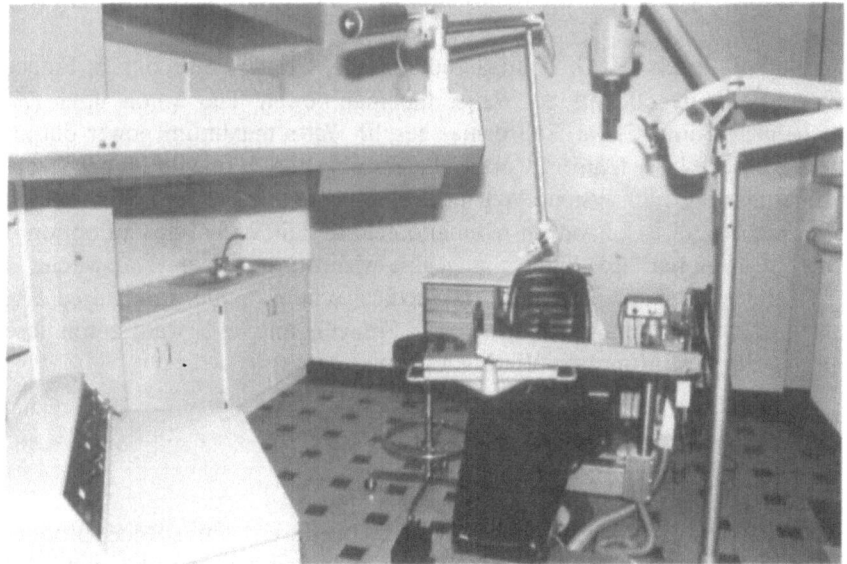

Fig. 3.4. Dental laser room. The CO_2 laser with its articulated arm is ready for dental treatment.

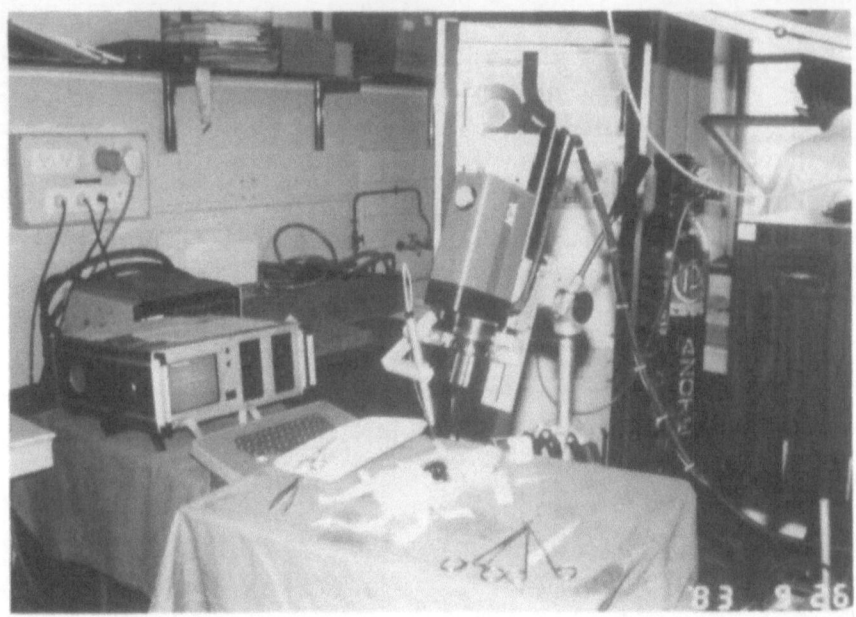

Fig. 3.5. Animal laboratory at the medical school. The laser beam is focused via a handpiece on the liver of a rat. An infrared camera records the liver surface temperature. The Quantel prototype Nd:YAG laser is driven by a microcomputer.

a maximum power output of 30 Watts continuous wave (CW), or 250 Watts pulsed at 500 Hertz. The second CO_2 laser source is a waveguide (Optrolas, Lille, France). The maximum power is 20 Watts. The laser is hand held and the beam is directly aimed at the treatment site without transmission system (Fig. 3.6).

The Nd:YAG lasers (YAG Medical 100 and 101, CILAS, Marcoussis, France) have respectively 50 and 80 Watts maximal power. The argon laser (770 Lasersonics, Santa Clara, California) has 10 Watts maximum power output. The Argon-dye laser (Aurora Cooper Lasersonics) has a maximum power of 7 watts using the Argon system. When the alternative tunable dye system is used, the power output is 1.5 watt at 630 nanometers. This system has an option of either green or red laser light, changeable with only the flip of a switch.

Two other lasers are located at the medical school: a 500 watt pulsed YAG laser (prototype from Quantel, Orsay, France), and a 5 watt argon laser (Spectra Physics, Mountain View, California).

1.3. Laser Accessories

Optic fibers for Argon, Nd:YAG and dye lasers are special products manufactured at the Laser Center. Different endoscopic laser probes and handpieces are adapted to each medical application. For external use (Dermatology,

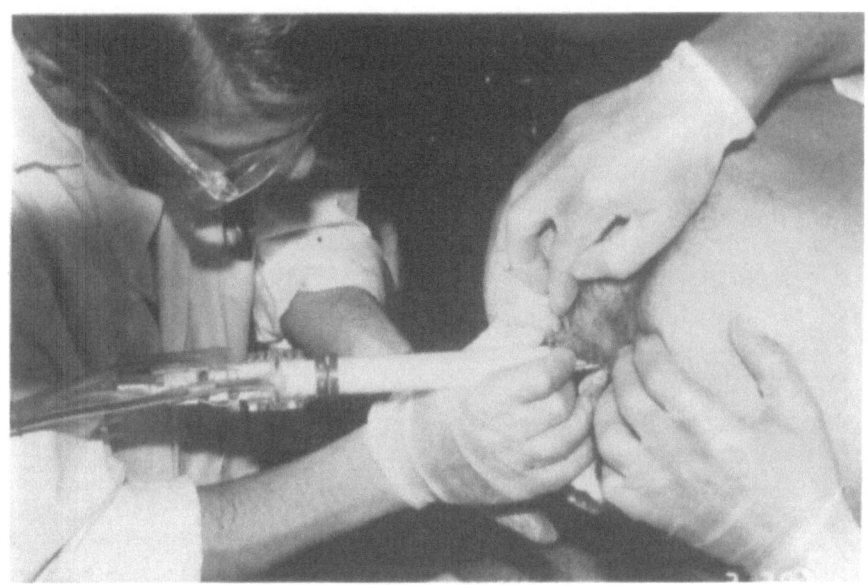

Fig. 3.6. Hand held waveguide CO_2 laser. Treatment of anal condylomata.

Gynecology), the hand-pieces are equipped with four different lenses, easily changeable without adjustments (Fig. 3.7).

Four spot sizes are available: 0.2 mm, 1.2 mm and 2.5 mm for the Argon laser and 0.4 mm, 1 mm, 2 mm, and 4 mm for the Nd:YAG laser (Fig. 3.8).

For digestive endoscopy, Argon and Nd:YAG laser probes have 1.6 mm external

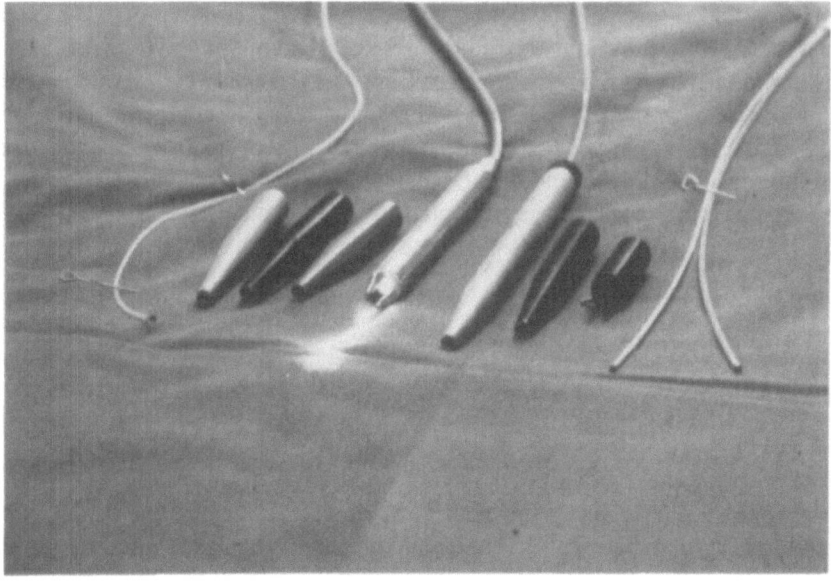

Fig. 3.7. Laser hand pieces for argon and Nd:YAG lasers.

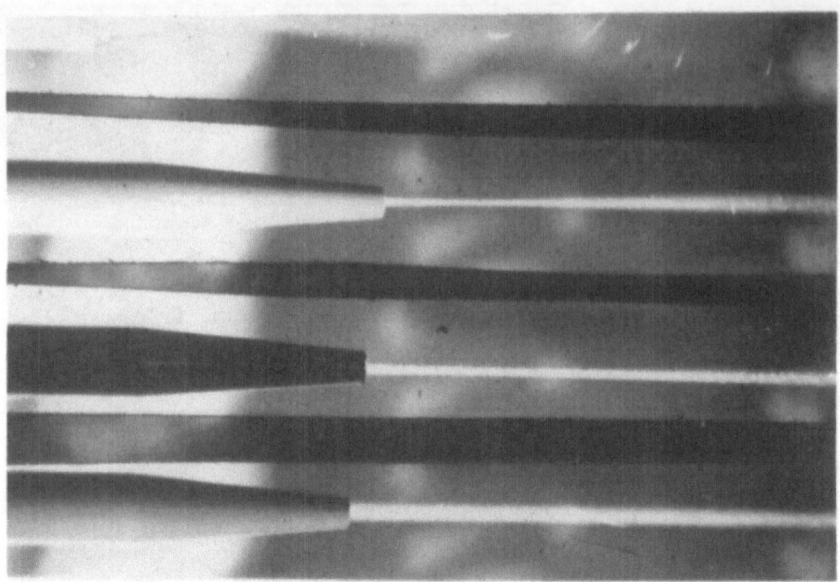

Fig. 3.8. Light dispersion from laser hand pieces.

diameter (compared to the 2.2 mm of commercial products). These same thin laser probes are also very useful in bronchoscopy. For urology, a special system was designed to replace the gas insufflated into the probe by water via a non-modified cystoscope.

All these fibers are coupled to the different lasers by the same type of connector (KMR standard, ATI, Evry, France). The high accuracy of this connector allows utilization of the same fiber on every laser in the Center (except CO_2 lasers) without any adjustment of the coupling system.

A robotized scanning handpiece has been especially developed in collaboration with the INSERM Unit 279 for the argon laser treatment of port wine stains. This system allows safer and faster treatments than the conventional technique by adjacent points.

Micromanipulators have been adapted to the operative microscope (OPMI 1, Carl Zeiss, Germany) for the use with CO_2 or argon lasers.

2. The laser unit organization and activity

2.1. The Permanent Staff

The staff of the Laser Center is composed of two nurses, three assistant nurses, one secretary, and three medical doctors: a resident, an assistant, and the director of the Unit. The director and the assistant are both gastroenterologists and carry out the digestive treatments. All the other treatments are performed by specialists from various departments coming to the laser center with their patients. Privileges are given after agreement between the chief of their department and the director of the Laser Center based upon experience and training of the laser user. Every staff member and user must be knowledgeable about the particular safety regulations concerning the use of lasers.

2.2. Scheduling Treatments

Central scheduling is organized by the secretary. Each specialist has a reserved time in the laser Center schedule. Cases are scheduled the week before. In case of vacancy or cancellation, the time slot is given to any doctor with another case.

2.3. Treatment Activity

There are four main specialties utilizing the operative theater and/or the argon-Nd:YAG laser room on a regularly scheduled basis: Gastroenterology (five half days), Dermatology (four half days), Gynecology (three half days) and Urology (one half day). General surgeons, oral surgeons, ENT specialists (for the Argon laser) use the center at least once a week. The dental room was opened March 1986. The oncology room will be opened for treatment soon. Other specialties from the Lille University Hospital have their own lasers: Ophthalmology (two Argon lasers and a nano second Nd:YAG laser), ENT (a 20 watt CO_2 laser), and Pneumology (a 50 CW Nd:YAG laser). They are in close contact with the Center for technical problems and sometimes come to the Laser Center for special indications. Table 3.1 lists the number of treatments performed at the Laser Center in the years 1983 to 1986.

Table 3.1. The number of laser treatments performed at the Lille Laser Center in the years 1983 to 1986.

	1983	1984	1985	1986
Dermatology	1,257	1,792	1,558	1,512
Digest. endo.	1,063	1,476	1,537	1,759
Plastic surgery	213	107	40	25
Gynecology	88	325	303	324
Urology	60	54	41	18
ENT				71
Dentistry				31
Angioplasty				9
Various surgery	89	68	53	13
TOTAL	2,770	3,822	3,532	3,762

3. Clinical research

The evaluation of the efficacy and the benefit to the patient of any new technique is very important. It will confirm some indications and suggest others be withdrawn. Photographic and video facilities are available at the Center. After each treatment a form has to be filled by the medical doctor. A computer system is being installed at the Laser Center wherein all patient files will be stored. As an example, indications of laser treatment in Gastroenterology have been modified since the beginning of the laser treatment activity. We are using the lasers less often for upper gastrointestinal active hemorrhages and more frequently for GI tumors. The technique itself can also change. We are disappointed by the results of the lasers in esophageal carcinoma as isolated treatment and we are using endoscopic dilatation more often before laser treatment. In Dermatology, tattoo removal by argon laser was disappointing so we changed to CO_2 laser with better results.

4. Experimental research

Basic research is carried out on thermal and photochemical laser effects. With the help of the Biomedical Technology Center (INSERM, Unit 279, Lille) we are testing the thermal effects on animal models of commercial and prototype laser systems. An infrared thermocamera (Aga 720) has been modified and coupled to a computer. This records the surface temperature of the tissue during laser exposure. The Laser Institute of the University of Utah has provided us experimental models of cancer in mice which are used at Lille for testing new photosensitizers synthesized by the INSERM Unit 201 PARIS.

5. Education

Education is accomplished in several ways. First, many specialists within the Lille Regional Hospital would not have begun laser work if the facilities and expertise had not been available to them. Secondly, didactic educational courses in digestive endoscopy and dermatology have been developed on a regional, national and international scale which have further disseminated the scientific knowledge gained at the Laser Center. Third, photographs and video movies reporting the Laser Center experience are presented in post graduate courses. Lastly, a group of individuals have shown interest and knowledge of laser work and have been allowed hands-on training at the Laser Center.

6. Maintenance of the Laser Systems

The director and the assistant of the Laser Center are able to solve most of maintenance problems such as recleaving the fibers or cleaning and adjusting the laser mirrors. Only for an electronic problem with the power supply is a serviceman of the laser manufacturers called for help.

7. Financial

The cost of any new treatment is a major problem all over the world. But each country has different health insurance systems which make comparisons difficult. In France, expensive treatments (like digestive endoscopic laser treatments) are covered 100% by the national health insurance. Cheaper ones like port wine stain treatments are covered at 80% and others like tattoo removal are not covered at all. All the treatment charges do not cover the expenses of the Laser Center and the hospital has to supplement from its general budget. The major expenses are the staff salaries which are 60% of the total budget for the Laser Center. A multidisciplinary Laser Center is a good way to decrease the part of the equipment in this budget but the salaries increase the Center's budget.

For some applications, comparisons have been made between the cost of standard treatment and laser treatment for the same disease. As an example, the treatment of a rectal villous adenoma by laser in our hospital is slightly cheaper than by surgery, even if ambulance transportation is taken into account. (Laser treatment is performed on an outpatient basis).

8. Future of the multidisciplinary Laser Center

At present, the utilization rate of the two main laser rooms (Argon-Nd:YAG and operative theater) is 80%. This is ideal, as it allows time for basic maintenance. The number of treatments performed in the Laser Center is now stable. New specialties like ENT (for coagulation of angioma in the nose), dentistry, and angioplasty balance the decrease of activity from others like plastic surgery. The treatment numbers will not increase indefinitively for two reasons. First, the high cost of the salaries will not allow the staff to grow. Secondly, the goal of the Multidisciplinary Laser Center is not to gather together all the laser activities of the hospital. Ophthalmologists, ENT surgeons, and bronchoscopists already have their own lasers. If a speciality has a large activity which can be performed with a single monodisciplinary laser, it will be better for this specialty (and also for the Laser Center) to buy a new laser. This could be the case for gynecology. A cheap CO_2 laser, especially adapted for colposcopy, should be manufactured soon. With such a laser, the gynecology department could perform all its routine cases, and it would allow the Laser Center to have more free time for other specialities. Gynecologists would still use the Laser Center for special cases, when they need another laser, as for endoscopic treatment of endometriosis.

In conclusion, the goals of the Lille Laser Center are routine cases when several lasers are required for the same specialty, evaluation of new indications until the specialty is research, education of new indications until the specialty is able to buy a well adapted laser, clinical and experimental research, education, and finally development or testing of new laser equipment.

4. LASER SURGICAL UNIT ORGANIZATION

JOHN A. DIXON

There is something about the medical mentality that abhors the word 'organization'. All you have to do to begin laser surgery is to attend a course, buy a laser, plug it in and go to work – right? Wrong! All of the factors in our health care delivery system are arrayed against such a simplistic (and effective) approach. The laser user will soon be descending into a morass of problems relative to maintenance, transport, FDA approvals, protocols, institutional review board reviews, privileges, amortization of equipment, billing, trouble shooting and educational concerns.

The inevitable problems of introducing new technology into the clinical setting may be considerably diminished by advance planning. This chapter will suggest a format for laser unit organization, a description of the specific function of such a centralized unit and some thoughts relative to future directions in laser unit organization.

An effective unit should be designed to effectively handle most functions and problems with minimum expenditure of staff time (1). In the laser field, the staff people involved are from various departments such as medicine and surgery, a director or administrator who oversees the unit, clinical and support staff and multiple users. A typical organizational format appears in Fig. 4.1. This structure allows for departmental and institutional directions or objectives to flow through the director of the unit with the advice of a laser committee. Implementation of such objectives can be instituted by clinical support staff or technical staff to facilitate the work of laser users.

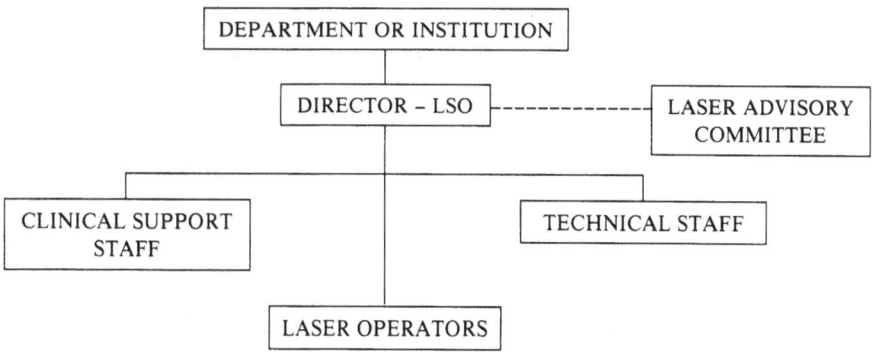

Fig. 4.1. Organizational chart for Medical Laser Unit.

D.M. Jensen and J.M. Brunetaud (eds), Medical Laser Endoscopy. 37-43.
© 1990 Kluwer Academic Publishers, Dordrecht

Conversely, problems or opportunities noted by the laser users can be channelled to the director of the unit who can then work through support staffs, the advisory committee or the institution in order to carry out the desired changes. Some specifics of operation, implementation and description of laser personnel follows.

Department or Institution – The parent organization of the laser unit can be a department such as the department of medicine or surgery or an institution such as a hospital or clinic body. In smaller institutions there will probably be a direct reporting relationship of the director of the laser unit to the hospital administrator or clinic director or other such official. In larger institutions, a clinical department may be responsible for the laser unit with input from other departments to the laser advisory committee. Institutional directions and goals are developed at this level.

Director-Laser Safety Officer – This person is the responsible administrative officer for the laser unit. In most cases the administrative and laser functions are combined. The director should have personal experience and interest in laser applications and be willing to spend the time to carry out the responsibilities necessary for the operation of the unit. Frequently, the director will be part-time in that position and have other clinical or administrative responsibilities. In larger institutions this will be a full-time job. The director is the hub of the entire operation. This person interfaces with the institution and departments through an advisory board, then directs the clinical and technical support staff to benefit laser operators. The medical specialty of the director is unimportant as long as the other criteria are met.

Laser Advisory Committee – This group is usually made up of representatives from those departments using the laser unit. Typically, surgery, medicine, obstetrics and gynecology, radiology, and ophthalmology will be involved. A representative of each of these departments meets periodically with the committee to advise the director of the unit on a myriad of considerations about privileges, equipment, research, etc.

Clinical Support Staff – These individuals report directly to the director and carry out the responsibilities to implement laser use. There is usually a head nurse who is responsible for scheduling, observation of safety factors, and directing the set-up and operation of the lasers. This person is usually charge of overall patient concerns such as electrocardiographic monitoring, monitoring of blood gases, and general items relative to clinical support.

In larger units, it is useful to have a medical technician working in the laser unit to assist in the ambulatory or general surgical operating rooms in the setting up and operation of laser, maintenance of equipment, dressing of fibers and preparation of endoscopic equipment.

Part-time technical support is also essential in the operation of the laser unit. Electricians and plumbers from the institution, such as the hospital, need to work closely with laser unit personnel for installation and maintenance of power and water supplies. Where multiple use of equipment is being implemented at various sites in the institution, support transportation mechanisms must be established as sensitive laser equipment may be easily damaged in transport. It is useful to have such individuals trained in the transportation of the unit rather than relying upon the nearest available person to move the lasers.

The Laser Operators Group – constitutes the actual users of the unit. Users may range from one specialty to as many as eighteen depending upon the size and complexity of the institution. Inasmuch as there are the ultimate consumers of the laser resource, the entire unit operation is geared to providing safe, economical, efficient support of their activities. A very sensitive ear should be constantly tuned to their needs.

Laser Unit Functions

Safety

The laser is unique among surgical instruments in that it poses hazards to the patient, operator and operating personnel. In large complex institutions, a 'piecemeal' approach to inservice education and safety such as might be mounted by a division or department is doomed to failure. There are always individuals who are not contacted by such compartmental safety programs and they will undergo exposure to laser radiation. The central laser unit through the laser safety officer has the responsibility of reviewing all sites in which lasers are operating and assuring compliance with ANSI and FDA requirements (2). All individuals who have contact with the laser at each of these sites must then be adequately trained with regard to safety precautions. Due to the constant turnover in hospital personnel, such educational programs must be ongoing as part of the routine orientation of each new employee or staff member.

Education, Credentialling and Coordination

There will inevitably arise the necessity for granting privileges to use the laser. With the number of procedures escalating at such a rapid rate, skill requirements are dynamic and must be constantly evolving. When training in use of lasers is well standardized, it will be relatively easy for each division or department to be responsible for its own granting of privileges. Until such time, it will be the responsibility of the central laser unit to review and grant privileges to the individual user. The director of the laser unit can act as staff to the laser committee in bringing together credentials and making recommendations about each application. Established specialty boards will likely soon include materials relative to the use of lasers and be of assistance to such committees.

With central scheduling of lasers, it is relatively simple to limit use of lasers to only those individuals who have privileges. Any controversies relative to use are immediately referred to the director who may request advice from the laser committee if necessary.

The high cost of certain uses of the laser makes central scheduling almost mandatory. While most operators are naturally acquisitive and possessive, joint usage is essential to keep cost per use down. Scheduling is usually done by the nurse or administrator in the director's office who blocks out the time for the use of each laser to the surgeon or operating room as needs become evident.

Central review and purchase of equipment is effective and facilitates application. If joint use and scheduling are to be employed, users and frequency of use must be carefully considered and allowed for in the purchase of new devices. Closely associated with this is the necessity for provision of adequate endoscopic and microscopic equipment to use with the lasers. In some instances, the laser may be introduced into the endoscopic suite. Frequently, however, endoscopic equipment must be provided at the laser unit and must be compatible with fibers used.

New procedures and applications are an every day part of the laser unit consideration. While initial applications may appear to relate to a single specialty, there are frequently implications and spin-offs involving other specialties. To have neodymium-YAG users such as pulmonologists, urologists, gastroenterologists and neurosurgeons communicating about new procedures is very helpful, promotes safety and reduces complications.

Periodic meetings devoted to research with lasers provides cross fertilization among disciplines. Traditional departmentalization frequently restricts such sharing of information which can be fostered by the laser unit. For instance, the various manifestations of Osler-Weber-Rendu disease are treated by opthalmologists, dermatologists, plastic surgeons, gastroenterologists, otolaryngologists and urologists. Joint research centered around laser treatment has brought about a better understanding of this disease and its treatment.

Record keeping is a vital function of the central laser unit. Many procedures still require completion of special protocol forms. Individualized informed consent forms must be completed. As these fall outside of the purview of the usual nursing procedure, the central unit must assume responsibility. Approvals by the Institutional Review Board, FDA, and laser manufacturers must be sought in certain cases. Photographic files must be maintained to document patient progress. Clinical assistance is frequently asked of the central unit for liaison with major operating room staffs where it is necessary to transport lasers, set them up, and assist in the laser surgical procedure. Night coverage by staff for emergencies involving lasers likewise must be provided for.

The laser unit becomes an important educational resource in many instances. Provision for photography, video recording and making of movies evolves because of the demands for inservice and graduate education. A central audiovisual laser library in larger institutions is maintained by the laser unit.

Postgraduate education for nurses, physicians and support personnel is facilitated and illustrated tours for visiting physicians are made more productive.

Because of the wide publicity given laser surgery, provisions must be made for screening the cards, letters, telephone calls and inquiries about the efficacy of laser application in a particular disease. Trained personnel in the laser unit may screen many of these contacts and see that appropriate referral is made for laser treatment. Sensitivity and compassion should be demonstrated toward the many individuals who seek the laser as a last resort in a far- advanced illness. An appropriately trained individual in the laser unit can greatly help with all the specialties.

Technical

There are a number of technical functions that are best handled collectively. Maintenance of lasers and trouble shooting of problems is a constant challenge. One or more assigned technical support personnel who deal with laser problems frequently can be more effective than the occasional technician. Contact is maintained with manufacturers to get lasers back on line as quickly as possible. The ability to recognize difficulties which may be resolved quickly by 'in-house' and those which require manufacturer's assistance is important.

Technical liaison with hospital electricians, plumbers and other service departments is frequently required in laser operation. Surges or changes in power or fluctuations in water supply will affect the function of lasers. Sometimes the addition of additional users to a circuit will cause problems that must be resolved by people aware of the entire utilities system.

Laser fibers of all types are subject to breakage, burning, melting and carbonization. It is possible to train technical personnel to repair laser fibers with available repair kits. This results in great monetary and time savings. A central technical person can frequently repair all fibers in a relatively short time at the end of the day.

Financial

Expensive laser equipment must be purchased and paid for according to standard business practices. One needs to look carefully at the probable number of treatments to be provided, the cost of the lasers, the probable useful life of each instrument and set up appropriate cost and billing practices. Such information frequently must be collected at a central site in the health care facility in order to adequately amortize equipment. It has been useful to separate equipment costs from physician's fees. Hospital financial officers are frequently able to quickly work out fair equipment costs which are readily accepted by third party payors.

The advent of many health plans and DRG's have required that someone carefully work through the total cost of laser use (equipment plus physician fees) to achieve reimbursement. The central unit staff is frequently in the best position to collect this information and present it to third party payors in a fashion that is understandable and most likely to receive favorable consideration.

Future Laser Organizations

It is obvious that increased usage by each specialty will change the functions previously described. An increased number of patients and standardization of techniques such as has occurred in opthalmology will result in dedicated units purchased by and used solely by that specialty. The specialty then becomes 'mature' in the sense of laser usage. Inservice laser safety programs have been established. Criteria and procedures for credentialing are well worked out and operating room personnel are fully acquainted with laser usage.

Fragmentation will no longer be the need for many of the centralized functions previously described. At this point, there will likely be certain residual functions left for the central laser unit. Some of these may be:

1. There will be the introduction of new laser wavelengths and technology. Well established laser users may feel erroneously prepared to use these modalities. There may be significant new problems introduced that need be addressed centrally.
2. Safety will always require supervision by central unit laser personnel. The rapid change in technical and support staff in multiple separate divisions can result in laxity and potential hazards. Such functions should be regarded as educational support as opposed to 'policing' action.
3. Central scheduling will still be necessary for some of the less frequent specialty users. It will be some time, for instance, before a Pulmonary Division can afford a dedicated full-time neodymium YAG laser for palliation of tracheobronchial tumors and will rely upon some sharing arrangement.
4. A central audiovisual library will continue to be useful. Lectures, training programs and courses given by the specialties frequently require basic illustrative material that can be centrally maintained.
5. There will be an important data collection function that will continue after many of the specialties become independent. Cost, morbidity and mortality figures can be best evaluated by central collection techniques.
6. A clearing house for research projects of an interdisciplinary nature will remain one of the most important functions of the central laser unit. Applications involving multiple organ systems frequently yield best to combined approaches. It is important for specialists to hear of developments in allied fields. Advances are frequently initiated by such interdisciplinary contacts. The central laser unit may act by providing the forum for such contacts and by supervising and assisting with research, laser equipment acquisition and use.

42

References

1. Dixon JA. In: Surgical Application of Lasers, Dixon JA: ed, New York: Year Book Medical Publishers, 1983: 2.
2. American National Standards Institute. Standard Z 136.1, New York, 1980.

5. GI ENDOSCOPIC HEMOSTASIS AND TUMOR TREATMENT – EXPERIMENTAL RESULTS AND TECHNIQUES

DENNIS M. JENSEN

Introduction

Lasers have been used for endoscopic hemostasis in gastroenterology (GI) for more than ten years and for GI tumor treatment for at least five years. Still many questions remain about the best techniques, indications, histologic and clinical results, and comparisons with standard treatments (often surgery) and with non-laser endoscopic techniques. Some important questions have been addressed and answered in careful laboratory studies. The purpose of this paper is to relate laboratory studies with lasers and non-laser endoscopic techniques to clinical questions concerning endoscopic control of GI hemorrhage and tumor treatment. Results and techniques will be related to the endoscopic treatment of bleeding peptic ulcers, esophageal varices, angioma, and GI tumors.

Methods

Endoscopes

For endoscopic experiments, therapeutic instruments with large (3.7 mm) bore suction channels or double channels facilitated simultaneous suctioning and coagulation. Large non-laser thermal probes (3.2 mm diameter) such as heater probe or bipolar electrocoagulation (BICAP) required large endoscopic channels.

Endoscopic Hemostasis Methods

Neodymium-Yttrium-aluminum-Garnet (YAG) Laser. For the author's experiments an 120 W YAG laser (Cooper Lasersonics, Sunnyvale, Calif.) with a 600 um quartz lightguide and coaxial CO_2 was used (1, 2). The power range is 0-120 W output from the lightguide tip and pulse duration 0-20 sec. This laser lightguide has a 9.5 degree full angle of divergence. Clinically relevant equipment settings (power, pulse duration, treatment distance, etc.) were used with each experiment. Whenever any endoscopic YAG laser treatments were

D.M. Jensen and J.M. Brunetaud (eds), Medical Laser Endoscopy. 45-70.

performed, a protective filter was placed over the endoscopic eyepiece. For open experiments protective goggles were worn by all personnel.

Argon Laser (ALP). For the author's experiments, either a 20 W Spectrophysics 171 argon laser or a 12 W 770 Spectrophysics argon laser (Cooper Lasersonics, Sunnyvale, Calif.) with 400 um quartz lightguide and coaxial CO_2 gas jet were used (2, 3). The argon lightguide has a 9° full angle of divergence. The power range for the 770 is 0-12 W and for the 171 is 0-20 W from the lightguide tip. A protective filter was placed over the endoscopic eyepiece whenever endoscopic argon laser treatments were performed. For open experiments protective goggles were worn by all personnel. Clinically relevant instrument settings were used with each experiment.

Monopolar Electrocoagulation (MPEC) was applied with a monopolar electrode (model CD-3L, Olympus Corporation, New Hyde Park, NY) and a standard Valleylab SSE2-K electrosurgical unit (Boulder, Colo.). Water was infused with a syringe through the center of the probe for irrigation (4, 5). In open experiments, a pressure gauge could quantitate the probe tip to tissue apposition pressure. An analogue computer quantitated joules of power delivered with each pulse for MPEC. Although many other types of MPEC electrosurgical units and probe configurations are commercially available, they were not evaluated in the experiments presented except hot biopsy forceps and the hydrothermal probe for the colon experiments and Olympus monopolar for colon and stomach.

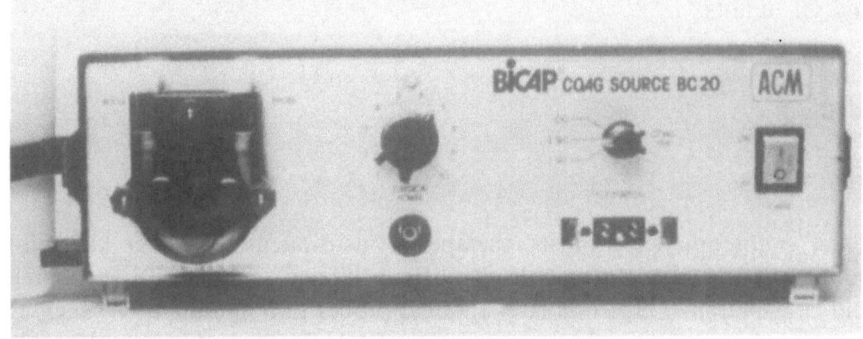

Fig. 5.1. BICAP 50 Watt generator (American ACMI).

Bipolar Electrocoagulation (BPEC) was applied with a prototype endoscopic unit whose probes were made by Medi-Tech (Watertown, Mass.) or a commercially available unit by American ACMI (Stamford, Conn.) – BICAP – see Fig. 5.1 (2, 4, 6). An analogue computer quantitated joules of power delivered with each pulse. Water was infused via a syringe through the center of the probe for irrigation. In open experiments, apposition pressure was controlled with a hand held pressure gauge. The irrigation and coagulation were performed via foot switch control with large (tip diameter 3.2 mm) or small probes (diameter 2.4 mm) – see Fig. 5.2.

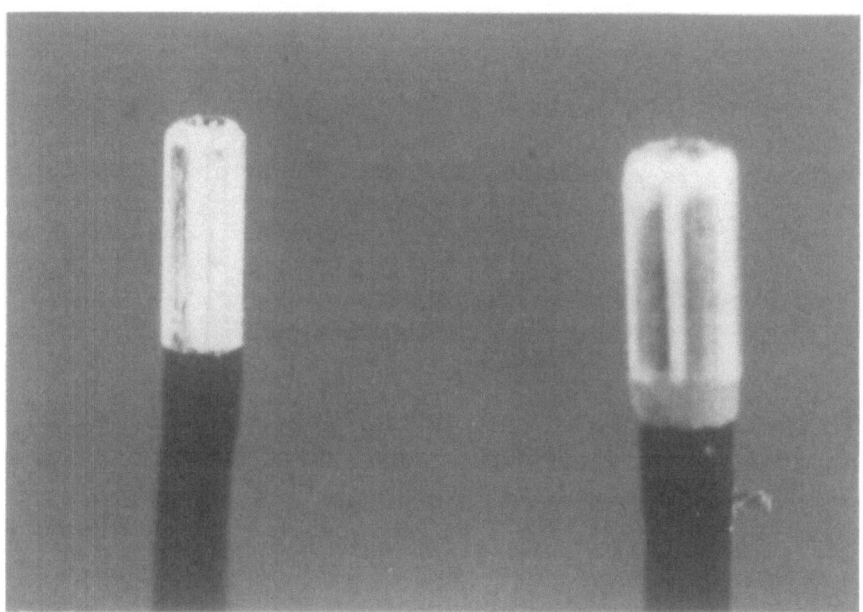

Fig. 5.2. BICAP coagulation probes, right is large (3.2 mm diameter) and left is small probe (2.4 mm diameter).

Heater Probe (HP) was applied with a prototype endoscopic HP (Auth, Seattle, WA) and a commercially available unit (Olympus Corp.) – Fig. 5.3 – with large (3.2 mm) or small (2.4 mm) probes – Fig. 5.4 – (8). Energy in joules per pulse was preset and simultaneous coagulation and washing were performed via foot switch control. For open experiments, apposition pressure was controlled with a hand held pressure gauge. For endoscopic hemostasis experiments, a two channel therapeutic endoscope was used. A commercially available heater probe unit is now being marketed by Olympus Corporation.

Sclerotherapy (SCLERO). For hemostasis with SCLERO, 2 ml of sclerosant was injected intravariceally using a 23-gauge needle in a flexible endoscopic catheter. Different, effective sclerosants were tested (9).

Ferromagnetic Tamponade. A 60 Hz, 208 V ferromagnetic tamponade system (Walker Scientific, Worcester, MA) was tested (8). The treatment distance from the ferromagnet to the tissue was approximately 6 cm and the power setting was 85% of maximum. The tamponade mixture consisted of 10 g of 325 mesh iron powder (Alfa Products, Danvers, MA), 1000 U of topical thrombin (Parke-Davis, Detroit, MI), 1 g carboxymethylcellulose, 1 ml of glycerin, and 10 ml of water. Five to seven milliliters were applied to the bleeding lesion with an endoscopic catheter, and the electromagnet was turned on for 10 min. After 10 min. the electromagnet was turned off and the tamponade mixture was washed from the lesion with water. Continued bleeding was assessed visually.

Electrofulguration was produced with a modified needle electrode and a Valleylab SSE2-K electrosurgical unit (Boulder, CO) in the pure coagulation

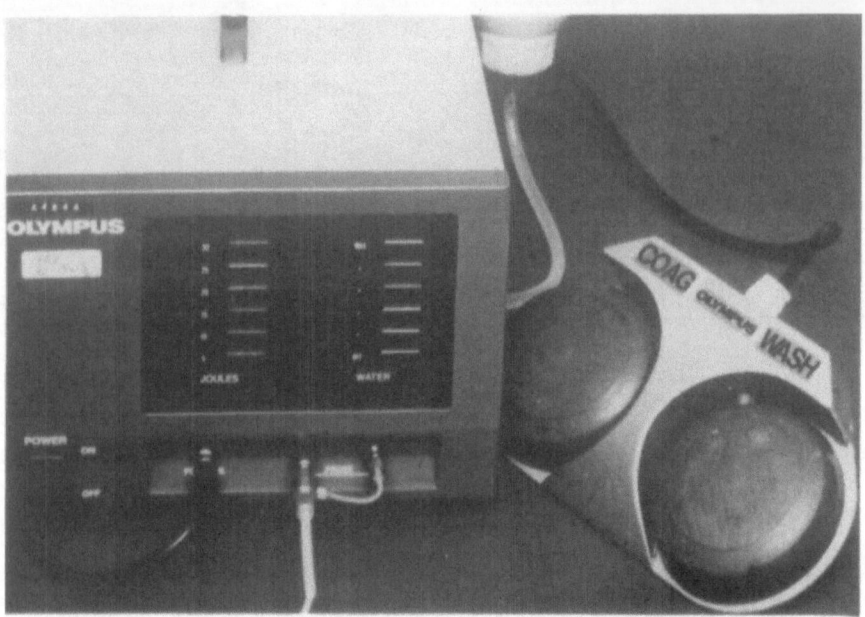

Fig. 5.3. Heater probe power unit with foot pedal (Olympus Corp.).

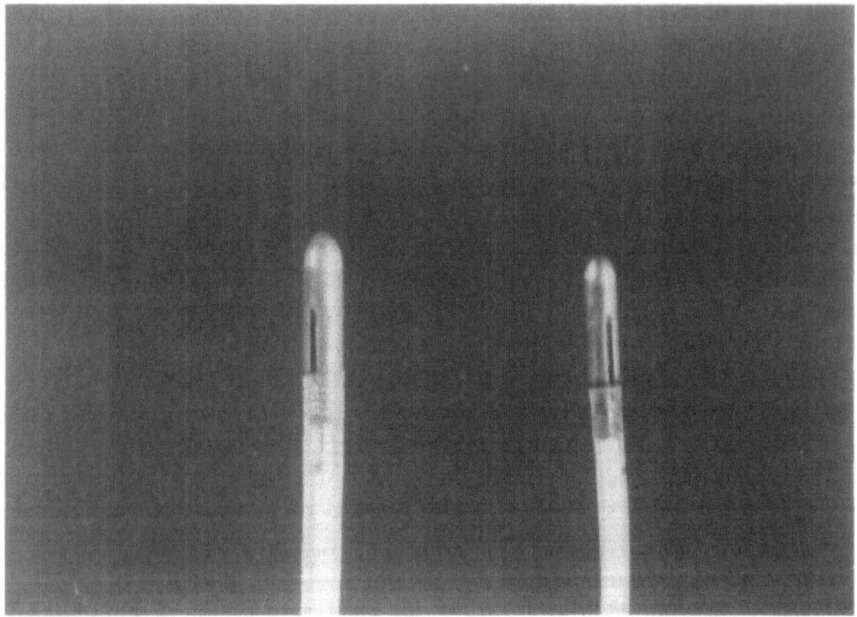

Fig. 5.4. Heater probe, right, is small (2.4 mm diameter), the left is large (3.2 mm).

mode (10). A hand held syringe was used to keep the target lesion wet during open experiments. Treatment distance was adjusted to produce sparking without tissue contact.

Hydrothermal Probe. A system of monopolar electrocoagulation that provided simultaneous water irrigation and coagulation ('the hydrothermal probe') was evaluated in the canine colon for safety and efficacy (11). This system is marketed by Karl Storz Corporation.

Animal Models

Standard Ulcer Models

The introduction of the 'standard ulcer-maker' by Protell et al. provided a mechanical model of acute, bleeding ulcers (12). Extensive studies in animals to evaluate the efficacy and safety of endoscopic hemostatic methods and to compare these methods under the same conditions have been reported.

This large suction biopsy capsule produced acute gastric ulcers approximately 10 mm in diameter and 1.5 mm deep, extending into the vascular submucosa. With heparinization, lesions continue to bleed unless effective treatment is applied. Standard ulcer bleeding rates have varied from 0.1 ml to more than 10 ml/min in our mongrel dogs. The induced ulcers have from 2 to 6 bleeding points around them; all of these must be treated to visually control bleeding in heparinized animals. Most investigators using animals define hemostatic efficacy as the ability of a treatment method to completely stop bleeding from acute standard ulcers in heparinized animals.

Using a standard ulcer-maker, several models are useful to evaluate hemostatic efficacy. A gastrotomy bleeding ulcer (open) model allows the best control. Fasted adult canines are anesthetized and endotracheal intubation is performed. The mucosa of the corpus of the stomach is exposed by a sterile laparotomy and anterior gastrotomy. Fluid losses are replaced with intravenously administered saline. Anticoagulation with sodium heparin, given intravenously in doses of 200 units/kg initially and 100 units/kg with each additional hour, prevents spontaneous clotting. Lesions made with a standard ulcer-maker continue to bleed from the vascular submucosa unless effectively treated. Bleeding rates can be estimated from direct collections of blood in graduated containers during a prescribed interval. Treated and control lesions can be observed directly for continued bleeding, and hemostatic efficacy can be determined. For later identification of ulcers, the nearby mucosa can be labeled, using metal clips or sutures.

Initial studies of a new modality are usually done using the gastrotomy bleeding model. Optimal conditions and techniques for the use of each hemostatic method can be determined. Also, any variables affecting hemostatic efficacy and acute tissue damage can be determined and controlled, for example, power setting, treatment distance, and pressure of apposition. After initial studies with this model, endoscopic studies are usually performed to validate hemostatic efficacy under conditions more like those in clinical UGI bleeding.

A clamped gastrotomy bleeding ulcer ('open-closed' endoscopic) model was conceived by Gilbert et al. (13). An atraumatic intestinal clamp is used to seal a small anterior gastrotomy after quantitation of bleeding from each standard ulcer. Animals are heparinized. After endoscopic treatment of each lesion, the clamp is removed and the ulcers directly inspected to confirm hemostatic efficacy and to determine acute serosal whitening or perforation.

We have produced acute ulcers extending into the submucosa via the operating endoscope and a large 'hot' biopsy forceps (Olympus Corp., New Hyde Park, NY) passed through the large channel (10). These are acute mechanical lesions created by cutting; no electrosurgical unit is employed. The advantage of this method is that lesions can be placed wherever the investigator desires. After randomization of such lesions, we have successfully labeled lesions with an endoscopic clipping device (Olympus Corp.) for later identification. In heparinized dogs, these lesions continue to bleed unless treated successfully.

This endoscopic bleeding ulcer model allows endoscopic testing of the efficacy of a method without operating on the animal. Many lesions can be made, treated, and labeled. Both control and treated ulcers heal within 3 to 4 weeks without causing untoward effects in healthy animals. The disadvantages are the lack of standardization of ulcers, the inability to quantitate bleeding, and, at times, the inability to identify ulcers for histologic identification 4 to 7 days later.

Safety

For studies that include delayed histologic assessment, the gastrotomy and abdominal incisions are surgically closed. Intramuscular antibiotics are administered postoperatively. The animals are then sacrificed after 4 to 9 days (usually 7) and the ulcers are identified. This is the time when tissue damage from thermally active treatment modalities is the most evident by histologic staining. Routinely recorded at autopsy are the presence of serosal changes (whitening or infection) overlying the ulcers, tacking of the omentum to ulcers, and intra-abdominal abscesses or other evidence of peritonitis or perforation. Also, the ulcers can be inspected after fixation and before multiple sectioning for evidence of full thickness injury.

Most investigators using the standard ulcer-maker in animals evaluated safety in terms of the maximum depth of histologic damage seen on tissue staining of ulcers treated 4 to 7 days earlier. The percentage of external muscle layer damage (EMLD) is usually determined, in addition to the frequency of full thickness (100% EMLD) injury for each treatment method. To make these evaluations of maximum depth of injury accurately, serial sectioning of tissue blocks was previously required. This was tedious and very expensive. Martin et al. reported a technique that eases this assessment (14). Using a device constructed from mounted razor blades, 1 mm slices of tissue are cut from fixed ulcers before paraffin embedding. With a dissecting microscope, the

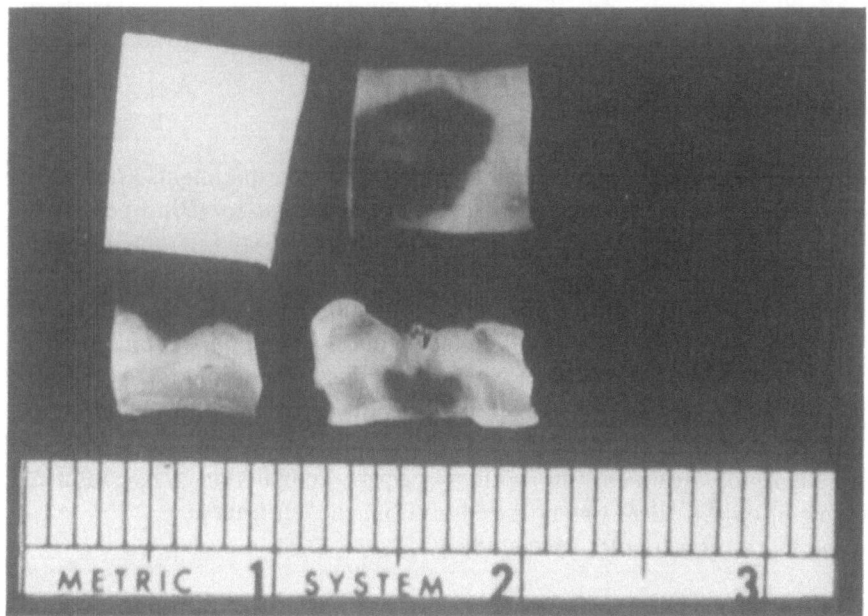

Fig. 5.5. Gross inspection of fixed gastric tissue seven days after thermal coagulation with BICAP (left) and YAG laser (right). The top shows the serosal aspect with hemorrhage after YAG treatment (right, YAG 50 Watts, 1 sec pulses, total 350 Joules, 4 mm spot) and normal appearance after BICAP (left, BICAP 15 Joule 1 sec pulses, 150 J total). The bottom shows the cut section for BICAP (left, limited injury) and YAG (right, full thickness injury).

section with the deepest damage is selected for microscopic examination after paraffin embedding, serial sectioning, and hematoxylin and eosin (H and E) staining. H and E sections are read in a coded fashion with the depth of tissue injury recorded as the percentage of damage using this method compared favorably with estimation of damage from microscopic examination of serially sectioned ulcers. Moreover, the method is easy and economical.

Advantages of Ulcer Models

These standard models are valuable in permitting assessment and comparison of hemostatic efficacy and resultant tissue injury from different treatment methods used under controlled conditions. Different investigators can compare results using these models. Randomized controlled studies can be performed for different methods in the same animals. The models permit investigators to determine the best instrument settings to use with each method and to define the variables affecting both hemostatic efficacy and tissue damage. Hemostatic efficacy and histologic injury can be quantified, whereas these measurements cannot be accurately made in human studies. Furthermore, any new or proposed endoscopic treatment method can be standardized, tested, and, if necessary, improved before human trials are begun.

Direct Arterial Coagulation

In order to determine purely vascular effects, these experiments assessed the ability of each device to directly coagulate an exposed artery (10). In each case, treatment was directed to a single spot on the artery. Usual instrument settings (i.e. those clinically used by experts) were employed for each device, with the exception of MPEC, which was applied with short pulses of less than 0.5 sec to minimize electrical sparking. Contact probes were applied with sufficient force (10-30 gm) to occlude the target artery, unless conditions were otherwise specified. Repeated treatment pulses were delivered until coagulation was obtained or a maximum of 10 pulses. Following treatment, the artery was severed at the treatment site with a scalpel. Coagulation was considered successful only if there was no bleeding from the cut artery.

The following variables were studied:

A. Arterial size. The outside diameter of intact mesenteric and serosal arteries was measured with a micrometer. Intact arteries of 0.25 to 2.5 mm diameter were treated with each device.

B. Active bleeding. To assess efficacy in treating a bleeding artery, active bleeding was produced by puncturing a 1 mm mesenteric artery with an 18 gauge needle. Treatment with each device was delivered directly to the bleeding site. Treatment was judged successful only if active bleeding was halted.

C. Contact probe treatment without vessel compression. Our usual technique in coagulation arteries with the contact probes (MPEC, BICAP, heater probe) involved pressing against the artery with sufficient force to occlude it prior to heat delivery. In this part of the experiment, the activated contact probes were applied with light touch (less than 10 grams of appositional force) to intact 1 mm mesenteric arteries.

D. Laser treatment with ancillary vessel compression. Clinically, endoscopic laser treatment is performed without mechanical contact with the tissue. In this part of the experiment, ancillary vessel compression was added to laser treatment by pressing a clear glass slide against the artery to occlude it, then directing the laser light through the transparent glass slide to heat the compressed artery.

E. Effect of high power density. This part of the experiment assessed the effect of treatment of an intact 1 mm mesenteric artery with each device using high power density setting.

Using a reproducible canine model of esophageal varices, several hemostatic modalities were tested and compared to determine which were most effective in stopping variceal bleeding (15). Methods tested were endoscopic sclerotherapy, ALP, YAG, MPEC, BPEC, FT, and HP.

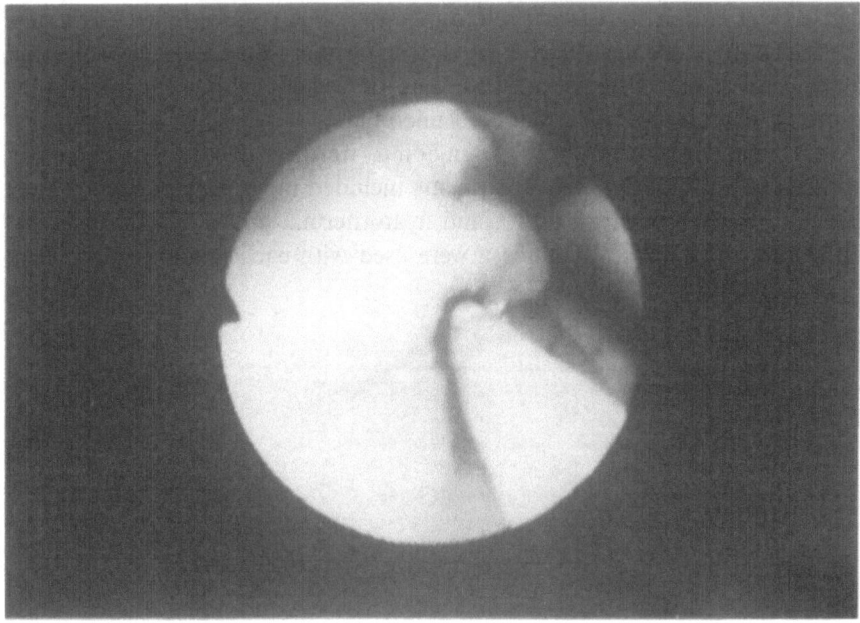

Fig. 5.6. Endoscopic photograph of a sclerotherapy needle in a canine esophageal varix for intravariceal injection.

Twenty dogs with two to four moderate to large-sized esophageal varices each were used for these studies (8). The dogs were anticoagulated with sodium heparin (200 U/kg initially, then 100 U/kg/h). During each experiment, three to six variceal bleeds were induced in each animal. To induce bleeding, the varix was punctured with a 19 gauge needle attached to an endoscopic catheter. The bleeding rate was quantified through a second large suction catheter connected to a calibrated vial. Each bleeding varix was randomized to control or treatment with one of the hemostatic modalities. A balloon cuff on the shaft of the endoscope cephalad to the varix served to increase intravariceal pressure and distend esophageal varices. It was also used with sclerotherapy to keep sclerosants in the injected segment and increase contact time. After successful hemostasis, a balloon cuff was inflated for 3 minutes cephalad to the treatment site to distend the varices and increase intravariceal pressure. This was used to test for rebleeding.

Adult mongrel dogs weighing between 40 and 60 lb. were used. Each dog was anesthetized with intravenous sodium pentobarbital and intubated. A sterile midline laparotomy was made. The right colon was mobilized and stool was milked gently out of the ascending colon (7, 11, 16). An atraumatic clamp was applied on either side of the selected segment, such that blood flow to this segment was impaired. A 10 cm colotomy was made on the antimesenteric side. The remaining stool was lavaged with sterile normal saline and gentle suction. For each animal, 10 different measurements of the colonic wall thickness at the colotomy were made with a standard micrometer.

To simulate treatment of colon angioma, normal mucosa was treated at laparotomy (11, 16). Different treatments included in the randomization were YAG, ALP, MONO, HP, BICAP, and hydrothermal probe. Standard clinical settings for coagulation of mucosa were used with each modality.

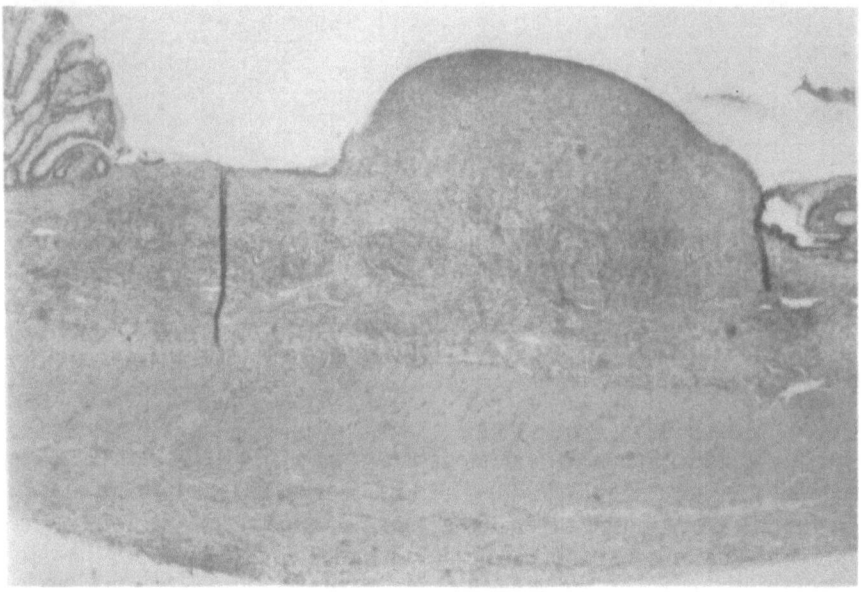

Fig. 5.7. Micrograph illustrating thermal damage only to the sub-mucosa after BICAP treatment of normal right colon mucosa to simulate an angioma (BICAP 20 Joules, large probe, total 200 J).

The surgery was done under sterile conditions. After mucosa treatment with each method, the mucosal lesions were labeled with silk sutures. After surgical closure, antibiotics were given for 48 hrs. At the time of autopsy 7 days later or when the animal appeared ill, the presence of abscess or perforation was assessed. The tissue damage was also assessed from 1 mm tissue sections and from coded histologic sections at 7 days. Colonic wall thickness (from mucosa to serosa) and depth of injury to normal mucosa treatment were estimated from these sections using a calibrated microscopic eyepiece.

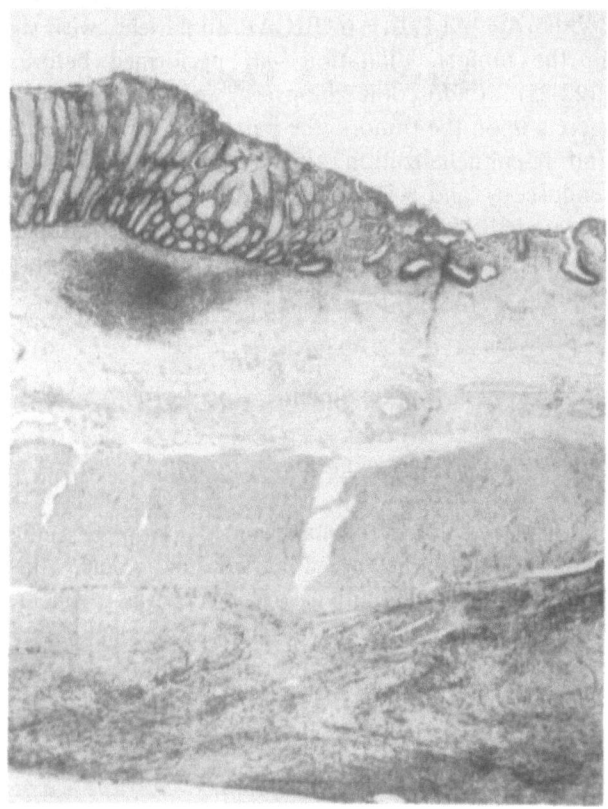

Fig. 5.8. Micrograph illustrating thermal damage through the entire colon wall seven days after YAG laser treatment of normal right colon mucosa (50 Watts, 0.5 sec pulses, 250 joules total, with a 4 mm spot).

Depth of Tissue Coagulation and Complications

For open (stomach, colon) and endoscopic (stomach) chronic animal studies, the depth of coagulation was determined. After fixation, hematoxylin and eosin staining, tissue coagulation was assessed from 1 mm tissue sections and from coded histologic sections. Bowel wall thickness (from mucosa to serosa) and depth of coagulation were estimated from these sections using a calibrated microscopic eyepiece.

Also, whenever follow-up endoscopies, second operations, or autopsies were done, the extent of ulceration, healing or re-epithelialization, or damage was assessed. The presence of perforation or abscess was also determined at surgery or autopsy.

Clinical Tumor Coagulation

Laser and other thermal methods were used for palliative endoscopic treatment of bleeding and/or obstructing GI tumors in patients who were not surgical candidates. Endoscopic coagulation rather than vaporization was the method used with YAG, ALP, HP or BICAP. In patients with significant gut stenoses from the tumors, dilatation was performed before endoscopic coagulation (22-25). Endoscopic biopsies were performed to evaluate coagulation effects upon the tumors, the pattern of coagulation for different modalities, and re-epithelialization after treatment. Luminal patency was recorded at endoscopy and with follow-up barium X-rays. The effect of palliation was graded by symptomatic and objective criteria. Adjuvant radiation and/or chemotherapy were also recommended as appropriate after relief of obstruction and control of bleeding (24, 25).

Results and discussion – Ulcer treatment

Efficacy During Endoscopic Coagulation – Standard Gastric Ulcers

Under similar experimental circumstances in randomized studies (1-8) done with an open model or the clamped gastrotomy model, the efficacy of endoscopic coagulation of standard gastric ulcers was excellent with argon laser (93-100%), YAG laser (90-100%), bipolar electrocoagulation (88-100% – Meditech probe; 90-100% BICAP probe), monopolar electrocoagulation (90-100%), and heater probe (90- 100%). Refer to Table 5.1.

Table 5.1. Efficacy for hemostasis of standard gastric ulcers.

	OPEN GASTROTOMY	ENDOSCOPIC OPEN-CLOSED
Control	0%	0%
Argon laser	100%	100%
(8-10 W)		
YAG laser	90-100%	93-100%
(50-90 W)		
Bipolar electrocoagulation	88-100%	97%
(Medi-Tech)		
Monopolar electrocoagulation	90-100%	100%
BICAP		
Small	90-100%	90-95%
Large	100%	100%
Heater Probe		
Small	90-100%	90-95%
Large	100%	100%

Efficacy is the percentage of ulcers with no more bleeding upon inspection after treatment. Twenty or more bleeding standard ulcers were randomized to control or each treatment method in heparinized dogs. Different results depended upon the specific setting used (1-8).

With the non-laser, contact probes (BICAP, HP, MPEC), larger diameter probes (3.2 mm diameter) facilitated treatment because they 1) coagulated better, 2) washed better, 3) tamponaded more efficiently, and 4) required fewer treatment pulses and less time for coagulation than with smaller probes (2.4 mm diameter). However, with active bleeding in this heparinized model, such treatment with large probes was greatly facilitated by a therapeutic endoscope (with 2.8 mm and 3.7 mm suction channels) which permitted simultaneous suctioning of blood or fluid and treatment.

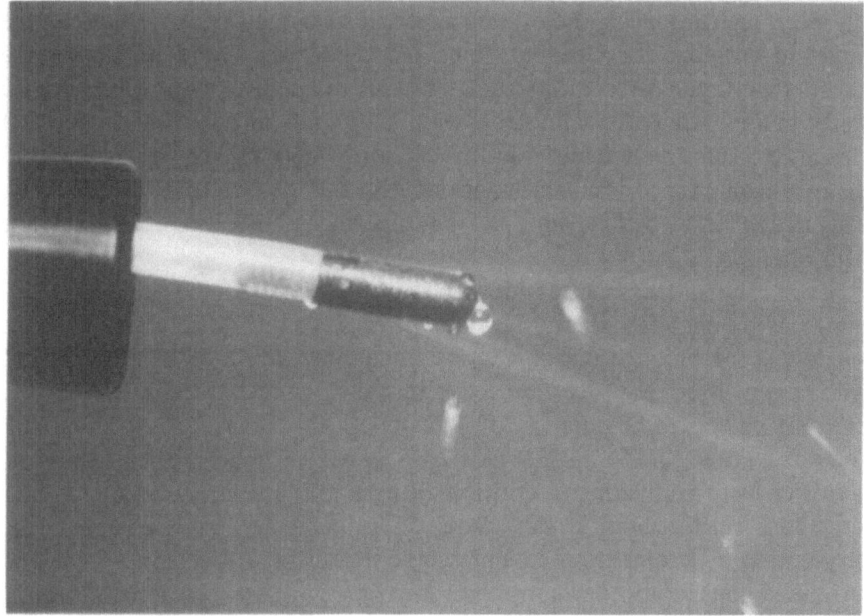

Fig. 5.9. Large heater probe with coaxial water irrigation via a therapeutic endoscope.

Treatment with single channel (3.7 mm) endoscope was much more cumbersome because the probes (particularly the large one) had to be removed from the suction channel whenever one needed to suction blood or fluid. With a single channel therapeutic endoscope, simultaneous treatment and suctioning with the 3.2 mm (large probe) were not possible and therefore endoscopic treatment was quite difficult for actively bleeding ulcers in the clamped, gastrostomy model. The therapeutic two channel endoscope also facilitated treatment with the lasers, particularly the removal of CO_2 gas that was used to blow away blood from the ulcer base prior to treatment.

Guidelines and Limitations for Endoscopic Ulcer Hemostasis with Argon Laser

The blue-green wavelength of argon laser is absorbed by hemoglobin or other red pigmented compounds. Although the argon laser could be efficiently transmitted through an endoscope with a quartz waveguide, this selective absorption by blood may limit the coagulation ability and influence the depth of tissue coagulation. Nevertheless, when careful guidelines for endoscopic use of argon laser were followed, treatment of bleeding lesions was quite feasible and effective (3).

The specific limitations and guidelines for endoscopic treatment of bleeding standard ulcers by argon laser are: a) treatment distance of 1-3 cm (lightguide tip to target); b) coagulation (whitening) of bleeding lesions rather than vaporization (producing holes); c) adequate CO_2 gas backpressure at the target to visualize the bleeding point and clear away blood that otherwise absorbs the argon laser energy; d) as en face orientation as possible; e) 8-10 watts output from the lightguide with $\leq 10°$ full angle of divergence; f) clearance of blood and clots from the bleeding target prior to treatment; and g) treatment directly on bleeding points and, if that is unsuccessful, coagulation immediately around the bleeding point (this can facilitate hemostasis).

A two channel therapeutic endoscope with standard (2.8 mm) and large (3.7 mm) suction channels greatly facilitated treatment by allowing simultaneous suctioning (of blood, fluid of CO_2 gas) and coagulation of bleeding lesions with argon laser. For the clamped gastrotomy model, localization of the bleeding point and preparation of it for treatment (clearing it of blood and fluid and getting in an en face position) was much more difficult than the actual endoscopic treatment. Position changes of the animal and target water irrigation of bleeding lesions were often necessary to accomplish the preparation of lesions prior to endoscopic treatment. All of these guidelines were used clinically in our controlled trial of argon laser for bleeding peptic ulcers and yielded excellent clinical results (17, 18).

Overall, using endoscopic argon laser with these guidelines for standard ulcer treatment afforded efficacy of 93-100% (refer to Table 5.1) compared with other methods. To achieve hemostasis in the heparinized standard ulcer model necessitated meticulous coagulation of 6-10 small vessels around the edge of the standard ulcer. Approximately 10% of standard gastric ulcers in heparinized dogs had high bleeding rates ≥ 5 cc/min and were difficult to control with endoscopic argon laser. Larger vessels (found histologically on serial sections) accounted for these higher bleeding rates and presumably the difficulty with endoscopic argon laser coagulation. In later experiments, tamponade with contact probes (particularly BICAP and heater probe) greatly facilitated treatment of such standard ulcers with high bleeding rates or large caliber mesenteric arteries (10).

Guidelines and Limitations for Endoscopic Ulcer Hemostasis with YAG Laser

The near infra-red YAG wavelength also can be easily transmitted endoscopically via quartz waveguides. Absorption of YAG energy by overlying clots, blood or fluid was less of a problem compared to endoscopic argon laser.

However, target treatment onto or near a bleeding point was necessary to avoid extensive tissue damage, to facilitate coagulation, and to avoid vaporization.

The technical factors in endoscopic YAG laser hemostasis such as the therapeutic, two channel endoscope and need to prepare the bleeding lesion prior to treatment were similar to argon laser treatment discussed above. However, specific guidelines and limitations differed.

YAG laser guidelines (1, 2) for endoscopic treatment of bleeding ulcers were: a) treatment distance of 1-4 cm; b) as en face an orientation as possible for treatment; c) high power (70-80 watts) and short pulses (0.5 sec) were very effective for coagulation; d) although less important for efficacy than argon laser, adequate CO_2 gas at the target blew away blood and reduced treatment time by allowing visualization of bleeding points; and e) edema developed after initial YAG laser shots, and could reduce bleeding as well as full thickness tissue injury.

The efficacy of endoscopic YAG laser for hemostasis of standard gastric ulcers was excellent (Table 5.1). The ulcers with high bleeding rates were easier to control with YAG than with endoscopic argon laser. However, more tissue injury resulted (Table 5.2).

Table 5.2. Histologic injury for standard gastric ulcer treatment.

	OPEN GASTROTOMY	ENDOSCOPIC OPEN-CLOSED
Argon laser	4- 8%	10%
(8-10 W)		
YAG laser	77-97%	43%
(50-90 W)		
Bipolar electrocoagulation	0-30%	17%
BICAP		
Small	5-20%	10%
Large	10-25%	20%
Heater probe		
Small	15-25%	15%
Large	15-35%	25%
Monopolar electrocoagulation	3-50%	53%
Control	0%	0%

Histologic injury was determined 5-7 days after treatment from serial tissue sections of the standard ulcers. Histologic injury is listed as the percentage of ulcers with 100% external muscle layer damage. No delayed perforations were noted. Twenty or more standard ulcers were randomized to control or each treatment. Different results depended upon the different settings used (1-8).

Also, other disadvantages of endoscopic YAG were similar to endoscopic argon laser: a) CO_2 gas for blowing away blood from the target was necessary for efficient coagulation but was inconvenient to remove, b) tangential treatment was ineffective, and c) tamponade of large vessels (>1 mm outside diameter) or heavy bleeders was not possible and therefore coagulation of them is difficult (10). There is a very impressive heat sink effect for arteries greater than 1 mm which makes coagulation with non-tamponade devices ineffective (see section on arteries). With the newer, contact thermal probes (BICAP and heater probe) these are no longer problems (refer to those sections).

Guidelines and Limitations of Endoscopic Hemostasis with Monopolar Electrocoagulation

For successful endoscopic hemostasis of standard ulcers, monopolar electrocoagulation standard probes, modified probes, or the hydrothermal probe all required more skill than any other thermal modality. Also, efficacy and tissue damage were much less predictable and controllable. An analogue computer did not alter patterns of tissue injury nor increase ease of endoscopic use (see Table 5.2).

Our monopolar probes often stuck to the mucosa during coagulation. Pulling them away from the lesion after coagulation often resulted in rebleeding at the site. Although constant water or saline irrigation facilitated visualization of the bleeding points, tissue coagulation and hemostasis were more difficult. Specifically, the hydrothermal probe was considerably less effective for standard gastric ulcer treatment than standard monopolar probes.

Specific guidelines for endoscopic monopolar electrocoagulation were: a) as en face as possible, although some tangential treatment was possible with our newer probes; b) 50-100 watts/pulse and short (0.5 sec) pulses facilitated treatment; c) target washing to identify the exact bleeding points, tamponade of these, and target coagulation are recommended; d) simultaneous suctioning (of blood and irrigation solution) and endoscopic coagulation were easier with a two channel endoscope than a single channel therapeutic endoscope.

When specific guidelines were used with monopolar electrocoagulation, efficacy for standard ulcer treatment was excellent (Table 5.2). Although tamponade was possible at endoscopy with MPEC, ulcers with high bleeding rates and those tangentially oriented were difficult to control. Also, tissue damage was extensive (Table 5.2). Monopolar electrocoagulation was also more difficult to use than the newer commercially available thermal probes (BICAP and heater probe). Training experienced endoscopists to use monopolar electrocoagulation for hemostasis was also difficult. It was the most difficult of all thermal coagulation devices to teach.

Guidelines and Limitations for Endoscopic Ulcer Hemostasis with BICAP and Heater Probe

For successful endoscopic hemostasis of standard canine gastric ulcers, BICAP and heater probe required less technical skill than argon laser or monopolar electrocoagulation but more than YAG laser. However, the current commercially available BICAP and heater probes for clinical use are easier to use than their counterpart prototype laboratory units. Coagulation efficacy was excellent (Table 5.1) and tissue injury was predictable.

For endoscopic hemostasis of ulcers, specific guidelines are: a) settings of 25-30 joules on the heater probe unit or dial setting of 6-7 on a 50 watt BICAP generator with 1 second pulses facilitate coagulation; b) washing with water before and, as necessary, between coagulation pulses helps localize bleeding points and treat them; c) firm tamponade directly on the bleeding points to stop them and then coagulation allowed control of even the heavy bleeders; d) tangential treatment is even easier than en face treatment; e) larger probes (3.2 mm) are more efficient for coagulation and easier for endoscopic hemostasis than small (2.8 mm) probes; and f) the two channel therapeutic endoscope with either 3.7 and 2.8 mm suction channels or two 3.7 mm channels greatly facilitated endoscopic hemostasis of active bleeders. These guidelines for endoscopic canine ulcer hemostasis with BICAP and heater probe have been applied clinically to active ulcer bleeding and the non-bleeding visible vessel with excellent results in a randomized preliminary trial (19) and an ongoing double-blind controlled randomized trial (20).

When specific guidelines were followed, efficacy of standard ulcer hemostasis was excellent (Table 5.1) and tissue injury was predictable with BICAP or heater probe. Among the coagulation units available, experienced endoscopists could be most easily taught to use these two devices compared to lasers, monopolar electrocoagulation or electrofulguration. Compared to neophytes, these endoscopists were skilled at the preparation of the lesion prior to coagulation and placement of the probe directly upon the bleeding lesion. Emergency endoscopy and endoscopic hemostasis of ulcers with any coagulation device required significantly more skill and experience than any elective endoscopy for diagnosis or treatment (18).

Depth of coagulation – stomach

Although somewhat variable, the depth of thermal coagulation of bowel wall or standard ulcers for clinically applicable settings of argon laser, heater probe, and bipolar electrocoagulation as judged by histologic examination 5-7 days after treatment is 1.7-2 mm. The coagulation depth for YAG laser under similar conditions is 2.5-3.5 mm and for MPEC is 2.0-4.0 mm. For any of these modalities, increased bowel distention or probe pressure increases the depth of coagulation, while edema, blood, or clots decrease the coagulation depth. Unlike the colon, full thickness (mucosa to serosa) coagulation of the stomach wall or standard gastric ulcers in dogs did not result in delayed perforations. However, vaporization of tissue in a standard ulcer base during treatment with either argon or YAG laser could worsen arterial bleeding (by eroding into an artery) or cause an acute perforation (a through and through hole). The coaxial CO_2 gas used with argon or YAG tended to aggravate the pneumoperitoneum whenever an acute perforation occurred during endoscopic treatment in the clamped gastrotomy model.

In healthy dogs, standard gastric ulcers treated with thermal coagulation devices healed somewhat slower than non-treated control ulcers. Three to four weeks were often required for re-epithelialization and 'healing' of the treated mucosa with greater depths or diameters of coagulation necrosis (such as after YAG or MPEC). Tended to heal slower than those treated with BICAP, heater probe or argon laser. Delayed perforations, bleeding or nutritional problems after such coagulation necrosis of the stomach were not noted in any healthy dogs as might be expected clinically in some ill patients.

Efficacy of mesenteric artery coagulation (10)

Tissue Erosion. At some instrument settings, YAG, argon, monopolar electro-coagulation and electrofulguration produced tissue and vessel erosion which interfered with effective arterial coagulation. In contrast, such erosions were not observed with any setting of BICAP or heater probe.

Coagulation Ability for Mesenteric Arteries. YAG was effective with arteries less than 0.5 mm in diameter, but ineffective with larger arteries. If the artery was first compressed with a glass slide, laser efficacy greatly increased and the power requirement decreased. Without vessel compression, argon laser, electrofulguration, monopolar electrocoagulation, BICAP and heater probe were not uniformly effective for coagulation of 0.5 mm arteries. However, consistent success was achieved even with 2.5 mm arteries when heater probe or BICAP were applied with sufficient force to tamponade arterial flow.

Coagulation of Serosal Artery. Each modality was applied to the mucosal surface of the small intestine in an attempt to coagulate a 0.25 mm artery located on the serosal surface. Each device was ineffective when applied without concomitant vessel occlusion by pressure. In contrast, when the contact probes were applied with sufficient force to occlude the target artery, consistent efficacy was noted with ease of such coagulation in ranked order: heater probe $\geq$ BICAP $\geq$ monopolar.

Summary Guidelines for Arterial Coagulation

By far the most effective method for coagulation of medium sized (≥ 1.5 mm) arteries was first to occlude the vessel by compression and then apply heat to seal it. Vessel compression eliminated the arterial heat sink and produced coaptation of vessel walls which facilitated thermal sealing. For the contact probes (monopolar and bipolar electrodes or heater probe), the depth of tissue coagulation was controlled by varying probe appositional force and coagulation of deep arteries was possible. Tissue erosion, noted at times with electrofulguration, YAG laser, argon laser, and monopolar electrocoagulation, interfered with effective coagulation of arteries and worsened bleeding. In contrast, heater probe and bipolar electrocoagulation did not produce tissue erosion at any instrument setting. The overall comparative ranking for efficacy and safety for arterial coagulation was heater probe $\geq$ bipolar electrocoagulation (BICAP) $>$ monopolar electrocoagulation $>$ YAG laser $>$ argon laser $>$ electrofulguration.

Esophageal varices (8)

Hemostatic Efficacy

The hemostatic efficacy for the different endoscopic methods and control in the heparinized bleeding canine esophageal varix study are summarized in Table 5.3.

Table 5.3. Effectiveness of endoscopic treatment for variceal hemostasis.

Method	Effectiveness	%
YAG laser	10/10	100%
Sclerotherapy	42/43	98%
Heater probe – Large	5/10	50%
Argon laser	4/10	40%
Ferromagnetic tamponade	3/10	30%
BICAP – Large	2/10	20%
BICAP – Small	2/10	20%
Monopolar electrocoagulation	1/20	5%
Control	0/25	0%

Effectiveness was the number of varices with hemostasis after treatment that did not rebleed with balloon distension proximal to the treatment site/total number of varices treated.

Both YAG laser and endoscopic sclerotherapy provided reliable hemostasis for acutely bleeding canine varices. Large heater probe controlled bleeding 50% of the time, and all other methods stopped bleeding in less than half the trials. Rebleeding after balloon inflation proximal to the coagulated bleeding site did not occur with YAG laser or endoscopic sclerotherapy treated varices but did occur with the other methods.

All the thermally active methods caused some esophageal mucosal damage. These lesions tended to be superficial with heater probe, BICAP and argon laser. Healing within 5-10 days was usual after these treatments. With monopolar electrocoagulation, deep ulcers and one variceal perforation resulted. YAG laser treatments were associated with ulcers that required more than 14 days to heal. All esophageal varices were still present on weekly follow-up endoscopies after treatment with ferromagnetic tamponade and all the thermal methods. The principal differences between YAG laser and endoscopic sclerotherapy were the ease of application of YAG laser, the higher frequency of esophageal erosions or ulcers with YAG laser, and the lack of variceal obliteration with YAG laser.

Summary Guidelines for Variceal Hemostasis

Based upon the lack of efficacy of monopolar electrocoagulation, bipolar electrocoagulation, heater probe, argon laser, and ferromagnetic tamponade in this model of bleeding canine esophageal varices, similar poor efficacy clinically with these devices would be predicted. Additionally, monopolar electrocoagulation is not safe enough to use in the esophagus because of the danger of deep ulcers and perforation of the esophagus or a varix. If a clinician chooses to control acute variceal hemorrhage with emergency YAG laser treatment, urgent sclerotherapy during the same anesthesia is highly recommended with sclerosis of all the distal esophageal varices. Because varices remain patent after YAG laser treatment, rebleeding could be predicted unless more definitive treatment is used.

Angioma

Bowel Wall Thickness

The bowel wall (serosa to mucosa) is thin throughout healthy, large (20-40 kg) dogs, and varies from 2-4 mm. The thinnest gut region is the cecum ($\leq$ 2 mm) and the thickest is the body of the stomach ($\geq$ 4 mm). The increasing order of bowel wall thickness is cecum < right colon < esophagus < duodenum < antrum of stomach < body of stomach. *Endoscopic distention* thins out the bowel wall and significantly increases full thickness injury with any thermal method including ALP and YAG laser.

The correlation between overdistention of the bowel and depth of tissue injury with thermal treatment is dramatic. Comparing the injury to the gastric wall after endoscopic argon laser, *overdistention* (but not to the point of cardiorespiratory distress) correlated with a significantly greater incidence of full thickness damage than *normal* endoscopic distention (3). While all other treatment parameters except distension were held constant, 16 of 22 ulcers treated during overdistention had full thickness damage compared to 1 of 22 ulcers with normal distention. Similarly, treatment with all other endoscopic thermal modalities (YAG laser, MONO, BICAP, heater probe, or electro-fulguration) in the distended bowel (stomach, colon, or small bowel) significantly increased the depth of tissue coagulation in our laboratory. This effect was independent of tissue vaporization and was thought to relate to thinning of the bowel wall and/or alteration in the circulation during distention.

Efficacy and Safety – Colonic Coagulation (7, 11, 16)

The efficacy of hemostasis for control of standard ulcer bleeding in the colon was BICAP ≈ argon laser > YAG laser ≈ monopolar electrocoagulation ≈ hot biopsy forceps > hydrothermal probe. Argon laser, BICAP, and heater probe applied to colonic mucosa (to mimic treatment of angioma) in clinically relevant device settings did not result in delayed (3-5 days) perforations of the colon (refer to Table 5.4). They appeared safe and effective for hemostasis of bleeding colonic angiomata of the colon.

Table 5.4. Colonic injury to normal mucosa for different modalities.

	n	Full thickness injury	Delayed perforations
Argon laser (6-10 W)	82	18-26%	0%
YAG laser (50-75 W)	30	89%	13-27%
Bipolar electro. (Medi-Tech)	27	11%	0%
BICAP			
Small (10-20 J)	45	17-25%	0%
Large (10-20 J)	45	23-38%	0%
Monopolar electro. (20-50 J)	60	27-47%	13-27%
Hot biopsy forceps (30-45 J)	30	45-85%	0%
Hydrothermal probe (25-75 J)	37	29-75%	0%
Heater probe			
Small (10-20 J)	45	0- 7%	0%
Large (10-20 J)	45	7-33%	0%

n = number of normal mucosal areas treated. Full thickness injury is the number of these with histologic injury through the external muscle layer 3-7 days after treatment. Delayed perforations were found 3-7 days after treatment. W is watts. J is joules per pulse. Different results depended upon specific device settings (7,11,16).

YAG laser and monopolar electrocoagulation, applied to colonic mucosa (to simulate angioma) resulted in delayed perforations of the colon up to 25% of the time. The margin of safety with these devices was significantly less than with argon laser, BICAP or heater probe.

With any thermal device used in the colon, thinning of the bowel wall with distention or increased probe pressure increased the frequency of full thickness injury, serosal whitening, and delayed perforations. The perforations generally occurred 3-5 days after initial coagulation and were associated with significant worsening of all animals' condition. At autopsy most such perforations were associated with focal or more generalized abscesses (refer to Table 5.4).

Coagulated standard ulcers or normal mucosa in the colon greatly increased in size and depth and required longer to heal (>4 wks) than similar treatment in the stomach, duodenum or esophagus. Delayed slough of coagulum re-epithelialization and healing occurred late. This appeared related to the fecal stream, the bacterial load as well as other factors such as motility.

Guidelines for Gut Angioma Coagulation

Because the right colon is so thin in healthy dogs (<2 mm) and in older or ill patients, and angioma are so common there, caution with coagulation during colonoscopy is urged. Based upon our laboratory results, post-coagulation syndrome, acute perforations, delayed bleeding from induced ulcers and delayed perforations will be more common after coagulation in the colon with YAG laser and any form of monopolar electrocoagulation (except hydrothermal probe) than argon laser, heater probe or BICAP. Overdistention or increased probe pressure must be avoided during colonoscopic coagulation with any thermal modality.

Although the stomach and duodenum are thicker than the right colon in healthy dogs (and patients), similar precautions about distention, probe pressure, and avoidance of vaporization are recommended for angioma treatment there also. In general, a significantly lower amount of thermal energy with each device is required for coagulation of mucosa (or non-bleeding angioma) than bleeding ulcers. Specifically, mucosal coagulation (vs. standard ulcer hemostasis) for YAG laser was 40-50 Watts (vs. 75-80 Watts); argon laser was 5-7 Watts (vs. 8-10 W); monopolar electrocoagulation 40-50 Joules (vs. 100-150 J); BICAP 10-15 Joules (vs. 25-30 J); heater probe 10-15 Joules (vs. 25-30 J).

These general guidelines have been applied clinically in non-randomized trials of UGI and lower GI angioma with argon laser and a randomized trial with heater probe and BICAP (21-23). The lessons learned from the laboratory studies have been directly applicable to the clinical applications for angioma coagulation.

GI Tumors

Thermal coagulation Depth and Healing

The depth of tissue coagulation 5-7 days after thermal coagulation was predictable for the UGI tracts of dogs. It was less predictable in the canine colon because of the added problem of delayed slough, apparent increase in size and depth 5-7 days after thermal coagulation, and delayed perforations of the colon particularly after YAG or monopolar electrocoagulation. In general the coagulation depth in increasing order was argon laser $\approx$ BICAP $\approx$ heater probe $<$ YAG $\leq$ monopolar electrocoagulation. Coagulation depth in the bowel with the touch probes (BICAP, heater probe, or monopolar) could be increased with more appositional pressure. Coagulation depth with YAG, argon laser and monopolar electrocoagulation could be increased by vaporization of the superficial tissue layer. In general this resulted after the power density was increased.

Tumor Coagulation

Endoscopic coagulation of bleeding and/or obstructing GI tumors has been effective with lower power ($<$ 50 W) YAG laser (24-27). Dilatation to relieve tumor obstruction before laser endoscopy facilitated YAG laser or BICAP tumor probe coagulation. Vaporization of cancers was unnecessary and more dangerous than coagulation of tumor, especially for tortuous strictures. Dilatation along with the delayed sloughing of coagulated tumor helped assure luminal patency in patients with either obstructing colorectal or esophageal cancers.

Guidelines for Tumor Coagulation

Depth of tissue coagulation and the concept of delayed tissue slough with larger and deeper ulceration in the colon can be applied clinically to endoscopic tumor coagulation. The maximal tissue effect, particularly in the colon is 5-7 days after thermal coagulation. An efficient schedule of tumor treatment clinically would take this into account.

Although non-laser probes for endoscopic tumor coagulation are not yet practical, a BICAP tumor probe is available for treatment of symmetrical, circumferential cancer strictures which are not sharply angulated (26-27). Dilatation followed by BICAP tumor probe coagulation over a guidewire are feasible for esophageal or rectal cancer palliation.

Summary

Lasers have been used for endoscopic hemostasis in GI for more than ten years and for GI tumor treatment for at least five years. Still many questions remain about the best technique, indications, histologic and clinical results, and comparison with standard treatment (often surgery) and non-laser endoscopic techniques. Some of these have been answered in laboratory studies. The purpose of this paper was to relate different laboratory studies with YAG or argon (ALP) lasers, heater probe (HP), bipolar (BICAP) or monopolar (MPEC) electrocoagulation, and sclerotherapy (SCLERO) to clinical questions concerning endoscopic management of GI hemorrhage and obstructing tumors.

HEMOSTASIS STUDIES. 1. *UGI Endoscopic Standard Ulcer Hemostasis* in dogs with thermal devices established guidelines and limitations for clinical hemostasis in our controlled trials of bleeding ulcers with ALP and HP or BICAP. 2. *Canine Mesenteric Artery Coagulation Studies* emphasized the importance of tamponade and avoidance of vaporization for effective hemostasis of arteries. In our controlled trial with HP or BICAP, tamponade before coagulation facilitates hemostasis for active ulcer bleeding. Effective coagulation and prevention of rebleeding of non-bleeding visible vessels are common with HP or BICAP rather than vaporization and precipitation of bleeding as are more common with YAG or ALP. 3. *Gut Distention or More Probe Pressure* increased coagulation depth of the canine gut wall with any thermal method. Avoidance of these clinically during treatment of acute ulcers or angioma can reduce complications. 4. *Variceal Hemostasis* in a canine model was easy with YAG, but not BICAP, HP, MPEC or ALP. Compared to SCLERO, YAG caused more mucosal injury and did not permanently obliterate the varix lumen. Clinically, definitive treatment (SCLERO or surgery) should follow successful YAG laser varix hemostasis or rebleeding will be common. 5. *Colon Hemostasis* of normal canine colonic mucosa (simulating angioma) or standard ulcers was safe with ALP, HP or BICAP but delayed perforations resulted with YAG or MPEC. One could predict that complications (such as post-coagulation syndrome, perforation, or delayed hemorrhage) after clinical colon coagulation would follow similar patterns.

TUMOR STUDIES 1. *Depth of Coagulation* in canine stomach or colon were similar: ALP $\approx$ < BICAP $\approx$ HP < MPEC < YAG. Delayed slough of coagulum and ulceration were evident in the colon and re-epithelialization and healing occurred later than in the stomach. Based upon the pattern of coagulation for different modalities, safe endoscopic treatment can be gauged by tumor size, location, and configuration. 2. *Tumor Coagulation* was effective for tumor destruction in human studies with histology follow-up. Vaporization of tumor was unnecessary and more dangerous for tortuous strictures. Clinically, we used lower power (< 50 W) YAG laser for coagulation after dilatation to relieve tumor obstruction. In our opinion these important lessons are relevant to GI endoscopic laser applications.

References

1. Johnston JH, Jensen DM, Mautner W, Elashoff J. YAG laser treatment of experimental bleeding canine gastric ulcers. Gastroenterology 1980;79:1252-1261.

2. Johnston JH, Jensen DM, Mautner W. Comparison of laser photocoagulation and electrocoagulation in endoscopic treatment of bleeding canine gastric ulcers. Gastroenterology 1982;82:904- 910.

3. Johnston JH, Jensen DM, Mautner W, Elashoff J. Argon laser treatment of bleeding canine gastric ulcers: Limitations and guidelines for endoscopic use. Gastroenterology 1980;80:708-716.

4. Protell RL, Gilbert DA, Silverstein FE, Jensen DM, Hulett FM, Auth DC. Computer-assisted electrocoagulation: Bipolar vs. monopolar in treatment of experimental canine gastric ulcer bleeding. Gastroenterology 1981;80:451-455.

5. Jensen DM. Endoscopic control of gastrointestinal bleeding. In: Developments in Digestive Diseases. Lea and Febiger Publishers. 1980, pp 1-27.

6. Machicado GA, Jensen DM, Tapia JI, Mautner W. Treatment of bleeding canine duodenal and esophageal ulcers with argon laser and bipolar electrocoagulation. Gastroenterology 1981;81:859-865.

7. Jensen DM, Machicado GA, Tapia JI, Mautner W. Comparison of argon laser photo-coagulation and bipolar electrocoagulation for endoscopic hemostasis in the canine colon. Gastroenterology 1982;83:830-835.

8. Jensen DM, Silpa ML, Tapia JI, Beilin DB, Machicado GA. Comparison of different methods for endoscopic hemostasis of bleeding canine esophageal varices. Gastroenterology 1983;84:1455-1461.

9. Jensen DM. Sclerosants for injection sclerosis of esophageal varices. Gastrointest Endosc 1983;29:315-317.

10. Johnston J, Jensen D, Auth D. Experimental comparison of endoscopic Yttrium-aluminum-garnet laser, electrosurgery and heater probe for canine gut arterial coagulation: Importance of compression and avoidance of erosion. Gastroenterology 1987;92:1101-1108.

11. Jensen DM, Tapia JI, Machicado GA, Beilin DB. Hydrothermal probe, hot biopsy forceps, and YAG laser for hemostasis in the canine colon. Gastrointest Endosc 1983;29:189.

12. Protell RL, Silverstein FE, Piercey JRA et al. A reproducible animal model of acute bleeding ulcer – the 'ulcer maker'. Gastroenterology 1976;71:961.

13. Gilbert DA et al. Animal endoscopic studies of CO_2 assisted argon laser photocoagulation preparatory to controlled trials in men. Gastroenterology 1978;74:1037.

14. Martin L et al. The multisection tissue slicer: A simpler technique for assessing the maximal depth of experimental injury. Gastrointestinal Endosc 1979;25:61.

15. Jensen DM, Tapia JI, Machicado GA, Tapia JI, Kauffman G, Beilin DB. A reproducible canine model of esophageal varices. Gastroenterology 1983;84:573-579.

16. Jensen DM, Tapia JI, Machicado GA, Beilin DB, Silpa ML. Comparison of electrocoagulation and heater probe for hemostasis in the canine colon. Gastrointest Endosc 1982;28:151.

17. Jensen DM, Machicado GA, Tapia JI, Elashoff J. Controlled trial of endoscopic argon laser for severe ulcer hemorrhage. Gastroenterology 1984;86:1125.

18. Brunetaud JM, Jensen DM. Current status of argon laser hemostasis of bleeding ulcers. Endoscopy 1985;18;Supplement 2:40-45.

19. Jensen DM, Machicado GA, Silpa ML. Argon laser vs. heater probe or BICAP for control of severe ulcer bleeding. Gastrointestinal Endosc 1984;30:134.

20. Jensen DM, Machicado GA, Kovacs TOG, Van Deventer G, Randall GM, Reedy T, Silpa M, Sue M. Controlled, randomized study of heater probe and BICAP for hemostasis of severe ulcer bleeding. Gastroenterology 1988;94:A208.

21. Jensen D, Bown S. Gastrointestinal angiomata: Diagnosis and treatment with laser therapy and other modalities. In: Fleischer D, Jensen D, Bright-Asare P, eds., Therapeutic Laser Endoscopy in Gastrointestinal Disease. Boston: Martinus Nijhoff, 1983, pp. 151-160.

22. Jensen DM, Machicado GA, Silpa ML. Treatment of GI angioma with argon laser, heater probe, or bipolar electrocoagulation. Gastrointestinal Endosc 1984;30:134.

23. Jensen DM, Machicado GA. Bleeding colonic angioma: Endoscopic coagulation and follow-up. Gastroenterology 1985;88(Part 2):1433.

24. Shindel N, Jensen DM, Sue M, Machicado GA. Palliation of obstructing GI tumors with

endoscopic lower power YAG laser. Gastrointest Endosc 1985;31(#2):158.

25. Jensen DM. Lasers in the GI cancer war and on other fronts. Gastroenterology 1984;87:974-976.

26. Jensen DM. Palliation of esophagogastric cancer via endoscopy. Gastroenterol Clin Biol 1987;11:361-363.

27. Jensen DM, Machicado GA, Randall GM, Tung LA, English-Zych S. Comparison of low power YAG laser and BICAP tumor probe for palliation of esophageal cancer strictures. Gastroenterology 1988;94:1263-1270.

6. UPPER GASTROINTESTINAL ANGIOMATA: DIAGNOSIS AND TREATMENT

DENNIS M. JENSEN AND GUSTAVO A. MACHICADO

Introduction

Acute or chronic upper gastrointestinal (UGI) bleeding and iron deficiency anemia may result from UGI angiomata. In this report, specific angiomatous lesions discussed are Osler-Weber-Rendu (O-W-R) telangiectasia and other angiomata. O-W-R syndrome, a disorder of dominant inheritance (1, 2), was diagnosed in our series (3) when patients had a positive family history; mucous membrane, tongue (Plate 1), and digital telangiectasia (Plate 2); and endoscopically documented bleeding from UGI telangiectasia (Plate 3).

Non-O-W-R angiomata were diagnosed when features of O-W-R syndrome were absent but UGI angiomata (Plates 4-6) were the source of UGI bleeding. The etiology of GI angiomata is unknown but several associated conditions have been recognized. These include valvular heart disease, increased age, collagen-vascular syndromes, renal failure, cirrhosis and previous radiation to the gut (2-4).

Abnormal mucosal and submucosal vessel proliferation characterize O-W-R telangiectasia and other angiomata. The terminology used to describe the endoscopic appearance of these *arterio-venous malformations* has not been standardized. Discrete mucosal lesions are often described by GI endoscopists as *telangiectasia, hemangioma, angioma, ectasia* or *AV malformations*.

Others describe discrete of diffuse lesions, particularly of the colon, as *angiodysplasia*. '*Watermelon Stomach*' (Plate 7) describes a more diffuse gastric lesion associated with chronic UGI bleeding (5, 6). *Phlebectasia* or *lymphectasia,* dilated veins and lymphatic channels, appear different endoscopically and pathologically. It may be difficult by endoscopic biopsy to document mucosal AV malformations because of crush or fixation artifacts. However, injection techniques or careful histology have been used to define the morphology in resected bowel, particularly for the colon (7). Many of our biopsies of obvious gastric angioma are not diagnostic, when standard tissue fixatives are used. However, occasionally characteristic thin walled vascular structures in a background of inflammation are evident (Plate 8). Endoscopic appearance of angiomata (Plates 3-6) are more characteristic than biopsies.

The incidence of O-W-R syndrome in the general population is about 5 in 100,000. In a large series of O-W-R patients, about one-third had severe gastrointestinal bleeding (1). There are no accurate estimates of the prevalence

D.M. Jensen and J.M. Brunetaud (eds), Medical Laser Endoscopy. 71-91.
© 1990 Kluwer Academic Publishers, Dordrecht

of a non-O-W-R angiomata in the general population as a source of significant GI bleeding. Non- bleeding angiodysplasia have been reported to be a common finding in surgically resected cecums and right colons of elderly patients when careful histologic examination and latex injections are performed (7). The prevalence of angiomata and O-W-R telangiectasia as a source for severe UGI bleeding in our series for a large Veterans Administration Hospital and University Hospital was 6-9%. Refer to Table 6.1.

Table 6.1. Final diagnosis for severe UGI bleeding in 200 consecutive patients at UCLA and Wadsworth VA hospitals (% of total).

	Wadsworth	*VA*	*UCLA*
Peptic ulcer		52%	49%
Duodenal	24	19	
Gastric	16	18	
Pyloric	10	10	
Marginal	2	2	
Varices		24%	20%
Esophageal	20	15	
Gastric	4	5	
UGI angiomata		9%	6%
Mallory-Weiss		7%	5%
Gastric erosions		2%	5%
Duodenal erosions		2%	0%
Tumors		2%	8%
Other		2%	7%

Traditional medical management of bleeding GI angiomata includes supportive care, transfusion, correction of coagulation of platelet abnormalities, and treatment of concomitant conditions such as cardiac, renal, or liver dysfunction. Other measures include surgical resection of involved bowel segments, angiographic embolization, and a trial of estrogens (1-2).

Methods

Diagnosis

Prior to endoscopic treatment of GI angiomata, important diagnostic considerations include their distribution, number, localization of the bleeding lesion, configuration, size and differential diagnosis.

Distribution. The majority of UGI angiomata or O-W-R telangiectasia in our patients are in the posterior aspect of the stomach corpus. Less common areas are the duodenal bulb, post bulbar area, and antrum. The esophagus and small bowel have been uncommon sources of bleeding (See Table 6.3).

Number. Often O-W-R telangiectasia and angiomata are multiple. If they are the source of UGI bleeding and occupy a large surface area or the entire circumference of the bowel segment, surgical resection rather than endoscopic coagulation should be considered. Individual or less extensive angiomata are amenable to endoscopic coagulation.

Localization of Bleeding Angioma. The segment of bowel with telangiectasia (O-W-R Syndrome) or individual angioma causing the GI bleeding should be localized prior to treatment. Emergency endoscopy and/or repeat elective endoscopy after the bleeding stops may be useful for localization of UGI bleeding angioma. Angiomata may be very difficult to distinguish from blood, submucosal lesions (Plate 5) or ulcers when there is significant, active bleeding. Whether the angiomata are incidental findings (8) or the source of significant bleeding needs to be determined prior to treatment. Our criteria for angiomata as the UGI bleeding site are: 1) active bleeding from the angioma; 2) some stigma of recent hemorrhage such as clot or erosion on the angioma and fresh blood nearby; 3) Hematemesis by history and negative panendoscopy except for non-bleeding angiomata.

Configuration and size often determine the choice of therapy and whether angiography or surgery should be considered. Small (less than 5 mm), flat, discrete angiomata are easier to treat than moderate (5-10 mm) or large (more than 10 mm) sized angiomata. Depressed angiomata may be mistaken for ulcers or erosions particularly if adherent clots are present. Large, elevated, or umbilicated (Plate 5) angiomata may have extensive submucosal or transmural vascular anastomoses. Angiography and surgical consultation should be considered prior to the endoscopic coagulation of such large, umbilicated lesions. Umbilicated angiomata are rare in our series of patients.

The *differential diagnosis* of small flat angiomata includes clot or adherent blood, suction artifact or erosion. Petechiae and submucosal or mucosal hemorrhages (Plate 9) related to thrombocytopenia, sepsis, severe coagulopathy, or renal failure can usually be distinguished by appearance and clinical history. If one is uncertain about the lesions, follow-up elective examination in a few days may be helpful. For moderate-sized or large angiomata, additional considerations include submucosal vascular tumors, trauma, focal inflammation, ischemia, endometriosis, or focal varices. Pre-treatment barium contrast studies and selective visceral angiography have been useful to exclude non-angiomatous lesions in some patients. Photographs for documentation are also recommended. For unconvincing or non-diagnostic lesions, repeat interval examination and photography are recommended for comparison. Directed biopsy of vascular lesions may be diagnostic because of the resultant increased bleeding and characteristic microscopic appearance (4, 9). Unless endoscopic treatment can be quickly applied, this approach is not recommended for diagnosis of suspected large angiomata. Small angiomata biopsied with either a standard or jumbo biopsy forceps do not bleed significantly in our experience unless they are umbilicated or have only a portion biopsied rather than complete removal with the first grasp. Even when the entire gastric angioma is biopsied, only about half the histologic specimens are diagnostic of AV malformations in our experience (10). The reasons for the disparity between this endoscopic prominence of angioma and the poor results of standard histopathologic techniques may relate to shrinkage of small vascular channels by different fixatives, deep location of the vascular abnormality, or lack of sensitivity of routine histologic techniques for demonstration of vascular abnormalities (10).

Techniques of coagulation

General

After determination of the limitations and guidelines for effective endoscopic use of all available thermal devices in canine studies (11-16), our CURE hemostasis study group evaluated argon laser, BICAP, and heater probe for treatment of GI angiomata. Patients with severe UGI bleeding or anemia and recurrent GI bleeding were treated (3, 17-22) if they met our criteria for bleeding from UGI angiomata (see Methods – Localization of Bleeding Angioma). Treatment of incidental UGI angioma in severe GI bleeders has been evaluated (8). We do not coagulate non-bleeding UGI angiomata found on routine panendoscopy in patients who do not fit our criteria for diagnosis of 'bleeding angiomata'.

Occasionally, when patients are referred for our evaluation with the diagnosis of 'UGI angiomata' and bleeding, we do not treat them endoscopically. Sometimes the lesions are so extensive (often contiguous or circumferential as in the cases of severe O-W-R syndrome or 'watermelon stomach') that patients are referred for surgical resection. Sometimes we cannot confirm the diagnosis and recommend re-evaluation of other therapy. In such patients who do not have other lesions such as erosions, ulcers, submucosal hemorrhages or underlying bleeding disorders which could account for the bleeding, we recommend repeat elective endoscopy with normal blood volume and limited intravenous anesthesia. GI angiomata can be easily missed or are less evident if blood volume is low or heavy sedation (particularly meperidine – Demerol®) is used during endoscopy or colonoscopy. Endoscopy with no intravenous medication, or only with a small dose of diazepam (Valium®) may make mucosal angiomata more evident compared to meperidine which seems to alter mucosal blood flow. Occasionally the only way to find small bleeding angioma (Plate 6) is to endoscope patients urgently, when they return with recurrent GI bleeding.

For endoscopic UGI hemostasis, a variety of endoscopes are useful and necessary. No single, currently available endoscope will allow the therapeutic endoscopist to reach or treat all UGI angiomata. The choice of endoscope depends upon 1) whether the case is an emergency or elective, 2) the size of the coagulation probes or laser catheters, and 3) the number, location, and size of the angiomata. For emergency cases, a large single suction (3.7 mm) channel (Olympus GIF-1T) or double (3.7 mm and 2.8 mm) channel therapeutic endoscope (ACMI AGT2 or Olympus 2T) is preferred (Fig. 6.1).

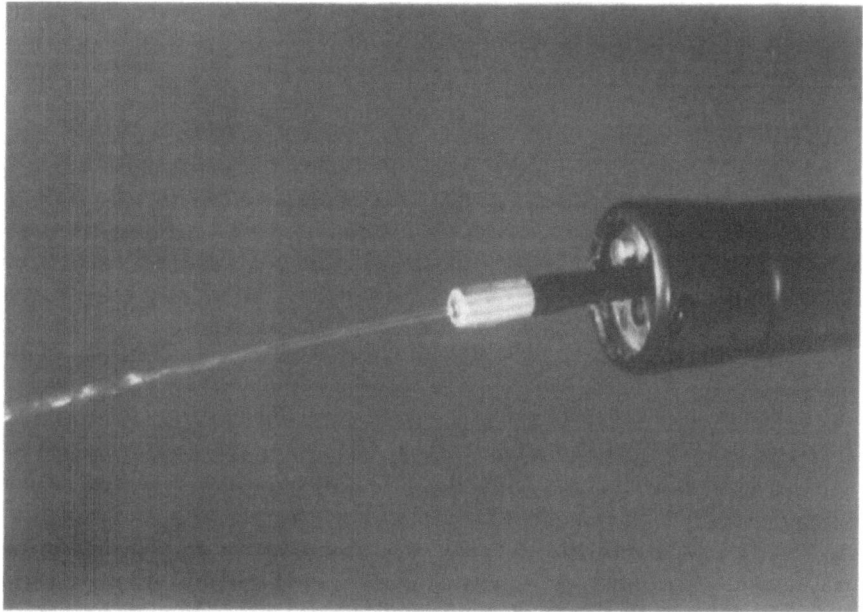

Fig. 6.1. Therapeutic two channel panendoscope (Olympus 2T10).

Simultaneous coagulation and suctioning (of air, fluid, blood) are feasible, particularly with the double channel endoscope. A large channel endoscope is needed for use of the large (3.2 mm) contact probes such as heater probe or BICAP. Such an instrument also facilitates suctioning of coaxial gas and avoidance of distention when a laser is used. Larger probes are preferred for coagulation of lesions larger than 4-5 mm in diameter.

Concerning video endoscopes, we are also using a variety of different instruments depending upon the location of the angiomata and size of the thermal probe to be used. At this time the therapeutic video endoscopes are not as versatile as standard fiberoptic instruments because of their larger size, longer non-flexible tip and lack of a two channel instrument. Nevertheless, for video documentation video endoscopes are superior.

Similar external diameter end-viewing (Pentax or Olympus) or oblique viewing (Olympus GIF-K) endoscopes are sometimes useful for elective coagulation of gastric or duodenal angiomata. For post-bulbar or fundal angiomata, a duodenoscope with a 2.8 mm suction channel such as the Olympus JF1T is very useful. Occasionally a longer end-viewing endoscope (such as the ACMI AGT2) or colonoscope (such as the Pentax FC-38LA) are useful for coagulation in the distal duodenum either during routine endoscopy or at surgery. The suction channel size must be selected to be able to through-put the laser catheter or contact probe. Although some laser catheters (1.7 mm diameter) can be passed through a pediatric endoscope (Olympus P3) or standard duodenoscope (Olympus JFB3), even small or BICAP probes (2.4 mm) will not pass through this small suction channel of 2.2 mm diameter. During a single coagulation session, two or more endoscopes such as end-viewing and side-viewing, may be necessary to reach and coagulate the UGI angiomata. Although lasers may be fired from a distance, contact probes must be touched on the angioma prior to coagulation. Changing of the endoscope, the probe size, or the patient's position may all facilitate placement of the probes upon the angioma to be coagulated.

General Treatment Measures After Endoscopic Treatment

Successful treatment of angiomata or telangiectasia depends upon coagulation of the abnormal vessels. Thermal damage results in mucosal and/or deeper damage. Coagulation necrosis occurs initially, followed by erosion or ulcer formation within 3-7 days. The more extensive the treatment (in surface area and depth), the more the tissue damage. For effective palliation, healing and re-epithelialization of the area with mucosa lacking the abnormal vessels is required. Adequate nutrition, oxygenation and supportive medical care are required to aid in healing these induced erosions and ulcers. We often use an H2 blocker (cimetidine, ranitidine or famotidine) or sucralfate after UGI angiomata treatment. Routine nasogastric tubes are not used. A program of careful follow-up must be developed for each patient with bleeding GI angiomata. The interval and extent of future endoscopic treatments will depend upon each patient's healing abilities, their rate of growth of new angiomata, and their ability to return for follow-up. Surgery to improve their underlying conditions (such as valvular heart surgery or renal transplantation) should also be considered in appropriate patients.

Coagulation units and techniques

Argon Laser

For endoscopic treatment of our first 24 patients with severe UGI bleeding from angiomata, we applied endoscopic argon laser with a Cooper Lasersonics model 770 unit (3, 14). The laser catheters were used with standard endoscopes (Fig. 6.2).

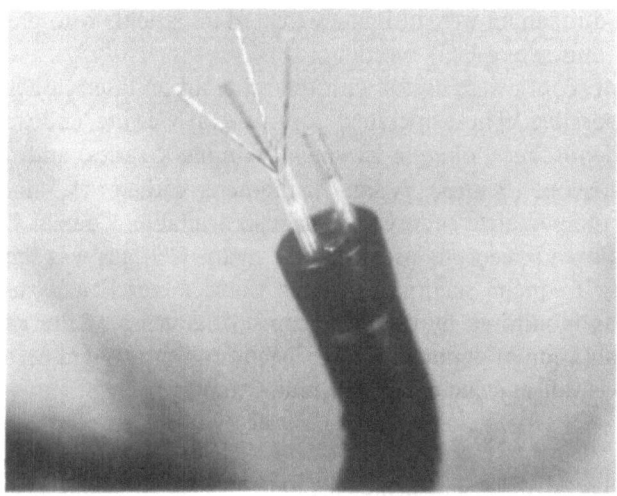

Fig. 6.2. Panendoscope with argon laser catheter in one channel and polyp grasper for clot removal down the other.

The full angle of divergence was 8-10 degrees, 5-8 Watts power output was used with low flow coaxial CO_2 gas, and separate water irrigation as needed. Prior to treatment the power output from the laser catheter tip and also the synchronized endoscopic filter were checked. A small area of normal gastric mucosa was coagulated to test the system prior to treatment of the lesion. If coagulation was not easy, the laser system was rechecked and the catheter changed if necessary prior to angioma coagulation. At a later time, we recleave or repair argon laser catheters rather than discard them. (See Brunetaud chapter).

Coagulation (whitening) of the entire angioma is the end-point (Plate 10). Vaporization is avoided. Treatment distance is 1-4 cm and can be gauged by experience or placing the catheter near the mucosa and withdrawing 1-4 cm. It is often possible to coagulate small flat lesions (smaller than 4-5 mm in diameter) with 3-4 pulses. If vaporization occurs, oozing bleeding is common but usually controllable with further coagulation. Washing the lesion to identify the bleeding is common but usually controllable with further coagulation. Washing the lesion to identify the bleeding point facilitates treatment of induced bleeding. For lesions larger than 5 mm, we coagulate the most dependent portion of the angioma first and then coagulate up the lesion. For multiple non-bleeding angiomata in a bowel segment, we coagulate the smaller lesions first in the dependent portions and then coagulate all others, finishing with the largest angioma. When an actively bleeding angioma is found, it is coagulated first. Washing with water and suctioning may be necessary to remove clots and blood that can obscure angiomata.

Argon laser treatment of multiple UGI angiomata was fast and easy. Except in emergency cases and those with more than 50 angiomata, we attempted to coagulate all angiomata in a single laser session. All the angiomata in the stomach and duodenum were ultimately treated in patients who presented with hematemesis and severe UGI bleeding.

Several endoscopes were useful with the same argon laser catheter to get as en face as possible. These included routine end-viewing endoscopes, side-viewing duodenoscopes, oblique viewing (Olympus K series) and rarely a thin caliber colonoscope (Pentax). A smaller diameter catheter (1.7 mm diameter) for use with the pediatric endoscope was also available. Coaxial CO_2 gas was used at low flow to keep the laser catheter clean. CO_2 gas was removed from the bowel by frequent suctioning rather than a recycling system. Gastric distention was monitored by the endoscopist (flattering of the gastric folds) and nurse (palpation of abdomen). Overdistention was avoided because it thins out the bowel wall and increases transmural damage.

Contact probes (BICAP and heater probe)

General

Probes were tested for functioning prior to endoscopic use. Specifically, the water jet irrigation and coagulation were checked. With a few drops of saline in a styrofoam cup and a low coagulation setting (2-3 on a 50 Watt BICAP generator vs. 10 Joules on the heater probe), heating and boiling of saline were verified. Malfunctioning, bent or damaged probes were replaced. Endoscopic coagulation of normal gastric mucosa was confirmed prior to treatment of the angiomata.

For urgent hemostasis, two channel therapeutic endoscopes (Fig. 6.1) and large probes (3.2 mm) were often selected. These instruments allowed removal of fresh blood, small clots and water from target irrigation. The actively bleeding angioma was coagulated first and then all other angiomata in the area.

For elective coagulation, endoscopy with a large (3.7 mm) or standard (2.8) channel instrument was done. The choice of instrument depended upon factors discussed previously. When large lesions were suspected, the large channel instruments and probes were preferred. These larger probes coagulate better, cover more surface area, wash better, and often induce less bleeding because fewer pulses are required. Also, the heat per unit area of coagulation is less with the larger than the smaller contact probes. This reduces the risks of transmural injury or perforation in elderly patients with thin gut walls.

Our technique for active bleeding angioma is to identify the focal bleeding point (usually a small arteriole near the center), apply gentle tamponade (not firm like chronic ulcers), and coagulate with 2-3 pulses. For elective coagulation, light contact is used directly on the angioma prior to coagulation.

For angioma less than 2-3 mm in diameter, small probes (2.4 mm diameter) are adequate for coagulation. Usually 2-3 pulses suffice. For larger lesions (larger than 3 mm), larger probes are preferred. For larger angioma (bigger than 5 mm), if the whole angioma cannot be covered by the probe, the most dependent portion of the angioma is coagulated first and then we proceed up the angioma. Whitening the entire angioma is the end-point (Plate 10). Unlike colonic angioma, feeding vessels are rarely evident for UGI angiomata. When present, feeding vessels are tamponaded gently and coagulated at the perimeter of the angioma. This will blanch the angioma and facilitate coagulation. Tangential (with one side) coagulation was excellent as was coagulation with the tip of either BICAP or heater probe. However, contact was required.

Target irrigation can be used as needed with either BICAP or heater probe. This is useful for visualization during active bleeding or for clearing small clots. Although a two channel instrument will permit simultaneous coagulation and suctioning, use of a single channel endoscope will necessitate removal of the contact probe before suctioning blood, clots, or a significant amount of fluid. Even with a small probe (2.4 mm) down a large single channel endoscope (such as Olympus GIF-1T), the suctioning capacity is inadequate to permit simultaneous suctioning of blood or fluid and coagulation.

Bipolar (BICAP) electrocoagulation

Coagulation of UGI angiomata was done with BICAP 50 watt generator (American ACMI, Stamford, CT). Large (3.3 mm) or small (2.4 mm) diameter probes were used at settings low enough to cause mucosal coagulation. (See Chapter 5 for a description and pictures of probes and power units.) These were adjusted for the probes while testing them on normal gastric mucosa but generally setting were 1 sec pulses and 2-3 on the dial. Rarely were higher settings necessary for angiomata coagulation (Plate 10), unlike bleeding peptic ulcers. Light touch was used and target irrigation as necessary. For BICAP, tangential coagulation is even better than coagulation with the tip (en face) although both are effective. If coagulum build-up on the probe occurred or sticking, the probe was removed and mechanically cleaned with a wet 4x4. After use, probes were cleaned mechanically with a 4x4, mild soap, alcohol and sterile water. For sterilization they were soaked in solutions such as glutaraldehyde. All fluid is blown out and probes are air-dried and re-used until either they will no longer coagulate effectively or they are severely bent. Worn out BICAP probes are replaced rather than repaired because they are much less expensive than laser catheters or heater probe. A different set of probes (large and small) are available for different patients with known or suspected infections: AIDS, hepatitis B, or severe leukopenia. Besides mechanical cleaning after coagulation in such patients, these probes and endoscopes are gas sterilized.

Heater probe

Although we previously used a prototype unit (Auth, Seattle) with large (3.2 mm) and small (2.4 mm) probes, the heater probe is now commercially available (see chapter 5 for descriptions and pictures of the heater probe unit). Similar to BICAP, the probes are tested ahead of time and generator settings are set low enough (usually 10-15 joules) to endoscopically coagulate normal gastric mucosa. Rarely are higher settings required for coagulation of UGI angioma. Gentle contact pressure was applied with techniques, probe size, and endoscope choice as described for BICAP. Target irrigation is used only as needed because suctioning subsequently is required to remove the pool of water before efficient coagulation can be performed.

After 10-15 coagulation pulses, sticking to the lesion and coagulum build-up on the probe are often encountered. Then the probe should be removed and mechanically cleaned with a wet 4x4. Further coagulation is then feasible.

For probe cleaning and storage, refer to the BICAP section. Heater probes are used until they bend or do not coagulate effectively anymore. Although these probes are relatively expensive, it is not currently possible to have them repaired.

Our results

Argon Laser

Non-O-W-R Angiomata. Fourteen patients with a mean age of 65 years and with more than 200 units of blood transfused prior to treatment had 120 UGI angiomata treated. Their predisposing medical conditions included valvular heart disease in five, cirrhosis in two, radiation treatment of a pancreatic malignancy in one and significant renal disease in two. All patients had failed medical management prior to endoscopic coagulation including treatment with iron and transfusions in all and estrogen-progesterone compounds in others. During the follow-up period of 36 months (mean), the mean stable hematocrit (while on iron replacement) rose from 24 to 35. The growth of new bleeding lesions varied from three months to 45 months in this patient group. During the follow-up period compared with the same time period before argon laser treatment, there was a reduction in emergency admissions for GI bleeding, total transfusions, and surgery. (See below – overall follow-up).

Osler-Weber-Rendu Syndrome. Ten patients, with a mean age of 63 years and more than 460 units transfused before treatment had 659 telangiectasiae treated with argon laser. They had also failed medical management prior to endoscopic coagulation. Five had valvular heart disease. The mean stable hematocrit (on iron replacement) in this group rose from 25 to 37 over the follow-up period of 30 months. Based on this time interval, a program of elective endoscopy and laser treatment was followed for each patient. During the follow-up period compared with the same interval before argon laser treatment, there was a reduction in total transfusions, admissions for GI bleeding and surgery.

Complications and conclusions

There have been no complications of endoscopy or argon laser in these patients with UGI angiomata. Argon laser is safe and effective for the treatment of endoscopically accessible angiomata of UGI tract. Although oozing type bleeding was common during coagulation of large lesions, it could be controlled in every case with further coagulation. Anemia, delayed bleeding, post-coagulation syndrome, perforation or any other complications were not seen.

Heater Probe or BICAP

We have used endoscopic heater probe or bipolar electrocoagulation (BICAP) to treat UGI angiomata in eleven patients with O-W-R syndrome and thirty-four with non-O-W-R angioma. All patients had failed medical management. Concomitant diseases of moderate or severe nature were present in most of these patients: 80% had heart disease, 25% had renal disease, and 20% had chronic liver disease. All had endoscopic documentation of bleeding from GI angioma before enrollment in a program of endoscopic treatment and follow-up.

Non-O-W-R Angiomata. Thirty-four patients with a mean age of 66 years and during initial treatment and follow-up, more than 250 UGI angiomata were coagulated. There were no major complications. However, large angiomata commonly bled with probe contact or during treatment but this could be controlled with further coagulation. In no patient was transfusion required because of induced anemia. During the follow-up period compared with the same interval before endoscopic treatment, there were significant reductions in total transfusions, admissions for GI bleeding, and surgeries. The mean hematocrit rose significantly.

O-W-R Syndrome. Eleven patients with O-W-R syndrome had a mean age of 65 years and recurrent UGI bleeding from telangiectasias. During initial treatment and follow-up, more than 600 telangiectasias were coagulated. There were no major complications although controllable bleeding from touching and treatment of large GI telangiectasia was common. In no cases was induced bleeding severe. Anemia or transfusions did not result. During the follow-up compared with the same interval before treatment there was a significant reduction in transfusions and admissions for GI bleeding along with a significant increase in mean hematocrit. See the general results and discussion section.

General results and discussion

Endoscopic Results

The predominant size and location of the bleeding angiomata were recorded for each patient. These are shown in Table 6.2.

Table 6.2. UGI angiomata sizes.

DIAMETER		PREVALENCE
Small	≤ 5 mm	63%
Medium	6-10 mm	30%
Large	11-20 mm	6%
Giant	> 20 mm	1%

The majority were small (less than 5 mm-63%) or medium (5-10 mm - 30%), rather than large or giant (larger than 10 mm). During diagnostic examinations, active bleeding was uncommon for UGI angiomata (14% of cases), whereas stigmata of recent bleeding (affixed clots, erosions on the angioma and adjacent fresh blood) or clean angioma were common. The predominant location for the angiomata considered the bleeding site is given in Table 6.3.

Table 6.3. UGI angiomata location.

SITE	PREVALENCE
Esophagus	0 %
Fundus	6 %
Posterior body	53 %
Antrum	6 %
Prepyloric area	3 %
Duodenal bulb	15 %
Second duodenum	12.5%
Third duodenum	1.5%
At Billroth II anastomosis	2 %

Although occasional angiomata were found in the esophagus, particularly with O-W-R syndrome, they were not thought to represent the bleeding point in any patient and were not coagulated. The most common locations were the posterior body of the stomach (53%), duodenal bulb (15%), and second portion of the duodenum (12.5%). The antrum (6%), pylorus (3%), third duodenum (1.5%) or at the BII anastomosis (2%) were uncommon locations.

Palliation Results – General

For each patient, outcomes were compared for equal periods of time before and after endoscopic coagulation. Data are presented in Table 6.4 for 21 O-W-R patients and 48 non-O-W-R patients.

Table 6.4. UGI angiomata-palliation results.

	2 Yrs before	2 Yrs after
Mean number of patients		
O-W-R	21	21
NON-O-W-R	48	48
Mean number of bleeds		
O-W-R	5.2	2.2*
Non-O-W-R	3.7	1.4*
Mean units RBC transfused		
O-W-R	19.3	7.8*
Non-O-W-R	10.7	4.5*

*p <0.05 After compared to Before treatment

For both groups, there was a significant decrease in the number of GI bleeds (hospitalizations) and RBC units transfused after endoscopic coagulation compared with before. There were no differences among the coagulation devices (argon laser, heater probe or BICAP) in these overall outcomes. However, for the O-W-R patients, argon laser was easier and less time was required for coagulation session than with the contact devices (BICAP and heater probe). With argon laser, lesions could be treated for a distance and contact was not required as was necessary with heater probe or BICAP. Most of our O-W-R patients had several hundred telangiectasia and required several coagulation sessions. For these O-W-R patients, approximately one-third the treatment time was required for argon laser vs. the contact probes. Nevertheless, contact probes are effective and with a deliberate and persistent approach, hemostasis and good palliation can be achieved with BICAP and heater probe.

Palliation Results – Cost

We also estimated the direct cost of care of patients with bleeding GI angiomata. Similar to the improvements in other outcomes such as the frequency of UGI bleeds, hospitalization, and transfusions, there has been a significant reduction in the direct cost of care of these patients with endoscopic coagulation and follow-up (23).

Risk Factors

In our clinical experience there are several prognosticators for poor outcome (19-22). These are listed in Table 6.5.

Table 6.5. Risk factors for poor outcome – GI angiomata.

Uncooperative patient
Abnormal bleeding
  – Pre-malignancy
  – Drug related
  – Idiopathic thrombocytopenia purpura
End-stage underlying disease
  – Heart failure
  – Renal failure
  – Connective tissue disorder
  – Malignancy
SP radiation
Severe catabolism
Very extensive bowel lesions
  – O-W-R telangiectasia
  – Watermelon stomach
  – Right colon
  – angiomata

Uncooperative patients or those unlikely to return for medical or endoscopic therapy should not be considered for endoscopic palliation. Because medical follow-up is required as well as further endoscopies, such patients will do poorly. Rebleeds will recur before effective treatment can be planned or administered. In most patients slow rebleeding and positive stool hemoccults precede overt bleeding and anemia. Follow-up will not be possible in this group of uncooperative patients.

Patients with any of these risk factors seem to fare poorly no matter what form of treatment for gut angiomata is chosen: medical, surgical, pharmacologic, or endoscopic. Rebleeding or continued bleeding frequently occur. In such patients, the safest form of palliation must be selected. Although experience is somewhat limited, we have noted 3-6 cases of each prognosticator in our series of patients with UGI and lower GI (See chapter 8) angiomata. Compared to patients without these risk factors, short (less than 60 days) and long-term (greater than 60 days) outcomes are poor in terms of continued bleeding or rebleeding. Several prognosticators deserve further comment.

Endoscopic treatment is not recommended as palliation for patients who may worsen as a result of this treatment. Patients with irreversible thrombocytopenia or qualitative platelet abnormalities and prolonged bleeding times, patients with very severe acute or chronic heart failure or renal failure, or patients not expected to survive for 30 days because of end-stage underlying medical conditions are poor candidates for endoscopic palliation. They may worsen in the short term because of the endoscopy itself or the induced ulcerations which can cause delayed bleeding or another complication. They often do not heal the induced ulcers well, nor survive to benefit from the longer term palliative effect. Recurrence rates of new angiomata may be high in patients with end-stage heart, renal or connective tissue diseases.

On the other hand, if underlying medical-surgical conditions can be effectively reversed, then gut angiomata may not bleed and may not require endoscopic palliation. This seems to relate to the pathophysiology of bleeding gut angiomata. For example, we have treated five patients with valvular heart disease, severe heart failure, and severe GI bleeding from gut angiomata whose GI bleeding and need for endoscopic palliation remarkably changed after successful heart valve surgery. Improvement in their cardiac functional status inversely related to reduced genesis of new GI angiomata and rebleeding. In our experience, worsening heart failure or renal failure in GI angiomata patients tends to increase their frequency of new gut angiomata and rebleeding.

The prognostic factors listed in Table 6.5 are independent of treatment chosen for management of the bleeding angioma whether endoscopic (laser vs. contact probe), surgical, pharmacologic or medical. The palliative treatment does not determine outcome in these patients but rather the underlying medical-surgical conditions do. When one is planning, evaluating or comparing palliation efficacy of different treatments for gut angiomata, these risk factors must be taken into account.

Discussion and results of other investigations

Bowers and Dixon (24) treated eleven patients with UGI angiomata and recurrent GI bleeding. Two patients had O-W-R syndrome. Associated conditions included aortic stenosis in 46%, renal failure in 23%, arteriosclerosis in 15% and essential thrombocythemia in 7.5%. Lesions were treated with argon laser and 3-4.5 watts were applied in 1-5 sec. pulses. The eleven patients with 105 lesions of the stomach and duodenum were treated in 16 sessions during the mean follow-up period of 6 months. Five patients had angiomata in both the upper and lower GI tracts. In comparisons at 1, 3, and 6 months pre- and post-treatments, the frequency of bleeding episodes and transfusion rates were reduced. There were no complications.

Waitman et al. (25) used argon laser at 7.5 watts to treat 50 patients with GI hemorrhage secondary to angiomata. No complications occurred. After treatment, two-thirds of the patients had complete cessation of hemorrhage during follow-ups of 6 months to 4 years. One third had decreased GI bleeding and transfusion requirement but required further treatments. One of the 50 patients with GI angiomata required surgery for a bleeding jejunal angioma.

Rogers (9,26) reported successful treatment of 50 patients with GI angiomata using a hot biopsy forceps (monopolar electrocoagulation). One patient with a lesion on the ileocecal valve could not be coagulated and required surgery. The distribution of lesions was 44 colonic, 5 gastric, and 2 duodenal. Thirty-nine of the 51 patients (76%) had some type of associated cardiac, vascular, or pulmonary disease. Five patients were followed for more than 5 years and 2 of these had recurrent GI bleeding from angioma. No complications were reported.

Young et al. (27) treated multiple gastric O-W-R lesions (average 6/patient) in 3 patients with endoscopic sclerotherapy. Sodium morrhuate was injected submucosally. Transient bleeding was a complication from two lesions. Endoscopic evaluation at 6 months revealed no telangiectasia and the patients had no recurrent bleeding.

Johnston treated 440 angiomata in 22 patients with a YAG laser (28). Good outcomes with a reduction or complete control of GI bleeding resulted in 19 patients. Delayed massive hemorrhage 7 to 16 days after YAG laser coagulation occurred in 3 patients (13.6%). Surgical pathology revealed bleeding from induced ulceration of the treatment sites. Johnston cautioned that the risk of delayed bleeding should be weighed against the potential benefit of YAG treatment for GI angiomata.

Rutgeerts treated 482 GI angiomata with YAG laser in 50 patients (29). The lesions were located in the UGI tract alone in 25 patients, in the lower GI tract alone in 31 patients and in both UGI and LGI tracts in 3 patients. In 30% of patients mild bleeding occurred during treatment but was controlled by further coagulation. YAG laser treatment reduced the bleeding rate from GI angiomata during the follow-up period of up to 18 months. The results were disappointing in 4 O-W-R patients and 3 angiomata patients with Von Willebrand's disease. Ten percent of all the study patients developed severe complications including severe pain during treatment, chronic duodenal ulcer, delayed severe bleeding or perforation. Endoscopy 1 week after YAG laser treatment always revealed ulcers, some which were large or deep. The authors recommended limiting YAG exposure to 200 joules per lesion in one session, particularly with extensive colonic angiomata.

Bown et al. treated 18 patients, 8 with O-W-R and 10 with non-O-W-R angiomata and severe O-W-R bleeding (30). Beginning in 1979, they applied argon laser with 5-6 watts and 1-3 sec. pulses to obliterate the mucosal component. After 1981 they coagulated angiomata with YAG laser at 60-70 watts and 0.5 sec. pulses. They limited energy exposure on any one lesion and resumed treatment two or more weeks later. Surgical resection was performed in patients whose bleeding could not be controlled endoscopically or for severe delayed bleeding as a complication. The mean follow-up is not stated but data are given only for 3 and 6 months. One patient was followed for up to 5 years.

The mean number of laser sessions to complete the initial laser treatment was 5 for O-W-R, 3 for single angioma and 2 for multiple non-O-W-R angiomata. 78% (14/18) of their patients benefited from the laser palliation during the short follow-ups at 3 and 6 months. However, 22% (4/18) were considered *failures* and required surgery for continued bleeding (3) or severe delayed bleeding (1 patient).

No complications occurred with argon laser, although the authors reported that only superficial coagulation was possible. Based upon their concept that deeper submucosal vessels are more important for angioma treatment than the mucosal component, they changed to YAG laser. YAG laser was associated with aggravated bleeding in 3 patients and severe delayed bleeding in 1 patient who required surgery for hemostasis. Complications occurred in 22% of patients treated with YAG laser. In spite of the increased risk of complications, Bown et al. favor the YAG laser for UGI angiomata hemostasis because of the deeper coagulation potential. Their current technique with YAG laser is to treat around the edge of the angioma rather than in the center in hopes of coagulating feeding vessels. They have not prospectively compared this YAG laser technique with any other methods in terms of safety or efficacy.

General discussion

The pathophysiology and etiology of gut angiomata may be related to altered circulatory status as suggested by several factors: 1) the common distribution of GI BICAP angiomata in 'watershed areas' of the cecum and posterior gastric corpus; 2) the common association with valvular heart disease; and 3) the improvement or worsening of GI bleeding relative to heart failure (3, 22). In our experience, overt GI bleeding is often associated with increasing size of GI mucosal angiomata; with medication such as anticoagulants, aspirin, or non-steroidal anti-inflammatory drugs; and with worsening cardiac dysfunction.

Accurate clinical data on complication or perforation rates for different thermal methods during or after angiomata treatment are not available. However, several important lessons have been learned from reported animal studies (11-16). Histologic studies in dogs have revealed that the relative *depth of penetration* and resultant *histologic damage* for endoscopically treated gastric ulcers in increasing order is argon laser ≤ bipolar electrocoagulation ≤ heater probe < YAG laser < MPEC. We have found similar relative damage for treatment of normal mucosa (simulating mucosal lesions such as angioma) for the canine stomach, duodenum, esophagus, right colon and cecum.

The *relative thickness* of normal canine bowel in decreasing order is: stomach > esophagus > duodenum > right colon > cecum. These approximate the normal human bowel relationships. Age, atrophy, or acute ulceration may decrease wall thickness. Chronic inflammation, tumor or edema may increase bowel wall thickness. Angiomata in patients do not usually increase in the bowel wall thickness. *Distention* of the stomach during endoscopic coagulation (15), as well as distention of any hollow viscus significantly increases the incidence of transmural thermal injury. For distensible mucosal lesions such as angiomata, treatment after overdistention should be avoided. The location of angiomata may influence ones choice of endoscopic coagulation method. Gastric angiomata are often in the posterior aspect of the stomach. Deep injury from treatment may result in penetration rather than free perforation. Angiomata in the cecum, right colon, or duodenum are often anterior so that transmural injury can cause free perforation or post-coagulation syndrome. A careful choice of endoscopic coagulation method and avoidance of distention are recommended.

Although endoscopic coagulation techniques are promising, there are several limitations. These techniques are palliative for gut angiomata. Follow-up must be empirically determined for each patient. It depends upon the 1) underlying etiology: O-W-R versus non-O-W-R angioma; 2) the severity and extent of the GI lesions and 3) the severity of concomitant medical-surgical disease. The benefit to the patient depends upon careful localization of bleeding sites rather than treatment of non-bleeding angiomata. Patients with circumferential, transmural A-V malformations or extensive, contiguous angiomata may not be candidates for endoscopic palliation.

The advantages of YAG and argon lasers for GI angiomata treatment are listed in Table 6.6.

Table 6.6. Advantages of lasers for GI angiomata treatment.

---

* Non-touch technique
* Faster for multiple lesions
* Elective coagulation is easy
* Low power is feasible for coagulation
* Catheter use feasible with different endoscopes
* Laser catheter re-use and repair are feasible

Because laser coagulation can be performed as a non-touch technique with a movable catheter (Figs. 6.2. and 6.3) from a distance, it can be easier and faster than contact probes. Particularly, elective laser sessions in patients with multiple angiomata such as O-W-R syndrome are efficient. The same laser catheter can be used with several different endoscopes. Unlike the contact probes which wear out and cannot be repaired, laser catheters can be recleaved and/or repaired for re-use. Lower power argon (4-7 watts) or YAG (30-50 watts) are feasible for coagulation of all angiomata cases. This is in contrast to emergency hemostasis of actively bleeding ulcers or Mallory-Weiss tears which are the only treatments requiring higher power argon (8-10 watts) or YAG (75-100 watts) lasers for successful hemostasis. Because lower power lasers are also useful for elective tumor coagulation, it may be possible in the future to have less powerful, less expensive, and smaller lasers. For example, multipurpose mid-power range (60 watt) YAG lasers are now being marketed for considerable less cost than the high power (about 100 watts) models. These 60 watt YAG lasers have less electrical (single phase, less amperage) and water cooling requirements, and are smaller and more portable than their high power counterparts. These YAG lasers should be feasible for elective tumor and angiomata coagulation. Mid-power argon lasers (4-7 watts) are not currently marketed but high power systems are available.

The disadvantages of argon and YAG lasers for GI angiomata treatment are listed in Table 6.7.

Table 6.7. Disadvantages of lasers for GI angiomata treatment.

* Vaporization into vessels can occur and precipitate bleeding
* Tangential treatment is difficult
* Inconvenient for emergency ICU cases
* Distention and pneumoperitoneum from gas insufflation occur
* Delayed perforation, post-coagulation syndrome or delayed hemorrhage or chronic ulcers may occur after YAG

Some are more important than others, especially for neophytes. Some disadvantages are preventable. Vaporization into gut angiomata and precipitation of severe bleeding should be avoided. One can do this by decreasing the laser power density by increasing the treatment distance and/or decreasing the laser power. The resulting coagulation effect on normal gastric mucosa needs to be verified before further angiomata treatment. Overdistention should be avoided by careful monitoring endoscopically (of gastric folds, organ size, etc.), reducing coaxial gas flow, and frequently suctioning out CO_2 gas. Overdistention prior to any form of endoscopic thermal coagulation significantly increases transmural coagulation compared to normal distention. Thinning out the wall thickness, causing ischemia, and reducing the blood flow may contribute to the increased damage related to overdistention. Tangential treatment can be obviated by use of a more flexible end-viewing endoscope or use of side-viewing or oblique-viewing endoscopes. Some investigators have introduced laser catheters which radiate laterally or obliquely (31). Because of the deeper tissue coagulation with YAG laser, there is a greater inherent risk of delayed perforation, post-coagulation syndrome and delayed hemorrhage compared to all other thermal devices except monopolar electrocoagulation. Until such time as tissue temperature can be monitored, this effect cannot be controlled. Repeated coagulation or widespread coagulation of contiguous angiomata with YAG laser should be avoided. This is particularly true in bowel areas that are anterior in location, thin walled (from distention, age, or atrophy), or damaged already (from prior ischemia or radiation).

Limitations of endoscopic coagulation and conclusions

Whether the benefit to the patient of endoscopic treatment of GI angiomata outweighs the effort, expense and risk need to be determined for each coagulation method and patient. Except for our own estimates of cost savings (23), there are no actual economic data available to compare the impact of endoscopic vs. routine management. Based upon our large experience with UGI angiomata, argon laser, heater probe, and bipolar electrocoagulation (BICAP) appear to be safe and effective for endoscopic palliation and can reduce the direct cost of care. We have not had any major complications.

Some investigators also report favorable results with YAG laser and monopolar electrocoagulation. However, the frequency of significant complications, particularly delayed ulceration and bleeding, has been as high as 10-20% in some reports of YAG laser treatment for UGI angiomata (28-30). It is unknown whether more experience or different techniques of YAG application such as reduction of the output energy or limitation of the total energy applied to a bowel segment will reduce this high complication rate. Because of its heating characteristics, YAG laser results in deeper coagulation and resultant ulcers than argon laser, heater probe, or BICAP. Based upon animal data (11-16) and reported clinical experience, more complications from endoscopic YAG coagulation of UGI angiomata are to be expected compared with BICAP, heater probe, and argon laser as more patients are treated.

More than any other factor, the prognosis of the patient and the presence or absence of clinical risk factors (Table 6.5) determine the patient's outcome. Like other non-endoscopic treatments of UGI angiomata, endoscopic treatment is palliative. Until the etiology and cure for angiomata are understood, such treatments, if safe and effective, are reasonable. Endoscopic therapy with lasers or other devices is not miraculous for most angiomata patients. Concomitant medical conditions must be treated simultaneously to optimize the palliative effect of endoscopic coagulation.

References

1. Smith CR, Bartholomew LG, Cain JC. Hereditary hemorrhagic telangiectasia and gastrointestinal hemorrhage. Gastroenterology 1963;44:1-6.
2. Ertan A, Hollander A. Vascular malformations of the gastrointestinal tract. Survey of Digestive Diseases 1985;3:42- 48.
3. Jensen DM, Machicado GA, Tapia JI et al. Endoscopic treatment of hemangiomata with argon laser in patients with gastrointestinal bleeding. Gastroenterology 1982;82:1093.
4. Weaver GA, Alpern HD, Davis JS et al. Gastrointestinal angiodysplasia associated with aortic valve disease: part of a spectrum of angiodysplasia of the gut. Gastroenterology 1979;77:1-11.
5. Cherry R, Lough JO, Jabbari M, Daly DS, Kinnear DG, Goresky CA. Gastric antral vascular dysplasia (the watermelon stomach): a cause of chronic upper gastrointestinal bleeding. Gastrointest Endosc 1983;29:2:193.
6. Gilliam JH, Geisinger KR, Wu WC et al. The 'Watermelon Stomach' morphologic diagnosis by endoscopy. Gastro 1985;88(Part 2):1394.
7. Mitsudo SM, Boley SJ, Brandt LJ et al. Vascular ectasias of the right colon in the elderly: a distinct pathologic entity. Human Pathology 1979;10:585-600.
8. Jensen DM, Machicado GA. Endoscopic treatment of incidental angiomata in patients with severe gastrointestinal bleeding. Gastrointest Endosc 1985;31(:2):158.
9. Rogers BHG, Adler F. Hemangiomas of the cecum: colonoscopic diagnosis and therapy. Gastroenterology 1976;71:1079-1082.
10. Randall GM, Jensen DM, Slodownik E, Weinstein WM. Endoscopic biopsy for diagnosis of gastric arteriovenous malformations. Gastroenterology 1987;92(#2):1588.
11. Jensen DM. Endoscopic control of gastrointestinal bleeding. In: Development in Digestive Diseases. Vol III. ed. J. Edward Berk, Lea and Feiger, 1980:1-27.

12. Johnston JH, Jensen DM, Mautner W. Comparison of laser photocoagulation and electrocoagulation in endoscopic treatment of bleeding canine gastric ulcers. Gastroenterology 1982;82:904-910.

13. Machicado GA, Jensen DM, Tapia JI, Mautner W. Treatment of bleeding canine duodenal and esophageal ulcers with argon laser and bipolar electrocoagulation. Gastroenterology 1981;80:708-716.

14. Jensen DM, Machicado GA, Tapia JI, Mautner W. Comparison of argon laser photocoagulation and bipolar electrocoagulation of endoscopic hemostasis in the canine colon. Gastrointest Endosc 1981;27:131.

15. Johnson JH, Jensen DM, Mautner W, Elashoff J. Argon laser treatment of bleeding canine gastric ulcers: limitations and guidelines for endoscopic use. Gastroenterology 1981;80:708-716.

16. Johnston JH, Jensen DM, Mautner W, Elashoff J. YAG laser treatment of experimental bleeding canine gastric ulcers. Gastroenterology 1980;79:1252-1261.

17. Jensen DM, Machicado GA, Tapia JI, Mautner W. Endoscopic treatment of telangiectasia with argon laser photocoagulation and bipolar electrocoagulation in patients with chronic gastrointestinal bleeding. Gastrointestinal Endoscopy 1980;26:200.

18. Jensen DM, Machicado GA, Silpa ML. Treatment of GI angioma with argon laser, heater probe, or bipolar electrocoagulation. Gastrointest Endosc 1984;30:134.

19. Jensen DM, Machicado GA. Bleeding colonic angiomata: Endoscopic coagulation and outcome. Gastrointest Endosc 1986. In Press.

20. Jensen DM, Machicado GA. Bleeding colonic angiomas: Endoscopic coagulation and follow-up. Gastroenterology 1985;88(Part 2):1433.

21. Jensen D, Bown S. Gastrointestinal angiomata: diagnosis and treatment with laser therapy and other endoscopic modalities. In: Fleischer D, Jensen D, Bright-Asare P, Eds. Therapeutic Laser Endoscopy in Gastrointestinal Disease. Boston: Martinus Nijhoff 1983:151-160.

22. Smith JW, Jensen DM. Gastrointestinal angiomas. Postgraduate Medicine. 1987;82:171-181.

23. Jensen DM. Gastrointestinal angiomata: Current diagnosis and treatment. In: Therapeutic Gastrointestinal Endoscopy. An Information Resource Manual. Publisher: American Society of Gastrointestinal Endoscopy 1987;11-15.

24. Bowers JH, Dixon JA. Argon laser photocoagulation of vascular malformations in GI tract: short term results. Gastrointest Endosc 1982;28:2:126.

25. Waitman AM, Grant DZ, Chateau F. Argon laser photocoagulation treatment of patients with acute and chronic bleeding secondary to telangiectasia. Gastrointest Endosc 1982;28:2:153.

26. Rogers BHG. Endoscopic electrocoagulation of vascular abnormalities of the gastrointestinal tract in 51 patients. Gastrointest Endosc 1982;28:2:142.

27. Young W, Gibbert V, Feinstat T, Trudeau W. The recurrent upper gastrointestinal bleeding in hereditary hemorrhagic telangiectasia (Osler's disease) successfully treated by endoscopic sclerotherapy. Gastrointest Endosc 1982;28:2:148.

28. Johnston JH. Complications following endoscopic laser therapy. Gastrointest Endosc 1982;28:2:135.

29. Rutgeerts P, Van Gompel F, Geboes K, Vantrappen G, Broekaert L, Coremans G. Long term results of treatment of vascular malformations of the gastrointestinal tract by Neodymium YAG laser photocoagulation. Gut 1985;26:586-593.

30. Bown SG, Swain CP, Storey DU et al. Endoscopic Laser Treatment of Vascular Abnormalities of the Upper Gastrointestinal Tract. Gut. In Press.

31. Hashimoto D, Takami M, Idezuki Y. Prismatic tip lateral radiation probe in YAG laser endoscopy. Gastrointest Endosc 1985;31:153.

7. LASER TREATMENT FOR VASCULAR MALFORMATIONS OF THE DIGESTIVE TRACT

J.M BRUNETAUD, V. MAUNOURY, D. COCHELARD,
A. CORTOT AND J.D. PARIS

Vascular malformations (VM) of the gastrointestinal tract (GI) can be responsible for acute digestive hemorrhage or chronic anemia. The treatment was previously surgical but now is more conservative with endoscopic hemostasis (1). We report our 8.5 year experience with endoscopic laser treatment at the Lille Laser Center.

Patients and method

Patients

Sixty-seven patients (32 males and 35 females) were referred to the Laser Center for endoscopic treatment of a VM. Thirty-nine presented with a recent active hemorrhage and 28 with chronic anemia from GI blood loss. The VM was considered as the cause of the digestive hemorrhage because 1) stigmata of hemorrhage at the VM were seen during endoscopy, or 2) VM were the only abnormality found during repeated endoscopies for multiple digestive hemorrhages.

The patients were divided into five groups (Table 7.1). Group 1 and 2 had an upper GI VM (group 1: no familial history, group 2: Osler-Weber-Rendu syndrome, O-W-R). Group 3 and 4 patients had colonic VM (group 3: right colon, group 4: left colon). Group 5 patients had a blue rubber bleb nevus syndrome (B-R-B-N). This hereditary syndrome consists of cavernous angiomas distributed throughout the entire digestive tract along with non-digestive localizations such as the skin.

Table 7.1. The patients by localization and etiology.

	No.	Mean age	Localization	Etiology
Group 1	43	71	upper GI	isolated
Group 2	10	56	upper GI	O-W-R*
Group 3	8	71	right colon	isolated
Group 4	4	37	left colon	isolated
Group 5	2	13	entire tract	B-R-B-N*

* O-W-R is Osler-Weber-Rendu syndrome and B-R-B-N is blue rubber bleb nevus syndrome.

D.M. Jensen and J.M. Brunetaud (eds), Medical Laser Endoscopy. 93-98.
© 1990 Kluwer Academic Publishers, Dordrecht

Associated diseases or possibly precipitating medications were found in sixteen patients (24%) and included 3 with antithrombocitic and 2 with steroid treatment, 6 with chronic renal failure, 2 aortic valvular stenosis, one thrombocytopenia, one Von Willebrand's disease, and one portal hypertension.

The goals of the treatment were 1) to stop the blood loss and to prevent recurrence in group 1, 3 and 4 patients, and 2) to reduce the blood transfusion rate in the group 2 and 5 patients.

Methods

An argon laser (770, Cooper Lasersonics, Santa Clara, Calif.) was mainly used for coagulation of VM with a 4 watt continuous beam (spot size 2 mm, irradiance 125 W/cm². The Nd:YAG laser was used (YAG 101, Cilas Marcoussis, France) with a 50 W continuous beam (spot size 2 mm, irradiance 1600 W/cm²). The Nd:YAG laser was used in only 3 circumstances: actively bleeding VM in the upper GI tract, local recurrence after an argon treatment in the upper GI tract, and cavernous VM (Blue rubber bleb nevus syndrome) in upper and lower GI tract.

Olympus GIF Q and CF LBW3 endoscopes (Olympus Corp., Tokyo, Japan) were used for laser treatment. Nitrogen was used to protect the fiber tip. For upper GI endoscopy, the argon and Nd:YAG laser fibers were inserted in a 1.6 external diameter catheter. The small diameter of the catheter allowed the gas to escape through the biopsy channel of the GIF Q endoscope during the laser treatment. For lower GI endoscopy, a cannula was introduced in the rectum along side the endoscope to evacuate the gas.

Patients were treated without sedation and as outpatients, except when they were hospitalized for an active hemorrhage or for colonic preparation. The maximum number of VM were treated during each session. The treatment was temporarily interrupted when the treatment induced bleeding from the VM. The VM was further retreated when it had stopped bleeding spontaneously. The patients were re-endoscoped and retreated every two weeks until complete disappearance of the VM. Then they were clinically followed, except group 2 patients who were systematically re-endoscoped and eventually retreated every 3 months. These group 2 patients also bled frequently from VM in the nose and were treated with the argon laser by our ENT colleagues (2).

Results

Results are summarized in Table 7.2.

Table 7.2. Results of the laser treatment.

Group	Pts	Mean # of laser Rx*	Approx # lesions	Usual F/U interval	Mean F/U	Recurrence rate
1	43	2 (1-5)	< 5	6 mo	24 mo	12%
2	10	4 (4-5)	>10	3 mo	71 mo	66%
3	8	1	1	---	14 mo	12%
4	4	2	2	---	17 mo	25%
5	2	4	>10	---	---	100%

* Mean number of laser treatment sessions during the initial treatment.

Group 1 Patients

All 43 patients stopped bleeding after an average of 2 laser treatment sessions (range 1-5). No recurrence was observed in the 11 patients who were lost to follow-up after an average period of 10 months, and in the 5 patients who deceased from other causes after an average period of 9.5 months. Twenty-two patients are still being followed during an average period of 24 months. A recurrent hemorrhagic episode was observed in 5 of the group 1 patients (12%). Four were successfully retreated. A chronic anemia persisted in the fifth patient who was under antithrombocitic treatment.

Group 2 Patients

All the 10 patients stopped bleeding after an average of 4.3 laser treatment sessions (range 4-5). See Plate 11 in the atlas. Four patients were followed only for a short period. Six patients were followed for an average of 71 months. Recurrent hemorrhagic episodes were observed in 4 (66%) of these 6 patients despite frequent laser treatment. However, the treatment benefited these patients, because a major decrease in the required blood transfusions was observed. As an example, a patient had had 700 units of blood transfused before laser treatment and did not require any transfusions during the two years of follow-up.

Group 3 Patients

All the 8 patients stopped bleeding after only one laser treatment. See Plate 12 (Atlas). The average follow-up is 14 months. Only one patient with aortic valve stenosis rebled (melena) and the origin of the recurrent hemorrhage was not detected.

95

Group 4 patients

All the 4 patients stopped bleeding after an average of 2 laser treatment sessions. During the 17 month average follow-up, recurrent anemia was observed in 1 patient without finding the cause.

Group 5 Patients

All the cavernous angiomas located in the stomach, duodenum and colon were successfully treated in the 2 patients. See Plate 13 (Atlas). However, both continued to bleed from angiomas located in the small bowel. One patient was operated upon and we tried to coagulate the angiomas with the endoscope guided by the surgeon. But, most of the small bowel angiomas were transmural and endoscopic laser coagulation would have induced a perforation of the bowel wall. The angiomas were too numerous to be surgically resectable and no treatment was possible. See Plate 14 in the atlas.

Complications

One hundred and ninety-one endoscopic treatments were performed in the 67 patients with VM and only one complication was reported. A perforation of the colon resulted in a patient treated for an angioma of the cecum. The perforation was successfully treated by surgery.

Discussion

The diagnosis of a VM can be difficult. During emergency endoscopy, a VM can be hidden by the bleeding or by a clot (3, 4). Follow-up endoscopies may be needed after the hemorrhagic episode to confirm its existence. On the other hand, VM are frequently found during elective endoscopy, but are not always responsible for digestive hemorrhages. Angiomas are reported to be the cause of 2% (3) to 5% (5) of the upper GI hemorrhages. The O-W-R syndrome prevalence is about 5/100,000 but only one third will present a digestive hemorrhage (6). VM are reported to be responsible for 35% of severe colonic hemorrhages (7). The treatment of incidental angioma was found to have no influence on the patient's outcome (8). Therefore, the role of the VM in the hemorrhagic episode has to be established before treatment. In our experience, the treatment of VM was limited to VM with stigmata of hemorrhages seen during endoscopy or when VM were the only abnormality found during repeated endoscopies for multiple digestive hemorrhages.

Our patients were divided into 5 groups which corresponded to different pathogenesis. The origin of VM in group 1 and 3 is likely to be a degenerative disease (average age 71 years), and in group 4 a congenital disease (average age 37 years). The VM in group 2 and 5 are hereditary diseases.

The initial treatment has been successful in all our 67 patients. During follow-up, 7 of the 55 (13%) group 1, 3 and 4 patients had a recurrent hemorrhage. New VM were found in 4 of them (all in group 1) and were successfully retreated. In the 3 other patients the origin of the recurrent bleeding could not be identified and therefore was not treated. Two reasons can explain the high recurrence rate (66%) in the 6 group 2 patients who were followed. 1) Two of them were living far away from Lille and were not re-endoscoped every 3 months, but only after a new hemorrhage. 2) Even in the regularly treated patients, new lesions can appear between two treatments. However, all 6 patients benefited from the treatment and had their quality of life greatly improved as assessed by reduction in bleeding episodes and transfusion.

Argon laser treatment of VM was reported with similar results in 7 other studies with a total of 155 patients (1,7,9-13). A cecal perforation in a patient with pulmonary insufficiency (10) was the only complication.

Three studies (14-16) reported the Nd:YAG laser experience in 99 patients with VM. The immediate success rate was limited respectively to 82%, 78% and 86%. Most of the failures corresponded to complications. Two perforations and 8laser-induced hemorrhages required surgical treatment.

Endoscopic non-laser treatments exist. Bipolar electrocoagulation (BICAP, Circon- ACMI,. Stamford, Connecticut) and thermal coagulation (heater probe, Olympus, Tokyo) were reported to be very efficient and safe (12). Sclerotherapy is another modality of endoscopic treatment for VM (17), but has not been widely used.

In conclusion, argon laser photocoagulation is a safe and efficient method of treatment for digestive vascular malformations. In patients with O-W-R syndrome, repeated treatments are needed. Even so, total control of the hemorrhages may not be obtained. But, the quality of life of these patients still remains greatly improved. Several complications were reported in the literature with Nd:YAG lasers. Therefore, the use of Nd:YAG laser is strictly limited in our institution to 1) actively bleeding VM in the upper GI tract, 2) local recurrence after argon treatment in the upper GI tract, and 3) cavernous VM (Blue rubber bleb nevus syndrome) in upper and lower GI tract.

References

1. Sudry P, Brunetaud JM, Paris JC, Bretagne JF, Danielou Y, Bouret JF, Le Bodic MF, Le Bodic L. La photocoagulation par laser à argon des angiomes digestifs: à propos de quinze cas. Gastroenterol Clin Biol 1981;5:426-32.
2. Piquet JJ, Brunetaud JM, Mosquet L, Burny A, Ton J. Laser à argon et maladie de Rendu Osler. Journal Français d'Oto- Laryngologie, 1985;34:325-26.
3. Quintero E, Pique JM, Bombi JA, Ros E, Bordas JM, Rives A, Teres J, Rodes J. Upper gastrointestinal bleeding caused by gastroduodenal vascular malformations. Dig Dis Sci

1986;31:897-905.

4. Thompson JN, Salem RP, Hemingway AP, Rees HC, Hodgson HJF, Wood CB, Allison DJ, Spencer J. Specialist investigation of obscure gastrointestinal bleeding. Gut 1987;28:47-51.

5. Fleischer D. Etiology and prevalence of severe persistent upper gastrointestinal bleeding. Gastroenterology 1983;84:538-43.

6. Smith CR, Bartholomew LG, Cain JC. Hereditary hemorrhagic telangiectasia and gastrointestinal hemorrhage. Gastroenterology 1963;44:1-6.

7. Jensen DM, Machicado GA. Diagnosis and treatment of severe hematochezia – the role of urgent colonoscopy after purge. Gastroenterology 1988;95:1569-1574.

8. Jensen DM, Machicado GA. Endoscopic treatment of incidental angiomata in patients with severe gastrointestinal bleeding. Gastrointest Endosc 1985;31:158 (abstr).

9. Bowers JH, Dixon JA. Argon laser photocoagulation of vascular malformations in the GI tract. Gastrointest Endosc 1982;28,2:126 (abstr).

10. Cello JP, Grendell JH. Endoscopic laser treatment for gastrointestinal vascular ectasias. Ann Intern Med 1986;32:142 (abstr).

11. Jensen DM, Machicado GA, Reedy TE, Elashoff J. Bleeding UGI angioma: Endoscopic coagulation and outcome. Gastrointest Endosc 1986;32:142 (abstr).

12. Jensen DM, Machicado GA, Silpa ML. Treatment of GI angiomata with argon laser, heater probe, or bipolar electrocoagulation. Gastrointest Endosc 1984;30:134 (abstr).

13. Waitman AM, Grant DZ, Chateau F. Argon laser photocoagulation treatment of patients with acute and chronic bleeding secondary to telangiectasia. Gastrointest Endosc 1982;28,2:135 (abstr).

14. Johnston JH. Complications following endoscopic laser therapy. Gastrointest Endosc 1982;28,2:135 (abstr).

15. Bown SG, Swain CP, Storey DW, Collins C, Matthewson K, Salmon PR, Clark CG. Endoscopic laser treatment of vascular anomalies of the upper gastrointestinal tract. Gut 1985;26:1338-348.

16. Rutgeerts P, Van Gompel F, Geboes K, Vantrappen G, Broeckaert L, Coremans G. Long-term results of treatment of vascular malformations of the gastrointestinal tract by Nd:YAG laser photocoagulation. Gut 1985;26:586-593.

17. Young W, Gibbert V, Feinstat T, Trudeau W. The recurrent upper gastrointestinal bleeding in hereditary hemorrhagic telangiectasia successfully treated by endoscopic sclerotherapy. Gastrointest Endosc 1982;28,2:148 (abstr).

8. TECHNIQUES OF HEMOSTASIS FOR LOWER GI BLEEDING

DENNIS M. JENSEN AND GUSTAVO A. MACHICADO

Introduction

Careful localization of the bleeding lesions via emergency colonoscopy after purge or during elective colonoscopy is the most important part of hemostasis in the colon. Because of the higher potential for complications from hemostasis in the colon, only lesions with serious bleeding should be considered for coagulation. Incidental lesions should not be treated. Angiomata are the most common lesions responsible for severe lower GI (LGI) bleeding and these are amenable to endoscopic hemostasis with a variety of techniques (See Plate 15). The purposes of this chapter are to review our results and techniques for endoscopic hemostasis and to compare them with reported experiences of others.

Our methods and results

Severe Hematochezia – Diagnosis and Treatment

For patients with progressive, severe hematochezia, intensive care unit management is recommended. During stabilization, sulfate purge orally or per NG tube after metaclopromide will facilitate cleansing the colon and permit urgent colonoscopy (1). At the bedside, colonoscopy for diagnosis and therapy is feasible. In our series, 80 consecutive inpatients were referred for severe hematochezia because nasogastric aspiration, anoscopy, and sigmoidoscopy were non-diagnostic. Prior to purge and urgent colonoscopy, panendoscopy was performed in all patients. Table 8.1 lists the final diagnosis prior to treatment.

The majority of these patients (64%) with severe hematochezia required some intervention for hemostasis (surgery, therapeutic endoscopy or angiography). The minority of these patients (36%) were managed medically and did not require intervention for hemostasis.

D.M. Jensen and J.M. Brunetaud (eds), Medical Laser Endoscopy. 99-107.

Table 8.1. Final diagnosis of severe hematochezia. (80 patients.)

Colonic		74%
Angiomata		30%
Diverticulosis		17%
Active bleeding	8%	
Adherent clot	9%	
Polyps or cancer		11%
Focal colitis or ulcers		9%
'Blind' rectal lesions		4%
Bleeding polyp stalk		2%
Endometriosis		1%
UGI lesions		11%
Presumed small bowel lesions		9%
No site found		6%

Table 8.2. Intervention for control of severe hematochezia. (51 patients or 64% of total.)

Therapeutic endoscopy		31 (39%)
Endoscopic coagulation		24 (30%)
BICAP	14	
Argon laser	6	
Heater probe	4	
Endoscopic polypectomy		5 (6%)
Hemorrhoid sclerosis		2 (3%)
Surgery		19 (24%)
Therapeutic angiography		1 (1%)

Table 8.2 details the interventions for control of the bleeding in these patients. In general, whenever surgery was necessary, a limited resection was possible because the bleeding lesion had already been diagnosed by urgent colonoscopy.

During emergent colonoscopy, both effective diagnosis (74% of the cases had colonic lesions) and treatment (39% had therapeutic endoscopy) were feasible.

Elective treatment – LGI angioma

For most of our patients (about 70%) LGI bleeding is usually self-limited. Colonoscopy and endoscopic coagulation can be performed electively (2) rather than as an emergency. Many patients with self-limited LGI bleeding have non-angiomatous sources of bleeding such as polyps, cancers, colitis, or rectal lesions. These will not be discussed here.

For the first 51 consecutive patients who had severe bleeding (self-limited) and colonic angioma (Plate 16), 21 were female and 30 were male with a mean age of 67.6 years (range 27-92). Refer to Table 8.3 for a tabulation of associated conditions. 76% of the patients had one or more of these conditions.

Table 8.3. Associated conditions in 75% of patients with bleeding colonic angioma.

46%	CHF or severe coronary disease
37%	Valvular heart disease
19.6%	Chronic renal failure
12%	Cirrhosis
12%	Osler-Weber-Rendu Syndrome
8%	Collagen vascular disorder
2%	Prior abdominal radiation

For these patients the mean number of prior GI bleeding was 5.2 (range 1-30) and the mean number of units transfused was 17.6 (range 0-150).

Techniques for Coagulation

Whether for urgent or elective colonoscopy, our standard prep is sulfate purge (3). Thin caliber, large suction channel colonoscopes which permitted throughputting of large probes (about 3.2 mm in diameter) are used. See Fig. 8.1.

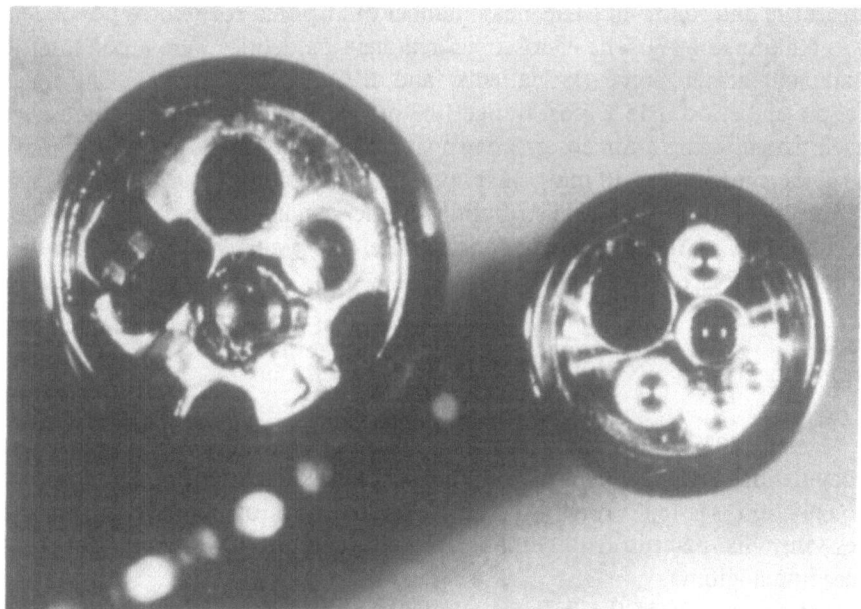

Fig. 8.1. Colonoscopes of Pentax (right) and Olympus (left) have large suction channels (3.7 mm diameter) which permit throughputting of large coagulation probes (3.2 mm diameter).

For hemostasis, our technique is to coagulate with a small probe (diameter 2.4 mm) lesions less than 2-3 mm in diameter and to directly coagulate (whiten) the entire angioma (See Chapter 5). For contact probes, light touch is used and washing to help differentiate blood from a vascular lesion. Settings of 2 or 3 (1 sec. pulses) on a 50 watt BICAP generator are used. For argon laser 6-8 watts at 1-4 cm treatment distance and low flow CO_2 gas is used. For heater probe, the generator setting is 10-15 joules. For YAG laser 40-60 watts and 0.5 sec pulses at 2-4 cm treatment distance and low flow CO_2 gas are recommended.

Large probes are recommended for lesions larger than 3-4 mm in diameter. When feeding vessels are present (See Plate 17), these are coagulated first next to the perimeter of the angioma. Then the angioma itself is coagulated from the most dependent portion. Induced bleeding is common although it can be easily controlled with further coagulation and washing. When active bleeding is present (Plate 15), target irrigation is used and the focal bleeding point is gently tamponaded and then coagulated. A large suction channel (3.7 mm) and the large probes facilitate treatment of the actively bleeding angioma or the large ones. Water irrigation along with coaxial gas is useful with the lasers.

Endoscopic Results

For the 51 patients with severe LGI bleeding and self-limited hematochezia, 338 colonic angioma were coagulated during 70 colonoscopies for initial treatment and follow-up. The mean number of angioma coagulated per patient was 6.6 (range 1-47). The endoscopic treatment modalities were argon laser (8 patients), heater probe (19 patients) and BICAP (24 patients). The mean follow-up period is 15.2 mos. (range 1-63 mos.). Angioma size was graded for each patient using a forceps of known size. 53% were small (less than 5 mm), 27% were medium (5-10 mm), 16% were large (10-20 mm) and 4% were giant (more than 20 mm). The distribution of the coagulated angioma was 39% cecum, 33% right colon or hepatic flexure, 5% transverse colon, 21% left colon, and 2% rectum.

Palliative Results

Overall, 80% of patients had their bleeding controlled with endoscopic coagulation. Fifty-five percent had no further bleeding after one colonoscopic coagulation session. Twenty percent required two or more colonoscopic sessions. Six percent required an UGI coagulation subsequently for UGI bleeding angioma.

Sixteen percent of the patients required surgery for severe rebleeding. Six percent had poor palliative results from surgery or colonoscopic coagulation. The overall palliative results are shown in Table 8.4. Each patient's course after colonoscopic coagulation is compared with the same number of months before treatment.

Table 8.4. Palliative results – coagulation of colonic angioma. (51 patients – mean F/U 15.2 months.)

	Before	After	P value
Mean Hct	26.7	35.7	<0.05
Mean bleeding episodes	5.2	1.0	<0.05

Factors associated with severe rebleeding during the follow-up period included incomplete initial colonoscopy (usually because of poor prep), failure of the patient to return for follow-up after stool hemoccults became positive, multiple or large angioma on initial colonoscopy, severe heart or renal failure, and an abnormal bleeding time. These factors were prognosticators independent of the kind of coagulation modality used.

Complications

There were no complications of urgent purge. However, some patients on dialysis for chronic renal failure retained significant fluid and were therefore dialyzed just after purge to avoid severe fluid overload.

Post-coagulation syndrome was diagnosed in 1 patient after heater probe coagulation and 1 after BICAP coagulation in the right colon. Both were treated medically. Both had multiple, right colonic, large angiomata all treated during a single treatment session.

Colonic ulcerations after treatment were common. Severe delayed bleeding (3-7 days after coagulation) was seen in two patients with abnormal bleeding times (1 each with BICAP and heater probe). Both patients required surgery for hemostasis. Post-coagulation syndrome, delayed bleeding or any other complication were not seen in any patient treated with argon laser coagulation.

Results of others – angioma

Rogers treated 51 cases of GI angioma with hot biopsy forceps, a type of monopolar electrocoagulation (4). Forty-four angioma were treated in the colon without complications. One lesion on the ileocecal valve could not be reached endoscopically and the patient underwent surgery. Two patients out of five followed for more than five years had recurrent hemorrhage due to angioma. These were successfully treated with repeat endoscopic electrocoagulation.

Bowers and Dixon used argon laser to treat 13 patients with lower GI bleeding from angioma (5). They coagulated 46 colonic angioma with 3-4.5 watt output and 1 to 5 second pulses. No complications occurred. Recurrent episodes of bleeding and transfusion were significantly diminished for at least

6 months after treatment.

Rutgeerts et al. coagulated 224 colonic angioma in 33 patients with neodymium YAG laser (5). The majority of the lesions were smaller than 1 cm in diameter and very few were larger than 2 cm. They applied 2-12 pulses of 0.5-1.0 second duration with a power output of 70 to 85 watts. Mild but easily controllable bleeding was induced with treatment in approximately 30% of the cases. Rebleeding and transfusions were significantly diminished post treatment. They reported a perforation rate for colon angiomata patients of 6%. They cautioned against applying more than 200 joules of YAG laser energy in the same area or retreatment of the coagulated area during the same colonoscopy.

Johnston reported three cases of delayed massive hemorrhage 7-16 days post YAG laser treatment of GI angioma (7). Surgical pathology revealed bleeding from induced ulceration at the treatment sites. He treated 440 angioma in 22 patients with YAG laser endoscopically. This represents a 13.6% rate of serious complications after YAG laser treatment of angioma. Johnston cautioned that the risk of complications such as delayed bleeding should be weighed against the potential benefit of YAG laser treatment of GI angioma.

Groisser treated 37 patients who had bleeding colonic angioma with YAG laser (8). Thirty-two (86%) had good results with decreased hospitalization and transfusion requirement. Five had rebleeding requiring other intervention. One was bleeding from an induced colonic ulcer and required surgery. Four others had suspected small bowel lesions. Five patients (13.5%) had serious complications after YAG laser treatment but did not require surgery. One had delayed bleeding from an induced colonic ulcer and required surgery.

Radiation proctitis and telangiectasia

There are a few cases of bleeding radiation proctitis and telangiectasia that have been treated with endoscopic coagulation. The technique by most endoscopists is to coagulate the focal, bleeding telangiectasia rather than the entire friable mucosa. Several treatment sessions are often required. Scarring or re-epithelialization with more normal tissue tends to occur over time. Caution is advised in circumferential treatment with YAG laser or monopolar electrocoagulation because strictures may result.

Brunetaud has treated five patients for bleeding radiation proctitis with endoscopic argon laser (9). Treatment parameters included 4-5 watts output, 1-4 cm treatment distance and coagulation of the bleeding telangiectasia. Good palliation has been achieved with a marked reduction in rectal bleeding and elimination of transfusions.

We have treated 4 patients with bleeding radiation induced rectal telangiectasia and proctitis. In two patients, each heater probe and BICAP have been used to coagulate the bleeding rectal telangiectasia (See Plate 18). Good palliation has been achieved without complications. A mean of 4 treatments was required for initial control of bleeding. New telangiectasia developed over time but follow-up every 4-6 months has prevented severe recurrent bleeding.

Dwyer (10) advocates a 'Z' pattern of treatment with YAG laser for rectal mucosa affected by radiation proctitis or telangiectasia. He claims that palliation is good and scarring results. Davis treated four patients with YAG laser radiation proctitis (11). While the 'Z' pattern of coagulation was used in two patients, two others had coagulation of the telangiectasia only. Both techniques provided good palliation without complications.

Discussion

Even though colonoscopy is still not recognized everywhere as a diagnostic and therapeutic tool in the management of severe ongoing colonic bleeding, our study of emergent colonoscopy in such patients demonstrates clearly that it is the diagnostic modality of choice as well as an effective therapeutic tool. Colonoscopy after a sulfate purge was used successfully and safely in 80 patients with severe hematochezia, the majority of whom had other serious medical problems. Colonoscopy could be performed at the bedside in an ICU setting in contrast to angiography or scanning.

A large percentage of the patients who present with severe lower GI hemorrhage are bleeding from colonic angioma which can be successfully coagulated endoscopically with YAG or argon laser, monopolar electro-coagulation, BICAP, or heater probe. Non-randomized reports by experts have reported complication rates of 0-5% for argon laser, 10-15% with YAG laser, 0-10% for monopolar, 0-4% for BICAP and heater probe.

No comparative studies among these various modes of coagulation exist in humans. We reported our experience in systematic comparative studies in the canine colon (12-14). For standard colonic bleeding ulcers as well as normal (non-ulcerated) mucosa to stimulate angioma coagulation, we compared the efficacy and tissue damage of different coagulation modalities. Refer to Chapter 5. The different methods included: YAG laser, argon laser, BICAP, heater probe, hydrothermal probe (HTP), monopolar electrocoagulation (MPEC), and hot biopsy forceps (HBF). In this model, argon laser, BICAP, and heater probe had 100% efficacy in controlling bleeding from heparinized standard ulcers whereas MPEC and HTP were effective 80% of the time. The least effective (less than 70%) were YAG and HBF.

More severe tissue damage resulted from YAG, HBF, HTP, MPEC treatment compared to argon laser, BICAP, or heater probe. This pattern of tissue injury was similar in both standard ulcers and normal mucosa treated. The normal mucosa was used to stimulate angioma. Delayed colonic perforation occurred 3-7 days after treatment in 13-27% of normal mucosal lesions treated with MPEC or YAG laser. No delayed perforations after mucosa treatment were found for argon laser, BICAP, heater probe, hot biopsy forceps or hydrothermal probe.

Based upon these randomized studies in the canine colon, one would predict a higher frequency of complications such as delayed bleeding, post-coagulation syndrome, and perforation with YAG laser and MPEC compared to argon laser, heater probe or BICAP.

Clinically, higher complications are being reported with YAG laser than the other modalities. The 13.5% complication rates of Grossier and 13.6% by Johnston after colon coagulation parallel the laboratory results for YAG laser. Efficacy has been otherwise good and 85-90% have good palliation after YAG laser coagulation of angioma.

Argon laser has been used safely and effectively in the colon for angioma coagulation by our group (1, 2, 15), Bowers and Dixon (5), and Waitman (16). No complications have been reported. This laser appears to be at least as effective as YAG and considerably safer. Delayed hemorrhage, perforations or post-coagulation syndrome have not been reported with argon laser treatment in the colon, whereas all have been reported after YAG laser treatment.

In experienced hands such as Rogers (4), hot biopsy forceps have yielded safe and effective results in the colon. However, others have reported post-coagulation syndrome, perforation and delayed bleeding after monopolar electrocoagulation in the colon. One would expect a greater frequency of these complications with MPEC than BPEC, heater probe, or argon laser based upon our animal colon data (12-14).

Although there is less experience with the cheaper, non-laser devices such as the heater probe and BICAP, they appear to be as effective as lasers for colonic angioma treatment or telangiectasia associated with radiation. Less frequent complications than YAG and MPEC for colonic angioma coagulation are being reported. Delayed bleeding or post-coagulation syndrome has occurred in less than 4% of our patients after heater probe or BICAP treatment of colonic angioma. No perforations have been reported.

In view of the laboratory and clinical data presented, we would recommend extreme caution in using YAG or MPEC in the colon and particularly in the cecum for angioma treatment. Whenever coagulation is to be performed in the colon, especially in the cecum, avoidance of distention or firm tamponade are recommended. Distention or too firm tamponade can thin out the bowel wall and increase the coagulation depth with any modality.

So far clinical experience with argon laser, BICAP, or heater probe has been more favorable then YAG or MPEC. The complication rates appear to be lower. Clinical results appear to correlate well with our laboratory experience in the canine colon. It is clear that more randomized and/or comparative clinical data should be obtained in order to find the best treatment methods which will benefit the patients the most with the least risk and cost.

Based upon our results with different techniques for colon angioma coagulation, the patient rather than the endoscopic treatment often dictates outcome (2). Patients with uncorrectable and abnormal bleeding times, severe renal disease, or severe heart failure often have poorer palliation results, higher complications rates, and faster recurrence rates of colonic angioma. The treatment modality does not determine outcome in these patients but rather other factors. These outcome parameters must be considered when one is evaluating and comparing palliation efficacy of different devices for hemostasis of colonic angioma.

References

1. Jensen DM, Machicado GA. Diagnosis and treatment of severe hematochezia – the role of urgent colonoscopy after purge. Gastroenterology 1988;95:1567-1574.
2. Jensen DM, Machicado GA. Bleeding colonic angioma: Endoscopic coagulation and follow-up. Gastroenterology 1985;88:1433.
3. Davis GR, Santa Ana CA, Morawski SG, Fordtran JD. Development of a lavage solution associated with minimal water and electrolyte absorption or secretion. Gastroenterology 1980;78:991-5.
4. Rogers BHG. Endoscopic electrocoagulation of vascular abnormalities of the gastrointestinal tract in 51 patients. Gastrointestinal Endoscopy 1982;28:2:142.
5. Bowers JH, Dixon JA. Argon laser photocoagulation of vascular malformations in the GI tract: Short term results. Gastrointestinal Endoscopy 1982;28:2:126.
6. Rutgeerts P, Van Gompel F, Geboes K, Vantrappen G, Broelkaert L, Coremans G. Long-term results of treatment of vascular malformations of the gastrointestinal tract by YAG laser photocoagulation. Gut 1985;26:586-593.
7. Johnston JH. Complications following endoscopic laser therapy. Gastrointestinal Endoscopy 1982;28:2:135.
8. Groisser VW. YAG laser treatment of colonic angiodysplasia. Washington Laser Symposium. April 18, 1985. Washington DC.
9. Brunetaud JM, Argon laser treatment of radiation proctitis. Third International Training Course in Laser Digestive Endoscopy. Sept. 5, 1985. Lille, France.
10. Dwyer R. YAG laser treatment of lower gastrointestinal bleeding. Washington Laser Symposium. April 18, 1985. Washington DC.
11. Davis RC. YAG laser treatment of radiation gastritis and proctitis. Tulane Medical School laser Symposium. October 19, 1984. New Orleans.
12. Jensen DM, Machicado GA, Tapia JI, Mautner W. Comparison of argon laser photocoagulation and bipolar electrocoagulation for endoscopic hemostasis in the canine colon. Gastroenterology 1982;83:830-5.
13. Jensen DM, Tapia JI, Machicado GA, Beilin DB, Silpa M. Comparison of electrocoagulation and heater probe for hemostasis in the canine colon. Gastrointestinal Endoscopy 1982;28:151-2.
14. Jensen DM, Tapia JI, Machicado GA, Beilin DB. Hydrothermal probe, hot biopsy forceps and YAG laser for hemostasis in the canine colon. Gastrointestinal Endoscopy 1983;29:189.
15. Jensen DM, Machicado GA, Tapia JI et al. Argon laser photocoagulation of bleeding colonic lesions (abstract) 20- 4. Laser Tokyo '81. (Proceedings of the 4th Congress of the International Society for Laser Surgery.)
16. Waitman AM, Grant DZ, Chateau F. Argon laser photocoagulation treatment of patients with acute and chronic bleeding secondary to telangiectasia. Gastrointestinal Endoscopy 1982;28:151-2.

9. TEN YEARS ENDOSCOPIC NEODYMIUM-YAG LASER COAGULATION IN GASTROINTESTINAL HEMORRHAGE

P. KIEFHABER, K. KIEFHABER, F. HUBER AND G. NATH

Introduction

Acute gastrointestinal hemorrhage is still an extremely dangerous complication of gastrointestinal diseases, severe general diseases, polytraumas, as well as a complication of operative and pharmacologic therapy. Modern hemostaseologists who like to highlight the difficulties in stopping acute gastrointestinal bleeding tend to quote the surgeon Ritter von Nussbaum, Munich, who said one hundred years ago: 'There is no better and no more reliable method to arrest bleeding than to close the hole from which the blood is coming out' (28).

When relating this to the present situation, it becomes clear that hemostatic therapy alone, such as substitution of clotting factors or platelets, is not sufficient to control gastrointestinal hemorrhage (41, 42). Pharmacologic agents such as vasopressin, glycylpressin, beta blockers, somatostatin or secretin are also not effective enough in stopping massive variceal or ulcer bleeding with a high degree of reliability (1, 2, 19, 35, 44, 46).

The real danger of treating patients for gastrointestinal bleeding is not adequately highlighted by showing the total mortality rate of about 10% (13, 30, 39) because the mortality rate of patients who need surgical therapy to control bleeding ranges worldwide up to 80% in bleeding varices and up to 65% in bleeding ulcers, including rebleeding episodes (9, 10, 14, 29, 43). Surgical experience and pathophysiological consideration resulted in a resolute approach in diagnosis and therapy: 'He who acts promptly helps twice' (3). That means prompt action helps in two ways. So it is essential to avoid a greater loss of blood volume and to prevent the transformation of hemorrhagic shock into irreversible states. This is especially important in cases of stuttered bleeding sites, because the shock event starts in the first minutes of every severe hemorrhage (24).

An endoscopic method which stops the bleeding immediately in conjunction with endoscopic diagnosis can break the vicious cycle of hemorrhagic shock effectively by reducing or avoiding most of the factors which aggravate the shock event: the prognostic important duration of shock and therefore consumption coagulopathy, the quantity of banked blood needed, and, especially, the amount of emergency operations. Such an endoscopic method must successfully stop all kinds of unselected and massive bleeding sites. The

D.M. Jensen and J.M. Brunetaud (eds), Medical Laser Endoscopy. 109-118.
© 1990, Kluwer Academic Publishers, Dordrecht

method has to be reliable for patients with severe underlying diseases as well as for patients with a high risk factor in emergency operations. Unlike other endoscopic methods (22, 23, 31, 32, 33, 34, 45, 47) for stopping bleeding such as injection or sclerosing, mono or bipolar electrocoagulation with or without water jet and heater probes, the Nd:YAG laser radiation offers the physical and endoscopic advantages of:

1. Application of energy without contact, meaning precision of aim especially in moving targets and in rather inaccessible areas.

2. A sufficient yet controllable depth of tissue coagulation.

3. The sealing of the defect with a glue like protein layer which covers the defect for days if pulses of 80-90W power output and 0.5 second duration of a Nd:YAG laser are used (15, 17, 18).

Techniques

A Neodymium-YAG laser of 100 Watt power output (Medilas, MBB, Munich) in combination with a flexible quartz light guide (Fig. 9.1) (Nath's triconic quartz fiber) (26, 27) inserted in a three channel endoscope (25) (Olympus, Tokyo) has been used for many years. At the endoscope tip the light guide is covered by an exchangeable quartz window, which protects the fiber. This window can be cleaned by the same washing system (water and air) which is used for cleaning the viewing optics. A suction-channel is installed for delivering pulsed coaxial CO_2 gas or water. In spite of its excellent physical qualities, the disadvantage was that the triconic quartz fiber broke too often, hence destroying the endoscope.

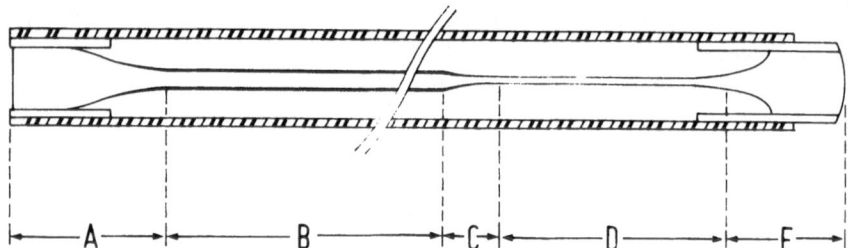

Fig. 9.1. Cross section of the triconical quartz fiber of Dr. Gunther Nath, Munich. A = Beam entrance cone, B = proximal long part of the fiber, C = diameter reducing cone, D = distal flexible short part of the fiber, E = beam exit cone.

A second type, a movable quartz silicon fiber (Dr. F. Frank, Dr. W. Rother, MBB. Munich) with a coaxial CO_2 gas for keeping the fiber tip clean is now in use. This gas assisted fiber can be fed into every conventional endoscope. In order to remove the CO_2 gas which lead to a painful distention of stomach and bowel as well as to respiratory problems, a two channel endoscope or an additional tube must be provided (38). On the other hand, and in contrast to the low divergence beam of the triconic fiber (26, 27), the use of the movable quartz silicon fiber is much more difficult; the problems are aiming and maintaining the power density in the cross section of the laser beam (Fig. 9.2). In small cavities, as for example in the duodenal bulb or in the area of esophageal gastric junction, the handling of the movable fiber tip and the bleeding defect can cause vaporization and result in aggravation of the bleeding. Unlike the three-channel endoscope, the aiming beam can only be seen from a distance of 1 cm when the cross section of the beam is larger. So the beam can more easily cover the cross section of the supposed underlying vessel (Fig. 9.3). In order to combine the physical and endoscopic qualities of the triconic quartz fiber and its low divergence angle with the non-fragile qualities of the quartz silicon fiber, we constructed a cylindrical lens of quartz which can be screwed into the endoscope tip in the same way as the first exchangeable quartz window.

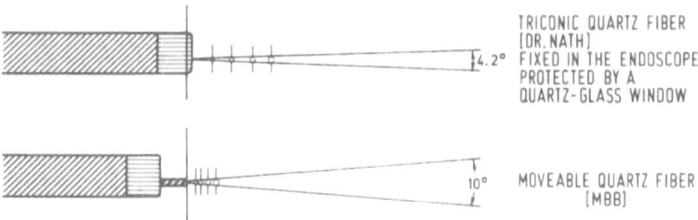

Fig. 9.2. The beam spreads of Nd-YAG laser radiation as emitted from the fiber tips of the two different laser transmission systems: the triconic quartz fiber (Dr. G. Nath, Munich) and the moveable gas assisted fiber (MBB). Spot sizes of the triconic quartz fiber at different distances from the fiber tip to the bleeding source with practicable variations.

So in combination with a newly designed three-channel endoscope (Olympus, Tokyo) an improved instrument can be presented. It has a white tip, a smaller diameter (1.2 cm) and a shorter bending radius of the endoscope tip compared to the TGF-2DL. Like the TGF-2DL Olympus endoscope, only small amounts of CO_2 gas are necessary and these are delivered by the third channel and can be removed by the open suction channel.

Indications

The indications for endoscopic Nd:YAG laser coagulation are as follows:
1. Acute gastrointestinal bleeding according to state Forrest I of esophageal and stomach varices; esophageal, stomach, duodenal and colonic ulcers; carcinomas and submucosal tumors; Mallory-Weiss tears; multiple erosions; angiodysplasias and Osler-Weber-Rendu hemangiomas.
2. In bleeding defects with recent signs of hemorrhage according to state

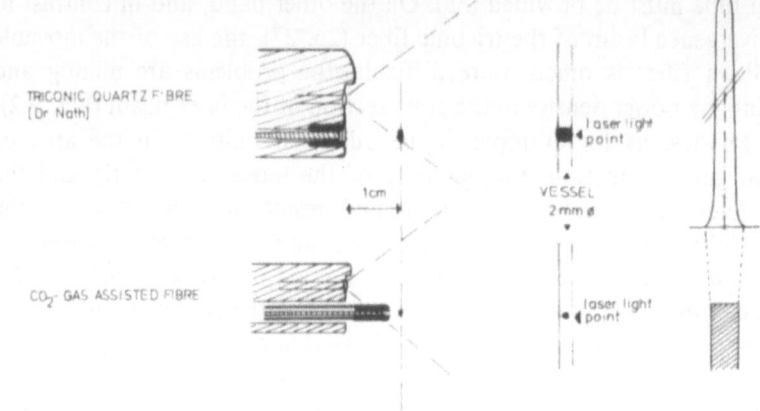

TRICONIC QUARTZ FIBRE
[Dr Nath]

1cm

laser light
point

VESSEL
2mm ⌀

CO₂ GAS ASSISTED FIBRE

laser light
point

Fig. 9.3. The triconic quartz fiber and the CO_2 gas assisted moveable fiber on endoscopic conditions at equal distance of the endoscope tip from the bleeding source, with regard to the coagulation effect in small cavities.

Forrest II, laser coagulation is indicated when the clot is red and blood is present in the stomach or in the duodenal bulb cavity. Coagulation is not indicated in the case of a black colored visible vessel (37).

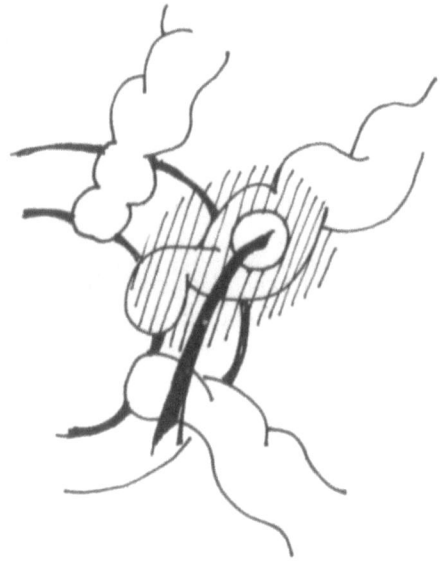

Fig. 9.4. Graphics of a bleeding esophageal varix. At first the hatched area should be irradiated with the Nd-YAG laser to reduce the blood flow of the surrounding vessels. At a second step the bleeding point itself should be coagulated.

In stopping active bleeding, the bleeding source has to be visualized exactly, even when using stomach lavage with large bore tubes or – in the case of overlying coagulated blood or large thrombus – with an endoscopic lavage of the bleeding site. In arterial spurting bleeding sites as well as in spurting variceal bleeding, the laser should be aimed first at the surrounding area in order to thrombose the feeding vessels and to cause edema. During the second step the bleeding point must be occluded (Plates 19-23 in atlas). Previous injection of soluted epineptivine 1:20 000 helps in inducing an endema.

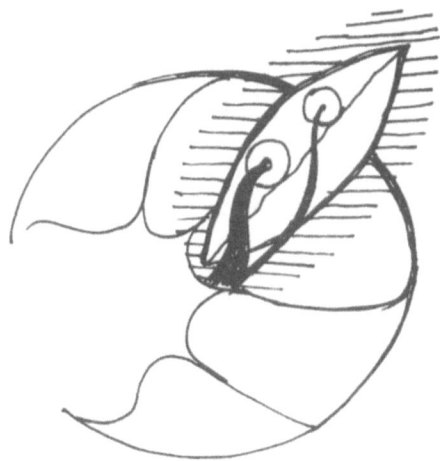

Fig. 9.5. Graphics of a bleeding Mallory-Weiss tear. At first the hatched area should be irradiated in order to occlude the vessels of the submucosa. At a second step the bleeding points themselves should be coagulated.

In the case of esophageal varices with recent signs of hemorrhage (state Forrest II) we perform sclerosing. Complications of sclerosing such as massive bleeding out of the injection channels (Plate 20 in atlas) or out of the so-called sclerosing ulcers, should be occluded by laser irradiation and not with balloon tamponade which has its own complications.

Parallel to the endoscopic procedure, it is essential to monitor and to treat the circulation as follows: continuous measuring of the pulse rate, blood pressure and ECG as well as the substitution of the volume by albumin solution, lyophilized or fresh frozen plasma, and fresh warm blood. With regard to unaltered platelets and non-fragile erythrocytes, fresh warm blood is most effective.

In the case of disturbed clotting factors, prothrombin complex, antithrombin III and factor XIII should be substituted (41, 42). General anesthesia to avoid aspiration is not necessary for all patients; but it is inevitable in cases when a stomach lavage is necessary for visualization of the bleeding site, or for restless alcoholics and patients with shock to have the opportunity of a better oxygen supply. To avoid rebleeding after laser coagulation, acid reduction with cimetidine or ranitidine plus pirenzepin is superior to treatment with a single medication (20).

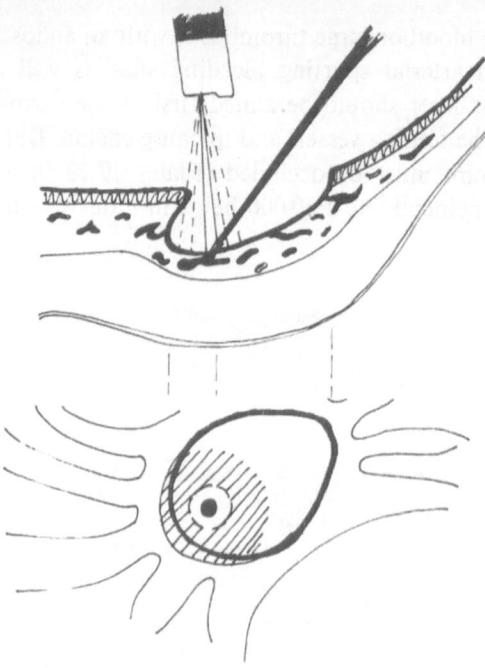

Fig. 9.6. Graphics of an arterial bleeding ulcer. At first the hatched area should be irradiated in order to occlude the vessels of the submucosa. At a second step the bleeding point itself should be coagulated.

Patients

Since 1975, of 2408 cases of emergency endoscopy 1058 (45%) have shown active arterial or venous capillary bleeding episodes in accordance with state Forrest I. This high percentage was due to numerous admissions of pre-endoscoped bleeding patients from over 30 hospitals. In most cases, patients were admitted with their 2nd-5th bleeding episode within days. Fifty-one percent of the patients were older than 60 years. In 505 bleeding episodes manifest shock with a shock index over 1 (Allgöwer) was registered. Three hundred sixty-six times blood replacement already exceeded 1500 ml within 12 hours before admission. In 331 bleeding episodes the hemoglobin had dropped down below 8gm%.

Results

Primary hemostasis was achieved in a total of 996 of 1058 bleeding episodes or 94%. The successfully treated bleeding episodes included 203 varices in esophagus and stomach (Plates 19-21 in atlas), and 125 Mallory-Weiss tears. Five hundred sixty-four ulcers in esophagus, stomach and duodenum (carcinomas included)(Plates 22-23 in atlas), 87 multiple erosions (Osler hemangiomas and angiodysplasias included) and 17 different bleeds in the colon.

Esophageal varices

Primary hemostasis in esophageal varices according to state Forrest I was 92% (203/219) by laser irradiation. Rebleeding was recorded in 48 of 150 cases. The rebleeding rate was reduced to 20% by consequent substitution of unaltered platelets, by fresh warm blood transfusions and infusions of fresh frozen or lyophilized plasma and sometimes clotting factors (prothrombin complex, antithrombin III and factor XIII). The rebleeding rate of 20% is not due to insufficient laser coagulation, because most bleeding sites are new ones, but to antibiotics which were necessary for a number of patients. Disturbed coagulopathy as a result of antibiotics is well known (6). Two perforations occurred. Unlike laser coagulation alone, the use of immediate sclerosing by injection of polidocanol (0.5 or 1%) – after stopping the acute bleeding by Nd:YAG laser coagulation – has reduced the mortality rate from 70% to 40% (24/60) over the last 5 years. In Child's groups A + B, the mortality rate was also reduced from 43% to 3.1% (1/33). The cases were not selected: Child A n = 8, Child B n = 25, Child C n = 27.

Bleeding Ulcers

Bleeding ulcers have been divided into the different types of bleeding ulcers of state Forrest I: acute and chronic ulcers. The cases of acute ulcers were caused by stress, drugs, tubes or vascular arterial malformations (ulcus Dieulafoy), whereas chronic ulcers resulted from peptic ulcer disease. The rate of primary hemostasis was 92% (425/462) in bleeding acute ulcers (state Forrest Ia + b) and 96% (97/101) in bleeding chronic ulcers (state Forrest Ia + b). The rebleeding rate of acute ulcers was reduced from 30.5 to 14% by regulation of coagulation factors. The rebleeding rate of chronic ulcers was 8% (7/86 patients) because in these cases the coagulability of the blood was seldom disturbed.

In 10 cases of bleeding acute ulcers, perforation occurred after laser coagulation, but at the same period there were 18 patients with perforation in acute ulcers without any laser treatment.

The rate of operations after successful laser coagulation of bleeding acute ulcers was reduced from 30% to 15% by a more precise indication for operation. In cases of bleeding acute ulcers the therapy after successful laser coagulation is predominantly conservative except in cases of large and deep-penetrating ulcers. In cases of bleeding chronic ulcers the therapy of choice after successful laser coagulation should be elective operation. However, only

50% of the patients agreed to be operated on for the first 4½ years and just 30% gave their consent over the last 5½ years.

Compared to surgical results the mortality rate in bleeding acute ulcers has been reduced from 58% (76/131) to 24% (31/128) in recent years. In bleeding chronic ulcers the mortality has been reduced from 25% (26/102) in resection and 15% (12/78) in vagotomy to 2.3%. For the last 5½ years no patient in the group of bleeding chronic ulcers has died after laser treatment (0/28) (15, 17, 18).

Conclusions

Endoscopic Nd:YAG laser coagulation of acute gastrointestinal hemorrhage has been tested and proved to be efficient by a university clinic and an associated large community hospital in the countryside. All gastrointestinal bleeding cases were unselected ones. In both hospitals high-risk patients with their 2nd-5th bleeding episode within days, old patients, post-operative patients – even from other hospitals – were admitted. Surgical patients and patients from the intensive care units of medical and surgical hospitals were included. The overall results in the primary hemostasis rates of each kind of bleeding source are remarkable. Similar success rates in primary hemostasis with the Nd:YAG laser and the reduction of the mortality rate have been reported on by R. Dwyer, H. Schönekäs, R. Sander and others (7, 16, 38, 40).

Controlled studies have been performed by I.A. MacLeod, P.R. Salmon. P. Rutgeerts, T. Ihre, and J. Escourrou (8, 11, 21, 36, 37). They have reported on the benefits of laser treatment in cases of group Forrest Ia+b and II when there was enough output power and a coaxial CO_2 gas. In group of Forrest II the benefit of laser treatment has been shown by the study of P.R. Salmon (37).

Nevertheless, controlled studies need the selection of cases. For ethical reasons high risk patients and patients whose operation are refused must not be randomized. Hence, in my view, controlled randomized studies of group Forrest I are not an adequate instrument to prove the efficiency of the method.

References

1. Becker B. Secretin in the treatment of acute gastric hemorrhage. Int Symposium Histamine H₂-Receptor Antagonists. Göttingen, 10-11/11/1977.
2. Bourroughs AK, Jenkins WJ, Sherlock S, Dunk A, Walt RP, Osuafor TOK, Mackie S, Dick R. Controlled trial of propanolol of recurrent variceal hemorrhage in patients with cirrhosis. N Engl J Med 1983;309:1539.
3. Buchborn E. Schock un Kollaps. In Handbuch der inneren Medizin, Springer Verlag, Berlin, Göttingen, Heidelberg, S.962, 1960.
4. Denck H. Zur Frage der zweckmäßigen Behandlung blutender Ösophagusvarizen. Wien klin Wschr 1963;76:274.
5. Denck H. Die endoskopische Behandlung von Oesophagusvaricen. Der Chirurg 1977;48:212.

6. Duda D, Heyes H, Wenske C. Antibiotika-induzierte Hämostase-störungen und Blutungsneigungen. Dtsch med Wschr 1984;109:388.

7. Dwyer RM, The technique of gastrointestinal laser endoscopy In: L. Goldman (ed.): The Biomedical Laser. Technology and Clinical Applications, Springer Verlag, New York, Heidelberg, Berlin 1981, S.255.

8. Escourrou J, Frexinos J, Bommelaer G, Edouard R, Rozental G, Ribet A. Prospective randomized study of YAG photocoagulation in gastrointestinal bleeding. In: K. Atsumi, N. Nimsakul (eds.), Laser-Tokyo '81, The 4th Congress of the International Society for Laser Surgery, Tokyo. 5-30.

9. Feifel G, Heberer G. Die Problematik der akuten oberen gastrointestinalen Blutung. Chirurg 1977;48:204.

10. Häring R. Chirurgische Notfallmaßnahmen bei der massiven Ösophagusvarizenblutung. Dtsch med Wschr 1977;102:289.

11. Ihre T, Johansson C, Seligson U, Törnsgen S. Endoscopic YAG laser treatment in massive upper gastrointestinal bleeding. Scand J Gastroent 1981;16:633.

12. Jessen K, Gilbert GA, Tytgat GNJ, Papp JP. Bipolare Elektrokoagulation bei aktiver oberer gastrointestinaler Blutung. Z Gastroenterologie 1983;21:268.

13. Jones FA. Problems of alimentary tract bleeding. Lancet I 1974;394.

14. Junginger Th. Gastrointestinale Blutung: Akute gastroduodenale Läsionen. Chirgische Therapie. In: J.R. Siewert, A.L. Blum, E.H. Farthmann, P.G. Lankisch (Hrsg.), Notfalltherapie (interdisziplinäre Gastroenterologie), Springer-Verlag, Berlin, Heidelberg, New York 1982;S.279.

15. Kiefhaber P, Nath G, Moritz K. Endoscopical control of massive gastrointestinal hemorrhage by irradiation with a high-power Nd- YAG laser. Progr Surg 1977;15:144.

16. Kiefhaber P, Moritz K, Nath G, Kreitmair A, Gorisch W. Endoscopic high-power Neodymium-YAG laser irradiation of acute gastrointestinal hemorrhage. In: I. Kaplan and P.W. Ascher (eds), Laser Surgery III, Part II. Proceedings of the 3rd International Congress for Laser Surgery, Graz 1979. OT-PAZ, Tel Aviv 1979, p.128.

17. Kiefhaber P, Kiefhaber K, Huber F, Nath G. Endoscopic applications of Neodymium-YAG laser radiation in the gastrointestinal tract. In: S.N. Joffe (ed.), Neodymium- YAG Laser in Medicine and Surgery. Elsevier, New York, Amsterdam, Oxford 1983, p.6.

18. Kiefhaber P, Kiefhaber F, Huber F. Der endoskopisch therapeutische Einsatz des Neodym-YAG Lasers bei der gastrointestinalen Blutung. Verdauungskrankheiten 1984;2:132.

19. Kohaus HM, Kautz G, Holzgreve A. Die unterstützende Therapie der akuten Ösophagusvarizenblutung mit dem Vasopressinderivat: Triglycyl-Lysin-Vasopressin (TGLVP). Intensivmed. 1982;19:30.

20. Londong W. Pharmakotherapie und Prophylaxe der akuten oberen gastrointestinalen Blutung. Z Gastroenterologie 1983;21:282.

21. MacLeod IA, Mills PR, MacKenzie JF, Joffe SN, Russel RI, Carter DC. Neodymium-yttrium-aluminiumgarnet laser photocoagulation for major hemorrhage from peptic ulcers and single vessels: a single- blind controlled study. Brit Med J 1983;286:345.

22. Matek W, Frühmorgen, Demling L. Blutende Magenläsionen endoskopisch gestillt – nur Notmaßnahme oder endgültige Therapie? Notfallmedizin 1982;8:463.

23. Matek W. Elektro-Hydro-Thermo-Sonde zur Therapie gastrointestinaler Blutungen. Z Gastroenterologie 1983;21:273.

24. Mittermayer C, Ostendorf P, Riede UN. Pathologisch-anatomische Untersuchungen bei der respiratorischen Insuffizienz durch Schock. In: Lichtmikroskopische und biochemische Analyse. Intensivmed 1977;14:252.

25. Moritz K. Tierexperimentelle Untersuchungen und Entwicklung eines Endoskops zur Anwendung von Laserstrahlen bei der endoskopischen Blutstillung im Gasrtointestinaltrakt. Inaugural Dissertation, Ludwig-Maximilians Universität München, Med Fak 1978.

26. Nath G, Gorisch W, Kiefhaber P. First laser endoscopy via a fiberoptic transmission system. Endoscopy 1973;5:208.

27. Nath G, Gorisch W, Kreitmair A, Kiefhaber P. Transmission of a powerful argon laser beam

117

through a fiberoptic flexible gastroscope for operative gastroscopy. Endoscopy 1973;5:213.

28. Nussbaum JN von. Über Blutverluste. In: Vom Fels zum Meer. Spemann's Illustrierte Zeitschrift für das Deutsche Haus. Verlag v. W. Spemann, Stuttgart 1 Band, S. 45 (1883/84).

29. Orloff MJ, Halasz NA, Lipman C, Schwabe AD, Thompson CJ, Weidner WA. The complications of cirrhosis of the liver. Ann Intern Med 1967;66:165.

30. Palmer ED. Upper gastrointestinal hemorrhage. Charles C. Thomas, Springfield, Illinois 1970.

31. Papp JP. Endoscopic electrocoagulation of upper GI hemorrhage. JAMA 1976;236:2076.

32. Paquet KJ, Oberhamer K. Sclerotherapy of bleeding varices by means of endoscopy. Endoscopy 1978;16:7.

33. Paquet KJ. Sklerosierung zur Prophylaxe einer Ösophagus-varizenblutung. Internist 1983;24:81.

34. Protell RL, Rubin CE, Auth D et al. The heater probe; a new endoscopic method for stopping massive GI bleeding. Gastroenterology 1978;74:257.

35. Reichlin S. Somatostatin. N Engl J Med 1983;309:1556.

36. Rutgeerts P, Vantrappen G, Geboes K, Broeckaert L. Neodym- YAG laser photocoagulation for hemostasis of gastrointestinal hemorrhage. Z Gastroenterologie 1983;21:263.

37. Salmon PR. Controlled tials of laser therapy in upper alimentary hemorrhage. 15 Jahrestagung der Deutschen Gesellschaft für gastroentorologische Endoscopie 8.-10.9.1983, Munich.

38. Sander R, Pösl, Spuhler A, Hitzler H. Der Neodym-YAG laser: Ein effektives Instrument für die Stillung lebensbedrohlicher Gastrointestinalblutungen. Leber Magen Darm 1981;11:31.

39. Schiller KFR, Truelove SG, Williams DG. Hematemesis and melena, with special reference to factors influencing the outcome. Brit Med J 1970;2:7.

40. Schönekäs H. Gastrointestinale Blutung: Ulcus ventriculi et duodeni. Endoskopische Therapie. In: J.R. Siewert, A.L. Blum, E.H. Farthmann, P.G. Lankisch (Hrsg.), Notfalltherapie (Interdisziplinäre Gastroenterologie), Springer Verlag, Berlin, Heidelberg, New York 1982, S. 205.

41. Schramm W. Multitransfusion – Pathophysiologie und praktische Konsequenzen. Dtsch Med Wschr 1980;105:1105.

42. Schramm W. Hemostaseologische Diagnostik und Therapie der akuten oberen gastrointestinalen Blutung. Z Gastroenterolgie 1983;21:253.

43. Schreiber HW, Kortmann KB, Schumpelick V. Indikationen zur operativen Therapie des peptischen Ulkus. In: W. Creutzfeld, M Classen (Hrsg.), Ergebnisse der Gastroenterologie. Demeter-Verlag, Gräfelfing bei München 1988. S. 147.

44. Shaldon S, Sherlock S. The use of vasopressin (Pitressin) in the control of bleeding from oesophageal varices. Lancet II 1960;222.

45. Soehendra N. Injektionsmethode zur Blutstillung im Gastrointestinaltrakt. Z Gastrenterolgie 1983;21:259.

46. Westaby D. Strategie in der Therapie der akuten Ösophagus-varizenblutung. In: K.J. Paquet, H. Denck, C.E. Zöckler: Die Ösophagusvarizenblutung. TM-Verlag, Bad Oynhausen, 1984. S.47.

47. Yamamoto H, Hajiro K, Matsui H, Tsujimura D, Yamamoto T. Endoscopic bipolar electrocoagulation for stopping gastrointestinal bleeding. Gastroenterol Jpn 1982;17:75.

10. ARGON LASER FOR SEVERE ULCER HEMORRHAGE: HEALTH AND ECONOMIC CONSIDERATIONS

DENNIS M. JENSEN AND GUSTAVO A. MACHICADO

Introduction

Upper gastrointestinal (UGI) bleeding is a common and often serious medical and surgical problem (1, 2). Fortunately, most patients hospitalized for UGI bleeding have spontaneous hemostasis and do not rebleed or require urgent surgery. In spite of improvements in endoscopic diagnosis, and medical-surgical care, the mortality rate has not changed in the last 30 years and remains at 8-10% (1-3). Nevertheless, clinical prognostic factors have been identified such as old age, concomitant medical-surgical illness, shock, multiple transfusions of blood, varices, malignancy, active bleeding at endoscopy and rebleeding in the hospital (1-4). Also, for peptic ulcers that have bled, endoscopic major (active bleeding or non-bleeding visible vessel) and minor stigmata of recent hemorrhage (flat red or black spot, grey slough, oozing from granulation tissue and non-bleeding clots) have been identified and used in some studies to randomize patients admitted for UGI hemorrhage (5-9). In controlled clinical trials, the control groups with minor stigmata have had very low rates of rebleeding such as 15-22% for non-bleeding adherent clots and 5-7% for non-bleeding spots (5-9). No improvement in outcomes of such low risk patients has been documented when they are treated by endoscopic argon or YAG laser in controlled randomized trials (5-10). On the other hand, several different controlled studies either with argon laser (7), YAG laser (8, 9, 11), monopolar electrocoagulation (12), or bipolar electrocoagulation (BICAP – 13) have reported significant reductions in rates of continued bleeding-rebleeding or emergency surgery for patients with major stigmata such as active arterial bleeding (7, 8, 11), bleeding from under an adherent clot (9), or a non-bleeding visible vessel (7, 8).

Only two previous controlled studies have included assessments of cost, one by Papp for non-bleeding visible vessels treated with monopolar electrocoagulation (12) and the other by Laine for active ulcer bleeding treated with BICAP (13). Both reported significant reductions in post-randomization cost of care for patients treated by endoscopic coagulation. Few studies have included an assessment of the patients who met clinical criteria but were excluded from randomization (6-8). None of the controlled studies reported to date have included patients whose severe ulcer bleeding began after admission for another medical or surgical problem. The purposes of the present study

D.M. Jensen and J.M. Brunetaud (eds), Medical Laser Endoscopy. 119-134.
© 1990 Kluwer Academic Publishers, Dordrecht

were to evaluate 1) the efficacy, safety, and economic impact of high power argon laser for endoscopic hemostasis of severe peptic ulcer bleeding in a controlled randomized, double-blind unicenter study, and 2) the reasons for exclusion and outcomes of patients with severe UGI bleeding assessed but not randomized in this study.

Methods

Definitions

Severe UGI bleeding was defined as a clinical presentation to an intensive care unit with hematemesis and/or melena; a fall in hematocrit of at least 10; and the requirement for three or more units of red cell transfusions for hemodynamic stabilization of patients. Patients with less severe bleeding were not assessed for this study.

Severe bleeding during hospitalization was clinically manifested by recurrent hematemesis and/or melena as well as hemodynamic instability twelve or more hours after initial bleeding and stabilization. Transfusion of two or more additional units of blood for hemodynamic stabilization was also required.

Active arterial bleeding was spurting bleeding at endoscopy.

A *non-bleeding visible vessel* was a raised 2-4 mm diameter red or brown area resistant to washing and usually in the center of the ulcer crater.

Entry criteria

All patients with severe UGI bleeding were assessed for this study. Both patients admitted to the hospital for severe UGI bleeding and those hospitalized previously for another medical or surgical problem who developed severe UGI bleeding while inpatients were included in this assessment.

All patients and their managing physicians were required to give informed consent for randomization, possible surgery, and transport to the laser endoscopy unit before entry into this study. Patients with severe bleeding and non-bleeding visible vessels at an initial endoscopy had to have severe rebleeding in the hospital prior to randomization in this study. All ulcer patients without spurting bleeding or those with non-bleeding visible vessels which did not rebleed were excluded from this study. The Human Subjects Research Committee at the West Los Angeles Veterans Administration Medical Center approved this study prior to initiation of it.

Endoscopic Equipment and Laser

A high power argon laser (Cooper Lasersonics Model 770, Mountainview,

CA) was used with 8-10 watts output from a 400 micrometer quartz lightguide with an 8-10° full angle of divergence. A synchronous endoscopic filter underfoot switch control protected the endoscopist's eyes during treatment. Coaxial CO_2 gas backpressure at a distance of 1.5 cm was calibrated before treatment to be 8 cm of water, as previously described (14, 15).

All patients had endoscopy with a therapeutic, two channel panendoscope (American ACMI AG2T, Stamford, CT or Olympus GIF2T, Lake Success, NY). These instruments had large (3.7 mm diameter) and standard sized (2.8 mm) suction channels. This facilitated simultaneous treatment and suctioning of blood, particularly with active bleeding. See Fig. 10.1 and also Fig. 6.2.

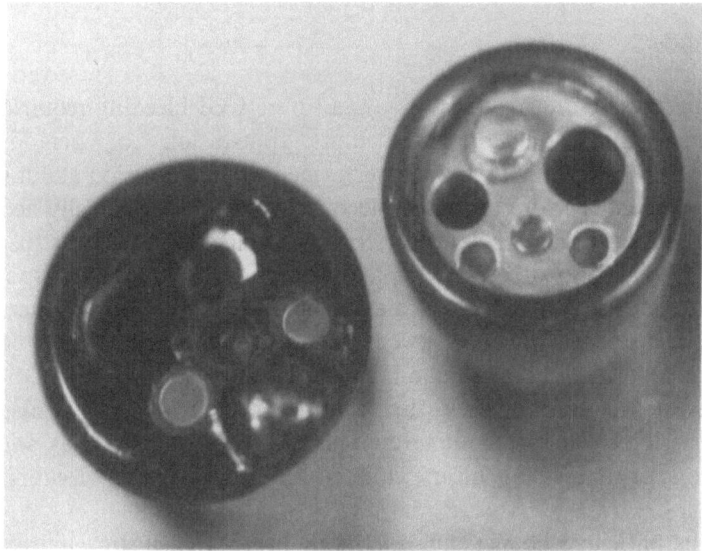

Fig. 10.1. Two channel endoscopes through which argon laser catheter could be placed down one channel and simultaneous suctioning of blood removed by the second channel.

Endoscopic Laser Technique

For patients randomized to laser treatment, vigorous water irrigation, change of position and/or a polyp grasper were used to remove clots and to localize the precise bleeding point immediately before laser treatment. Excess blood was suctioned. With the catheter tip 1-2 cm away, coaxial CO_2 gas was directed at the bleeding point to clear the area of blood. The laser was then fired in one second pulses at the bleeding point until hemostasis was achieved. If hemostasis of active bleeders could not be achieved with this technique, the ulcer base was washed, suctioned clear and the laser beam was circumferentially directed within 1-2 mm of the bleeding point. The goal was control of active bleeding. For ulcers with non-bleeding visible vessels, our technique was to treat circumferentially, 2-3 mm from the base of the non-bleeding visible vessel and finally to treat directly on top of it. The endoscopic endpoint was coagulation of the visible vessel and ulcer base 2-3 mm around the visible vessel.

Patients randomized to medical-surgical management had the aiming light shone on the ulcer from a distance of 5 cm or more, once active bleeding or a non-bleeding visible vessel was identified. Vigorous water irrigation of the bleeding ulcer or the polyp grasper were not used in these patients to remove clots and to localize the precise bleeding point before completion of the endoscopy. Laser and medical-surgical patients were observed via endoscopy for five minutes after randomization for continued bleeding or rebleeding.

Patient Management

All patients assessed for this study had severe UGI bleeding requiring ICU management and three or more units transfusion for hemodynamic stabilization. Urgent endoscopy was performed when a decision about surgery or other intervention for control of bleeding was deemed clinically necessary. Whenever patients met clinical entry criteria, a bleeding ulcer was suspected, and they gave informed consent for randomization, they were transported to the laser endoscopy unit for a diagnostic endoscopy with a therapeutic instrument. If endoscopic criteria were met and the laser aiming light could be aimed at the bleeding point or non-bleeding visible vessel, randomization was performed at the time of their first endoscopy. Patients with non-spurting ulcers or visible vessels without severe rebleeding were excluded as were non-ulcer lesions or inaccessible ulcers with active bleeding or non-bleeding visible vessels.

For other patients who met clinical criteria, urgent diagnostic endoscopy was performed in the ICU if 1) a diagnosis other than bleeding ulcer, such as varices, was suspected from the history, clinical and laboratory presentation, 2) the managing physicians-surgeons felt the patient was too sick and refused to give informed consent for the patient to be moved from the ICU to the laser endoscopy unit for randomization, 3) the patient refused randomization, or 4) the laser was not working. Refer to the Results section and Table 10.2.

All patients transferred to the laser unit for endoscopy and randomization had continuous monitoring, nursing care and transfusion as necessary. After the endoscopy for randomization, a nasogastric (NG) tube was placed for monitoring of further bleeding. Patients were returned to the ICU for further care. A written endoscopy report included 1) the diagnosis and nature of the bleeding (such as active bleeding or non-bleeding visible vessel), 2) whether the patient was randomized on the study, and 3) whether there was active bleeding at the end of the endoscopy. The randomization group (treatment vs. medical-surgical) was not revealed to the managing physician-surgeon team, the patient, or their family.

After endoscopy and randomization, all patients received cimetidine intravenously (300 mg every 6 hours) and antacids every 2-3 hours via a nasogastric tube. All patients were observed in an ICU for at least 24 hours. After transfer out of the ICU, they were allowed to eat and were placed on oral medications.

If any study patient had continued bleeding or had severe rebleeding after randomization and the managing physicians and surgeons determined that intervention for hemostasis was required, the treatment code was broken. After consultation with the therapeutic endoscopist, the managing physician-surgeon team could request repeat therapeutic endoscopy for laser treated patients or emergency ulcer surgery. Patients randomized to medical-surgical treatment who had continued bleeding or severe rebleeding could not be treated with laser and emergency ulcer surgery was recommended.

Cost Assessment for Study Patients

Although there were no bills available for our patients hospitalized at the West Los Angeles Veterans Administration Medical Center, we estimated post-randomization costs for each patient retrospectively. This was done by using the charges listed in Table 10.1. These would have been billed to similar patients at UCLA Medical Center for the same procedures, transfusions, surgeries, or hospitalization. No attempt was made to calculate other direct costs such as laboratory tests, pharmacy costs, or pathology fees. Also, we did not estimate indirect costs related to complications, surgery, or death (16). For each study patient, actual tallies were made of the post-randomization costs of care up until discharge or for 30 days (whichever came sooner), based upon Table 10.1 estimates. The mean and standard errors were then calculated.

Table 10.1. Estimated patient care costs in argon laser controlled study.

Emergency panendoscopy	$ 400
Emergency therapeutic laser endoscopy	$ 800
Emergency ulcer surgery	$ 4000
Blood transfusion/unit RBC	$ 125
ICU bed/24 hours	$ 800
Semi-private room/day	$ 300

These were the charges used to estimate the post-randomization costs for each study patients.

Randomization, Data Collection and Analysis

Randomization was performed during endoscopy after identification of spurting ulcer bleeding or a non-bleeding visible vessel after a severe rebleed. Ulcers must have been accessible to treatment before randomization. A sealed envelope was opened which designated endoscopic laser or medical-surgical treatment (no laser treatment). Cards had been previously made by a biostatistician using a random numbers table.

All patients assessed for this study had endoscopy. The outcomes of those not randomized were recorded. Ulcer study patients' data were entered onto standard forms. Patients were evaluated until discharge from the hospital or thirty days, whichever came first. Each patient was assigned an outcome score: 1 = uneventful recovery; 2 = minor rebleed with transfusion of three or less units after randomization; 3 = major rebleed with transfusion of three or more units, surgery or repeat laser treatment for hemostasis or major complication; 4 = death from any cause. Comparisons were made of their background variables and post-randomization outcomes using Student's t test, Fischers exact test and Wilcoxin Ranked Sum. A p value of less than 0.05 was considered to be a significant difference.

Results

Assessed Patients

Two hundred patients with severe UGI bleeding were assessed for this study. Table 10.2 lists the final diagnoses of these patients as established by endoscopy, surgery, and autopsy.

Peptic ulcers and varices accounted for the majority of diagnoses with prevalences of 52% and 24% respectively. UGI angiomata and Mallory-Weiss tears accounted for 9% and 7% of the final diagnoses. Gastroduodenal erosions and UGI tumors rarely were the cause of severe hemorrhage in our patients with severe UGI bleeding.

Table 10.2. Final diagnosis for severe UGI bleeding.

Peptic ulcer disease		52%
Duodenal	24	
Gastric	16	
Pyloric	10	
Marginal	2	
Varices		24%
Esophageal	20	
Gastric	4	
UGI angiomata		9%
Mallory-Weiss		7%
Erosions		4%
Gastric	2	
Duodenal	2	
Tumors		2%
Miscellaneous		2%

Final diagnoses were determined by endoscopy, surgery or autopsy in 200 patients with severe UGI bleeding requiring ICU admission and transfusion of 3 or more unit of blood. These are listed as a percent of the total.

124

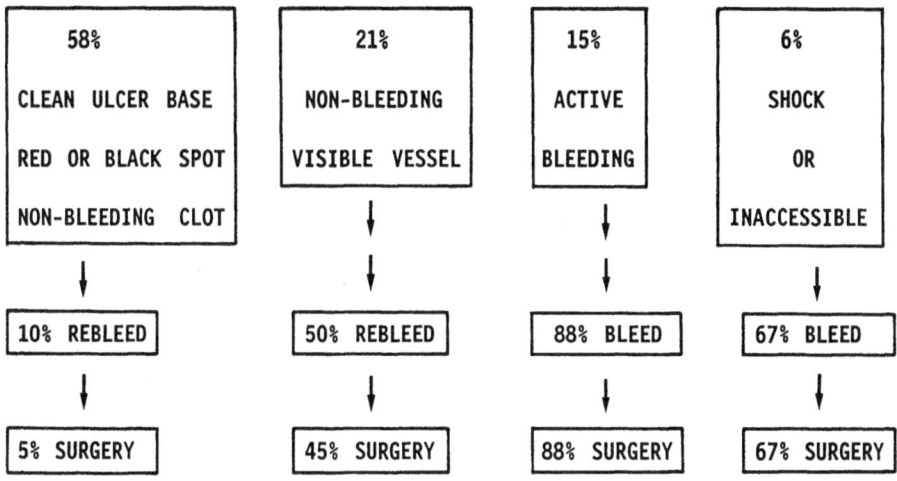

Fig. 10.2. A summary of the outcomes of 104 patients with severe peptic ulcer bleeding assessed for this study. Included are all patients both randomized and excluded with peptic ulcer bleeding. Topmost percentages are of the total number of patients. All other percentages are for that subgroup only.

For the patients with peptic ulcer as the final diagnosis, the outcomes are summarized in Fig. 10.2. The majority of ulcer patients who were assessed and endoscoped were excluded because they did not have spurting bleeding or severe rebleeding from a non-bleeding visible vessel. Fifty-eight percent had a clean ulcer base, a clean ulcer base but oozing from granulation tissue at the base (Plate 24 in the atlas), flat red or black spot or non- bleeding adherent clot. Only 10% of these rebled during hospitalization and 5% required surgery. In all only 6% of ulcer patients were excluded because of severe shock requiring emergency surgery (2 patients) or inaccessibility to endoscopy of the bleeding ulcer (4 patients) with severe deformity or clot. Two-thirds of these patients continued to bleed and required emergency surgery for hemostasis.

Twenty-one percent of all ulcer patients (22 total) had a non-bleeding visible vessel on initial endoscopy (Plate 25 in atlas). Overall 50% (11 patients) of these had significant rebleeding during hospitalization and therefore qualified for randomization. The reason for exclusion of five of these patients (45% of the total non-bleeding visible vessel patients excluded) are listed in Table 10.3. Emergency surgery was recommended by the managing physicians-surgeons to all these patients but one patient refused. Six of the 11 (55%) visible vessel patients with one episode of rebleeding were randomized in this controlled study.

Fifteen percent of the assessed ulcer patients (16 total) had active arterial bleeding at initial endoscopy (Plate 26 in atlas). These included only patients with active bleeding from the ulcer crater and not the granulation tissue on the

Table 10.3. Reasons for exclusion of patients with active bleeding or rebleeding from non-bleeding visible vessel.

	Non-bleeding visible vessel	*Active bleeding*
Patient refuses randomization	1	2
MD considers patient too sick to move to laser unit	3	3
Laser not operating	1	1
	5	6

The reasons that 5 patients with severe rebleeding from non-bleeding visible vessel or 6 patients with spurting arterial bleeding were excluded from randomization.

side. The latter were included in the first category of exclusions. Six of the active bleeding ulcer patients were excluded from the study. Refer to Table 10.3 for the reasons. Emergency surgery was recommended to these patients by the managing physicians-surgeons and was performed in all except one patient who refused surgery.

For the other excluded ulcer patients, the management depended upon the diagnosis and whether active bleeding was documented. The majority of ulcer patients did not have active bleeding or severe rebleeding and were treated medically. They were referred for surgery only for severe rebleeding, non-healing ulcers, or when malignancy was documented or suspected by endoscopic biopsies. Refer to Fig. 10.2.

Table 10.4 summarizes the rates of continued bleeding or rebleeding of all assessed patients by final diagnosis. All patients with severe rebleeding from focal bleeding sources were considered for therapeutic endoscopy. Varices rather than peptic ulcers most commonly accounted for recurrent bleeding (46% of cases), transfer back to an ICU, and intervention for hemostasis. For all patients assessed, surgery for hemostasis was performed in 27% and their overall mortality was 16%.

All patients with esophageal varices were evaluated for randomization in an ongoing controlled trial of sclerotherapy (17). All patients with UGI angiomata (18) and two patients with Mallory-Weiss tears which continued to bleed were treated successfully with argon laser. Patients with bleeding gastric varices were managed with vasopressin and tamponade tubes. If this management failed, shunt surgery was recommended. Patients with erosions were treated medically. Patients with UGI tumors were referred to elective surgery.

Study patients

The background patient characteristics are shown in Table 10.5. For these assessments, all argon laser treated patients were considered together and compared to all medical-surgical patients. There were no statistically significant differences between these subgroups in background characteristics.

Table 10.4. Frequency of continued bleeding or rebleeding.

Gastric or esophageal varices	46%
Peptic ulcer	
Gastric	30%
Duodenal	28%
Mallory-Weiss	14%
UGI angiomata10%	
UGI cancers	8%
Gastric or duodenal erosions	0%

The rates of continued bleeding or severe rebleeding during hospitalization for the 200 patients assessed are given as a percentage of the total for each diagnosis.

Table 10.5. Patient characteristics of argon laser controlled trial for severe ulcer bleeding.

	Argon laser	*Medical-surgical*
Total patients	7	9
*Mean age	60 ± 5	67 ± 4
*Mean units RBC transfused before randomization	8.1 ± 1.9	7.9 ± 1.3
Diagnosis		
DU	5	5
GU	2	4
Bleeding status		
spurting bleeding	5	5
non-bleeding visible vessel with one prior rebleed	2	4

*The means are given ± standard error. None of the differences were significant.

The outcomes of the argon laser treated and medical-surgical groups are presented in Table 10.6. The significant differences between laser treated and medical-surgical groups were in the mean units of RBC transfused after randomization (1.3 vs. 6.8), the need for emergency surgery (0 vs. 56%), and the mean for graded outcome scores. The mean cost of post-randomization care ($6850 vs. $12,342) and the rates of continued bleeding or rebleeding (29% vs. 78%) did not reach statistical significance because of the small sample size. Although there were two major complications and one death from bleeding in the medical-surgical group and none in the laser treated group, these differences were not statistically significant. Two major complications developed and both were related to severe rebleeding with hypotension and aspiration in one patient and hypotension and post-operative renal failure, CVA, and sepsis in another patient who died seven days after ulcer surgery.

In spite of the improvements in outcome for laser treated patients, argon laser was difficult to use via endoscopy for emergency ulcer hemostasis. Careful preparation of the bleeding point or non-bleeding visible vessel was necessary before treatment with removal of all overlying clots, blood and fluid. Near en face treatment position and avoidance of vaporization from too close treatment distance were also necessary for successful treatments. In order to

127

prevent overdistension of the UGI tract, CO_2 gas was only used during actual coagulation and the area was frequently suctioned.

All patients with active spurting bleeding had bleeding controlled with argon laser. One patient with non-bleeding visible vessel had moderate bleeding induced during treatment but this was controlled with further laser treatment. Five minutes after completion of laser treatment, all patients had no active bleeding, whereas all non-laser patients with active bleeding continued to bleed at this observation point. During the follow-up period, two laser treated patients rebled. After the code was broken and after a decision by the physician-surgeon team for emergency retreatment was made, one patient was successfully retreated with argon laser for a rebleed ten days after initial randomization. Although further rebleeding did not occur, he had elective ulcer surgery five days later because of the nature of his ulcer disease (silent, large with one severe rebleed while hospitalized) and severe pulmonary disease (steroid dependent). The other patient's rebleeding stopped with medical management. For the medical-surgical patients (see Table 10.6), 78% (7 of 9) had continued bleeding or rebleeding and 56% (5 of 9) required emergency surgery for hemostasis. The rebleeding of two medical-surgical patients stopped without surgery.

Table 10.6. Results – argon laser controlled trial for severe ulcer bleeding.

	Argon laser	Medical-surgical
Total patients	7	9
Continued bleeding or rebleeding	29%	78%
*Mean units transfused after randomization	1.3 ± 0.9	6.8 ± 2.2**
Emergency surgery for hemostasis	0	56%**
Major complications	0	22%
Deaths	0	11%
*Mean post-randomizationcost of care	$6850 ± 2294	$12,342 ± 3066

* Means ± standard errors are given. ** Significant differences between argon laser and medical-surgical groups.

Discussion

In order to evaluate the possible beneficial effects of argon laser for emergency hemostasis, a subgroup of patients with very severe ulcer hemorrhage was selected. Prior to the introduction of laser therapy in our hospital, emergency surgery would have been recommended for all these patients. The high rates of continued bleeding or rebleeding (78%), emergency surgery for hemostasis (56%), transfusion and mortality in the medical-surgical ('control') group are indicative of the severity of bleeding in the patients randomized. Although this was a small proportion of all the ulcer patients, a significant improvement in post-randomization outcome was documented.

Two other controlled studies of argon laser for severe ulcer hemorrhage have been previously reported. Swain et al. (7) reported a benefit for argon laser over sham treatment when several different subgroups of ulcer patients with non-bleeding stigmata of recent hemorrhage (spots or non- bleeding clots) were combined with active arterial bleeding, Swain et al. reported that the rates of permanent hemostasis for argon laser and sham were 43% vs. 0%; urgent surgery was 57% vs. 50%; and the mortality was 0% vs. 50%. For the subgroup of active bleeders, our results with argon laser were somewhat better. Initial hemostasis was achieved in 100% of our patients, 1 rebled (20%) but did not require surgery and healed with medical management. Swain et al. (7) randomized all patients with non-bleeding visible vessel at initial endoscopy before rebleeding occurred. They had less severe UGI bleeding clinically than our patients who were randomized with non-bleeding visible vessel after one rebleed. Their control patients had a rebleeding rate of 54%. Vallon et al. (6) reported no significant difference in outcome parameters after treatment of active arterial bleeders, non-bleeding visible vessels or other stigmata of recent hemorrhage. For the active arterial bleeders, their rates of emergency hemostasis with argon laser was 67% whereas 47% had continued bleeding and required emergency surgery.

The major differences of our randomized ulcer patients from those of the Swain (7) or Vallon (6) reports are: 1) the timing of diagnostic and therapeutic endoscopy, 2) severity of bleeding clinically, 3) the subgroups of ulcer stigmata at endoscopy which were randomized, and 4) inclusion of patients who developed ulcer bleeding while hospitalized in addition to those admitted with ulcer bleeding. Vallon and Swain performed endoscopy and randomization early, soon after patients presented with UGI bleeding, and before ICU care was initiated. Therefore, all patients were included in their study regardless of the clinical severity of UGI bleeding. They randomized both those whose bleeding was clinically self-limited as well as others whose bleeding may have been more severe. In contrast, all our assessed patients had very severe UGI bleeding clinically. They had endoscopy and randomization later and only after transfusions, ICU management and a clinical decision about the need for intervention had been made. We excluded from assessment all those patients hospitalized for self-limited UGI bleeding who did not require ICU management or transfusion of three or more units of blood. Vallon and Swain randomized patients with major (active bleeding and non-bleeding visible vessel) as well as minor stigmata of recent hemorrhage (red or black spots, oozing bleeding, non-bleeding clot). In contrast, we only included patients with spurting bleeding or those with a non-bleeding visible vessel who had severe rebleeding documented. We excluded all other patients even though they met clinical criteria.

The outcome of all assessed patients with minor stigmata of recent hemorrhage or clean ulcer bases was similar for the three argon laser studies. Ten percent of our patients in these categories had rebleeding and 5% had surgery (Fig. 10.2). These data also confirm the results of control group of

YAG laser patients recently reported by Swain et al. (8). Even in patients with clinically severe ulcer bleeding initially, there was such a low rate of rebleeding that patients with minor stigmata of recent hemorrhage (red or black spot, oozing from the edge, non- bleeding clot or grey slough) on initial endoscopy did not benefit from endoscopic coagulation (6-8). In our opinion, such patients should not be considered for therapeutic endoscopy unless they have severe rebleeding while hospitalized. Endoscopic coagulation with laser or other devices will only increase the cost of their medical care and put them at risk for complications of therapeutic endoscopy such as induction of severe bleeding which has been reported for argon (6, 7) and YAG lasers (8-10).

Vallon and Swain did not include patients who developed severe UGI bleeding while hospitalized for another medical or surgical problem other than UGI bleeding. We assessed such patients who developed severe UGI bleeding while hospitalized for another medical or surgical problem other than UGI bleeding. We assessed such patients who represented 14% of the total and 15% of all ulcer patients. These patients often had painless ulcers, were elderly, had other medical-surgical problems and were considered very poor surgical candidates. Among the randomized ulcer patients, 25% of the total (two laser, two medical-surgical) were in this category. Both 'control' patients required surgery for continued bleeding or rebleeding and one died. Both of the laser treated patients rebled but were managed without emergency surgery. One was successfully treated medically and the other was treated with repeat argon laser coagulation for hemostasis and later elective surgery. In our experience, this clinical subgroup of ulcer patients has the worst prognosis and often accounts for rebleeding and need for surgery or other intervention. Our findings confirm earlier reports (2-4). In our opinion further studies are indicated to evaluate the pathogenesis and treatment of this subgroup of patients.

In our opinion the effectiveness of argon laser for spurting arterial bleeding depends upon the experience of the therapeutic endoscopist and technique (15). In extensive experimental studies, we determined the guidelines and limitations of argon laser for endoscopic hemostasis (14, 15). Following these guidelines in the randomized clinical study required meticulous technique but resulted in excellent acute efficacy for bleeding ulcers in the present study and bleeding Mallory-Weiss tears and angiomata, in the excluded patients. In our experience, argon laser is the most difficult technique of all the thermal methods for emergency hemostasis including argon and YAG laser, heater probe, Bipolar electrocoagulation (BICAP) and monopolar electrocoagulation (19, 20, 24). Accessibility of the bleeding site, preparation of the bleeding site before treatment and actual treatment technique probably account for the different results reported. Swain did not report an initial hemostasis rate for accessible spurting ulcers (7). However, Swain's permanent hemostasis rate was only 43% with argon laser compared to 71% for our patients. By contrast Vallon had an initial hemostasis rate of 67% for bleeding ulcers (6). However, some of Vallon's ulcers randomized to argon laser were not accessible to laser treatment. For accessible ulcers with spurting bleeding, Vallon's initial hemostasis rate was 77%. In an uncontrolled study Brunetaud reported an initial hemostasis efficacy of 72% for ulcers with active bleeding (21).

Our overall rebleeding rate was 29% (2 of 7 patients) in laser treated patients. Both patients were in the subgroup with poor prognosis, deep and painless chronic ulcers which began bleeding while they were inpatients for a non-ulcer problem. The rebleeding rate for the ulcer patients in the Swain study was 33% and in the Vallon study was 44%. Brunetaud reported a rebleeding rate of 50% for selected patients treated with argon laser for active arterial bleeding (21). Brunetaud related rebleeding to the overall medical-surgical prognosis of the patients, the chronicity of the ulcer and slow healing rather than a difference in laser technique (15, 21). Undoubtedly, the size and location of the artery in the ulcer base also influence rates of initial hemostasis and rebleeding as reported by Swain (22) and Johnston (23).

In the present study, most patients who met clinical criteria for severe UGI bleeding did not meet our strict endoscopic criteria for randomization. Most patients were excluded because they had a non-ulcer lesion such as varices, angiomata or Mallory-Weiss tears. These were then assessed for other therapeutic studies to evaluate sclerotherapy (17), laser, or other thermal devices for control of active bleeding or prevention of rebleeding (18, 20, 24, 25). Among the patients with ulcers (52% of total), most were excluded because they had clean ulcer bases or other minor stigmata of recent hemorrhage (red or black spots, oozing from the side of the ulcer, grey slough, or non-BICAP clot). Most (90%) of these did not rebleed and only 5% required ulcer surgery during hospitalization. The most common reason for exclusion of the non-bleeding visible vessel patients was that rebleeding did not occur during hospitalization. The minority of ulcer patients who met clinical criteria were excluded because of uncontrolled shock or inaccessibility of the ulcer to firing the laser. Of all the ulcer patients assessed with severe bleeding, 29% had continued bleeding or rebleeding. Intervention (surgery or laser) was performed in 33%. The overall mortality for all patients (assessed and enrolled in the controlled ulcer study) was 11%. These data are similar to earlier reports (1-4).

Among the ulcer patients who met clinical and endoscopic criteria, the most common reason for exclusion was that the managing physicians-surgeons considered the patients too ill to move to the laser unit for randomization. Two other patients were excluded before transporting them to the laser unit because the laser was not operating. All these patients nevertheless were endoscoped in the ICU and could have been randomized there if portable coagulation devices had been available. A major limitation of any high powered laser is the lack of portability to the bedside. Both argon and YAG lasers have this limitation. In our hospital with several different medical and surgical ICU's, endoscopic treatment with a portable hemostasis device would have offered much more versatility than a laser. Currently, we are evaluating the efficacy and safety of two newer portable devices, heater probe and BICAP for such patients (20, 24, 25). Because of the portability and ability to coagulate tangentially, more high risk ulcer patients with active bleeding or non-bleeding visible vessels are accessible to treatment compared to non-portable lasers.

Recently, Laine reported the efficacy and feasibility of such bedside treatment with BICAP in a controlled study (13). He also reported a significant improvement in outcome of BICAP treated patients versus controls for actively bleeding ulcers in terms of a reduction in the rates of continued bleeding, transfusions, emergency surgery, and cost. In our preliminary studies of hemostasis with BICAP and heater probe for patients with spurting arterial bleeding from ulcers, initial efficacy was 93% and rebleeding rates were 24% and 17% respectively (25). More importantly, these portable devices were relatively easy to use, tamponade of active bleeders was feasible, and vaporization with worsening bleeding did not occur (13, 25-26). More recently, sclerotherapy of actively bleeding ulcers was reported to be inexpensive, portable, and effective in non-randomized studies (27-29). Chung et al. reported a controlled clinical study of epinephrine injection for active ulcer bleeding with significant differences in rates of continued bleeding, need for urgent surgery, and transfusion requirement for epinephrine injected ulcers versus control patients (30). These newer thermal and injection techniques offer major advantages over high power lasers for emergency hemostasis.

The limitations of argon laser for emergency hemostasis are a preferential absorption by blood, its high purchase cost and lack of portability, the need for careful training and meticulous technique, the inability to tamponade or treat tangentially, and the vaporization potential. YAG laser shares all these limitations except that it is absorbed less by overlying blood and it is somewhat easier to use (15). Good results have been reported by Swain et al. (8). For active arterial bleeding, hemostasis without rebleeding was observed in 80% (8 of 10) for YAG laser treated patients and 20% (2 of 10) of controls. When results of all subgroups with major and minor stigmata of recent hemorrhage were combined, the frequency of rebleeding was 10% in the laser group and 40% in the control group. They also reported significant differences in emergency surgery and mortality rates. Several other controlled studies reported reductions in continued bleeding or rebleeding rates for ulcer patients treated with YAG laser (9, 11). However, three other controlled trials with YAG laser reported no significant differences after YAG laser treatment (10, 31, 32).

Perhaps because of the variability of clinical results, the limitations of lasers for emergency ulcer hemostasis, the high cost of argon or YAG GI lasers, and the availability of newer devices which are portable and effective, neither argon nor YAG lasers are likely to gain popularity in clinical practice at most hospitals for emergency GI hemostasis in our opinion. Because of these factors, GI lasers are now being used less often for emergency hemostasis than for elective tumor palliation (15, 24, 33).

Our conclusions are that spurting ulcer bleeding and severe rebleeding from non-bleeding visible vessels were rare in patients assessed for severe UGI bleeding. Most of our patients with clinically severe ulcer bleeding could neither be included nor would benefit from argon laser treatment because they could not be moved to the laser unit for treatment or because they did not have stigmata appropriate for treatment (active arterial bleeding or severe rebleeding from a non-bleeding visible vessel). In spite of these limitations, argon laser treatment of ulcer patients with spurting arterial bleeding or severe rebleeding and non-bleeding visible vessels significantly improved the outcome compared to routine medical-surgical treatment. The introduction of cheaper, portable endoscopic hemostasis methods such as heater probe, BICAP or injection offer even more promise. A greater health and economic impact might be predicted if these methods prove to be at least as effective and safe as argon laser in the present study and ulcer patients at high risk for continued bleeding or rebleeding are selected for treatment. Specifically those patients would have clinically severe UGI bleeding and on endoscopy have major stigmata of hemorrhage. Randomized controlled clinical studies will be necessary to evaluate the health and economic impacts of these newer techniques.

References

1. Silverstein FE, Gilbert DA, Tedesco FJ et al. The national ASGE survey on upper gastrointestinal bleeding. Gastrointest Endoscopy 1981;27:73-102.
2. Avery Jones F. Haematemesis and melaena with special reference to causation and the factors influencing mortality from bleeding peptic ulcer. Gastroenterology 1956;30:166- 90.
3. Schiller KRF, Truelove SC, Gwyn Williams D. Haematemesis and melena with special reference to factors influencing the outcome. Br Med J 1970;2:7-14.
4. Allen R, Dykes P. A study of the factors influencing mortality rates from gastrointestinal haemorrhage. Quart J Med 1976;45:533- 50.
5. Storey DW, Bown SG, Swain CP et al. Endoscopic prediction of recurrent bleeding in peptic ulcers. N Engl J Med 1976;45:533-50.
6. Vallon AG, cotton PB, Laurence BH et al. Randomized trial of endoscopic argon laser photocoagulation in bleeding peptic ulcers. Gut 1981;22:228-33.
7. Swain CP, Bown SG, Storey DW et al. Controlled trial of argon laser photocoagulation in bleeding peptic ulcers. Lancet 1981;ii:1313-16.
8. Swain CP, Kirkhain JS, Salmon PR et al. Controlled trial of Nd-YAG laser photocoagulation in bleeding peptic ulcers. Lancet 1986;i:1113-7.
9. Rutgeerts P, Vantrappen G, Broeckaert L et al. Controlled trial of YAG laser treatment of upper digestive hemorrhage. Gastroenterology 1982;83:410-16.
10. Krejs GJ, Little KH, Westergaard et al. Laser photocoagulation for treatment of acute peptic ulcer bleeding. A randomized controlled clinical trial. N Engl J Med 1987;316:1618- 1622.
11. McLeod IA, Mills PR, MacKenzie JF et al. Neodymium yttrium aluminum garnet laser photocoagulation for major haemorrhage from peptic ulcers and single vessels: a single blind controlled study. Br Med J 1983;286:345-48.
12. Papp J. Electrocoagulation: Endoscopic control of gastrointestinal hemorrhage. In: Ed J Papp; Boca Raton, Florida: CRC Press. 1983;31-42.
13. Laine L. Multipolar electrocoagulation in the treatment of active upper gastrointestinal tract hemorrhage: A prospective controlled trial. N Engl J Med 1987;316:1613- 17.
14. Johnston JH, Jensen DM, Mautner W, Elashoff J. Argon laser treatment of bleeding canine gastric ulcers: Limitations and guidelines for endoscopic use. Gastroenterology 1980;80:708-16.
15. Brunetaud JM, Jensen DM. Current status of argon laser hemostasis of bleeding ulcers. Endoscopy 1986;18:Suppl 2:40- 45.

16. Jensen DM. Economic and health aspects of peptic ulcer disease and H2-receptor antagonists. Amer J Med 1986;81(Supp 4B),42-48.

17. Jensen DM, Silpa M, Reedy T et al. Controlled trial of sclerotherapy for bleeding esophageal varices in alcoholic cirrhosis. (Abstract) Gastroenterology 1986;90:Part 2:1476.

18. Jensen D, Bown S. Gastrointestinal angiomata: diagnosis and treatment with laser therapy and other endoscopic modalities. In: Fleischer D, Jensen D, Bright-Asare P, Eds. Therapeutic Laser Endoscopy in Gastrointestinal Disease. Boston: Martinus Nijhoff, 1983:151-60.

19. Johnston JH, Jensen DM, Mautner W. Comparison of laser photocoagulation and electro-coagulation in endoscopic treatment of bleeding canine gastric ulcers. Gastroenterology 1982;82:904- 10.

20. Jensen DM. Endoscopic control of gastrointestinal bleeding. In: Development in Digestive Diseases. Lea and Febiger Publishers. 1-27, 1980.

21. Brunetaud JM et al. Photocoagulation laser des hemorragies digestives graves du tractus digestif superieur. Acta Gastro-ent Belg 1982;45:47-54.

22. Swain CP, Storey DW, Bown SG et al. The nature of the bleeding vessel in recurrently bleeding gastric ulcers. Gastroenterology 1986;90:595-608.

23. Johnston JH. The sentinel clot and invisible vessel: Pathologic anatomy of bleeding peptic ulcer. Gastrointest Endosc 1984;30:313-14.

24. Kovacs TOK, Jensen DM. Endoscopic control of gastroduodenal hemorrhage. In: Annual REview of Medicine. Creger WP. Ed. 1987;38:267-77.

25. Jensen DM, Machicado GA, Silpa M et al. BICAP vs. heater probe for hemostasis of severe ulcer bleeding (Abstract). Gastrointest Endosc 1986;32:143.

26. Johnston JH, Jensen DM, Auth D. Experimental comparison of endoscopic neodymium-yttrium-aluminum-garnet laser, electrosurgery and heater probe for coagulation of canine gut arteries: Importance of compression and avoidance of erosion. Gastroenterology 1987;92:1101-8

27. Asaki S, Nishimura T, Satoh A et al. Endoscopic control of gastrointestinal hemorrhage by local injection of absolute alcohol: a clinical study. Tohoku J Exp Med 1983;141:373- 83.

28. Wordehoff D, Gros H, Stenzel M. Injection of non-variceal bleeding lesions of the gastrointestinal tract. Endoscopy 1985;17:129-32.

29. Soehendra N, Grimm H, Stenzel M. Injection of non-variceal bleeding lesions of the gastrointestinal tract. Endoscopy 1985;17:129-32.

30. Chung SCS, Leung JWC, Steele RJC et al. Epinephrine injection for actively bleeding ulcers: A randomized controlled study (Abstract). Gastrointestinal Endosc 1987;33,No2:146.

31. Escourrou J, Frexinos J, Bommelaer G et al. Prospective randomized study of YAG laser photocoagulation in gastrointestinal bleeding. Proceedings of Laser Tokyo 1981. Ed K Atsumi and N Nimsakul 1981;5-30.

32. Ihre T, Johansson C, Seligson V et al. Endoscopic YAG laser treatment in massive upper gastrointestinal bleeding. Report of a controlled randomized study. Scand J Gastroenterol 1981;16:633-40.

33. Jensen DM. Lasers in the GI cancer war and on other fronts. Gastroenterology 1984;87:974-76.

ATLAS OF COLOR PLATES

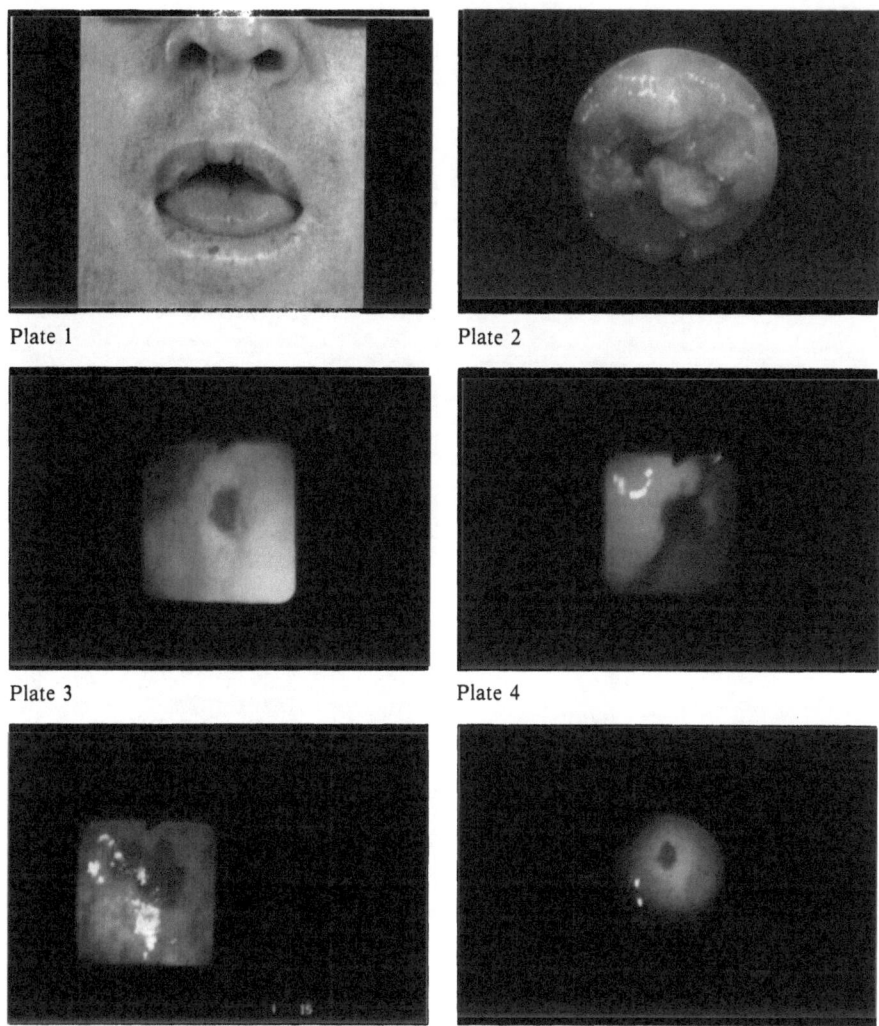

Plate 1

Plate 2

Plate 3

Plate 4

Plate 5

Plate 6

1. (Chapter 6) Telangiectasia of the lips and tongue in Osler-Weber-Rendu Syndrome.
2. (Chapter 6) Telangiectasia of the fingers in Osler-Weber-Rendu Syndrome.
3. (Chapter 6) Gastric telangiectasia in Osler-Weber-Rendu Syndrome.
4. (Chapter 6) Umbilicated gastric angioma.
5. (Chapter 6) Flat gastric angioma on atrophic gastric mucosa.
6. (Chapter 6) Flat gastric angioma with pale halo of mucosa.

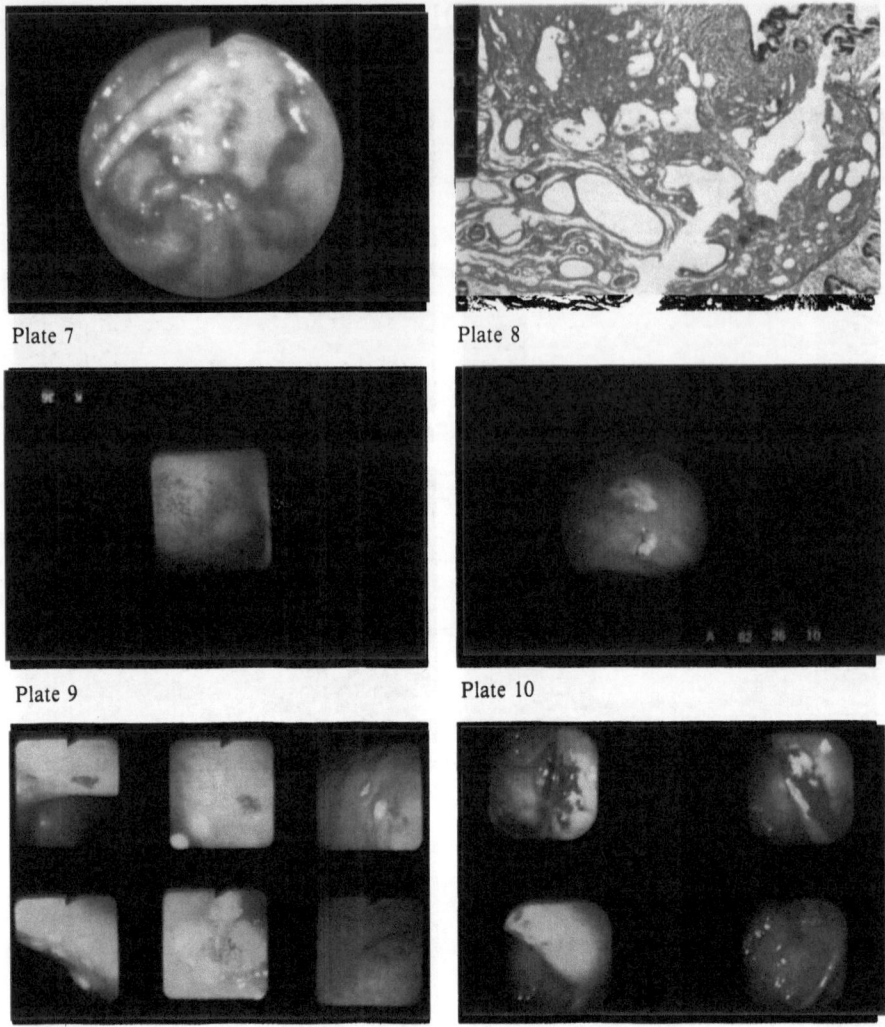

Plate 7

Plate 8

Plate 9

Plate 10

Plate 11

Plate 12

7. (Chapter 6) Watermelon stomach.
8. (Chapter 6) Dilated mucosal and submucosal vessels on endoscopic biopsy of gastric angioma.
9. (Chapter 6) Mucosal or submucosal hemorrhage must be distinguished from angiomata before initiation of treatment.
10. (Chapter 6) Gastric angioma after endoscopic coagulation.
11. (Chapter 7) Gastric Angioma before (left upper), during (middle upper) and after endoscopic coagulation with argon laser.
12. (Chapter 7) Cecal angioma, before (left upper), during (right upper) and 1 month after (left lower) endoscopic coagulation with argon laser via colonoscopy.

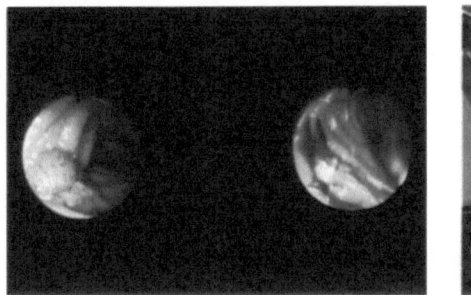

Plate 13

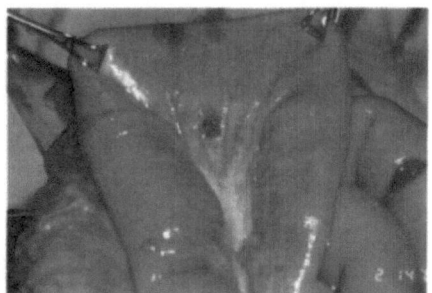

Plate 14

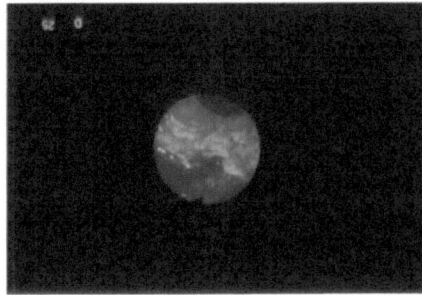

Plate 15

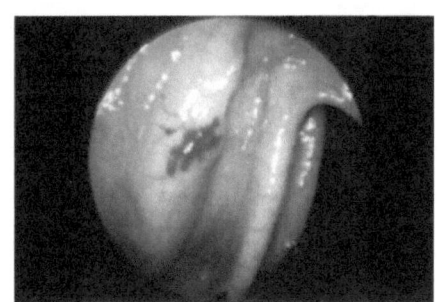

Plate 16

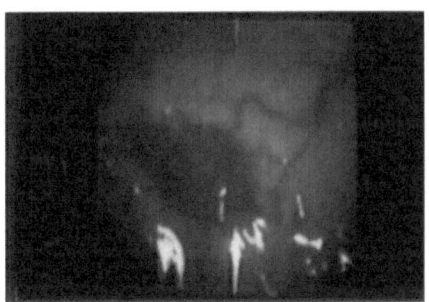

Plate 17

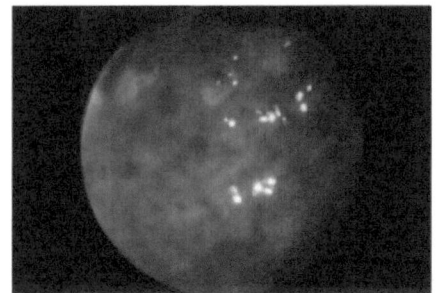

Plate 18

13. (Chapter 7) Duodenal blue rubber bleb nevis lesions before (left) and after endoscopic laser coagulation (right).
14. (Chapter 7) Blue rubber bleb nevis lesions at surgery
15. (Chapter 8) Actively bleeding cecal angioma.
16. (Chapter 8) Non-bleeding colon angioma.
17. (Chapter 8) Giant colon angioma with prominent submucosal feeding vessels.
18. (Chapter 8) Bleeding radiation induced rectal telangiectasias.

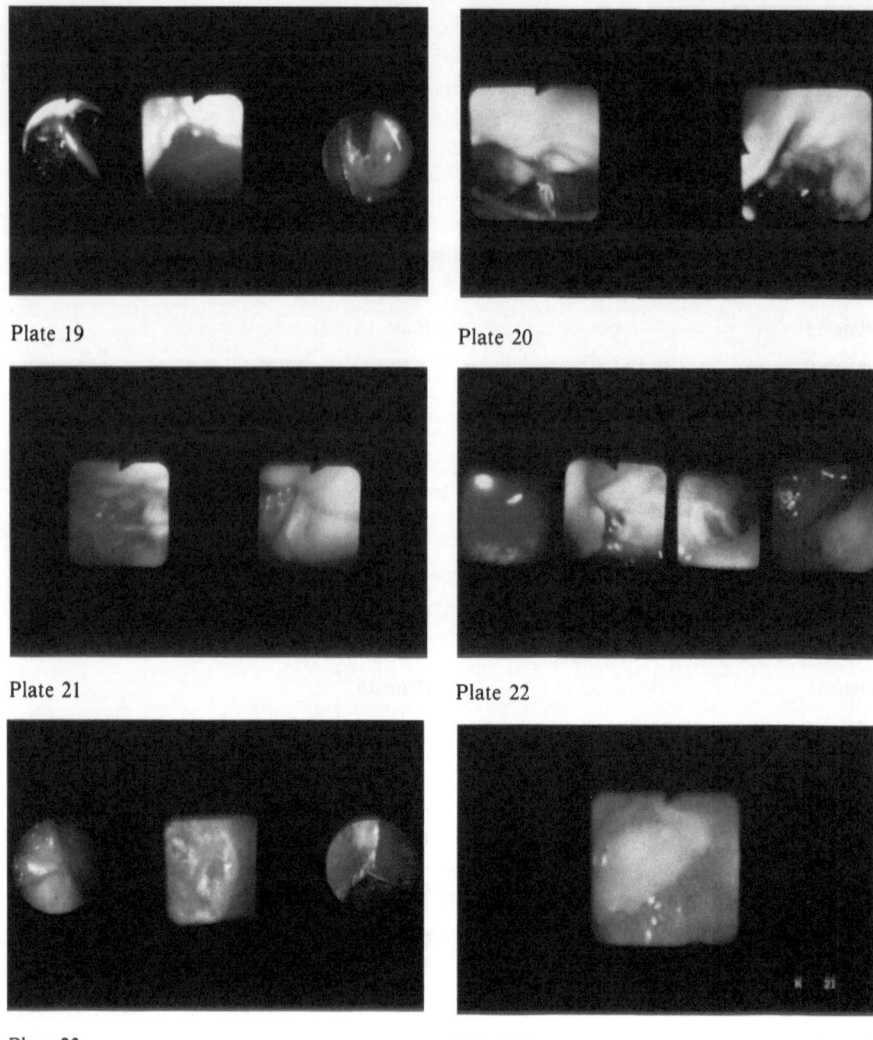

Plate 19

Plate 20

Plate 21

Plate 22

Plate 23

Plate 24

19. (Chapter 8) Spurting bleeding of a distal esophageal varix before (left), just after (middle), and on turn-around (right) following Nd-YAG laser coagulation.

20. (Chapter 9) Nd-YAG laser coagulation of a massive variceal bleed in the middle of the esophagus.

21. (Chapter 9) Nd-YAG laser coagulation of a massive variceal bleed in the distal esophagus. The patient later underwent elective portacaval shunting.

22. (Chapter 9) Nd-YAG laser coagulation of an arterial spurting acute ulcer in the duodenal bulb seven days after a cardiac valve replacement. Left is before treatment, left middle is immediately after Nd-YAG treatment, right middle is one week later, and right is six weeks later.

23. (Chapter 9) Spurting bleeding from an acute gastric ulcer. Left is before Nd-YAG laser coagulation, middle just after treatment, and right is six weeks later.

24. (Chapter 10) Ulcer with granulation tissue and oozing from the periphery. The patient was excluded from a laser randomized controlled trial (RCT) because of low risk of rebleeding.

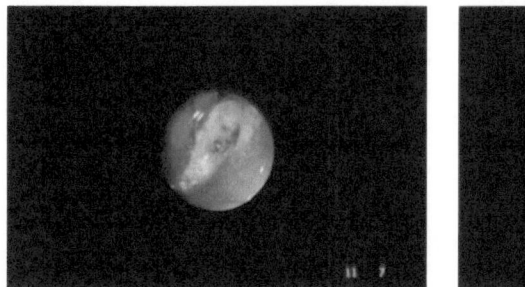

Plate 25

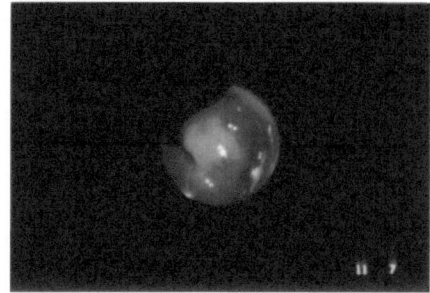

Plate 26

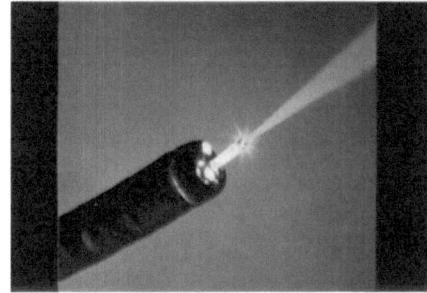

Plate 27

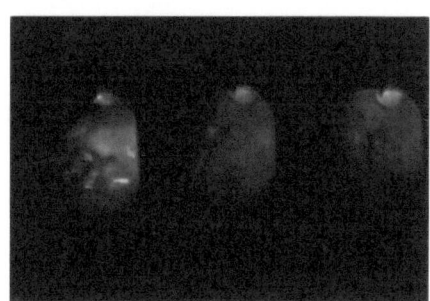

Plate 28

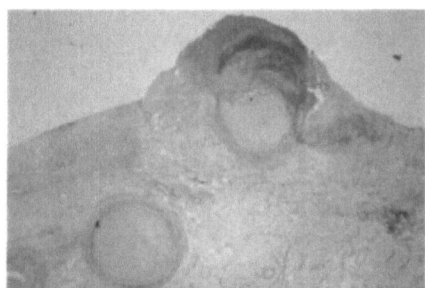

Plate 29

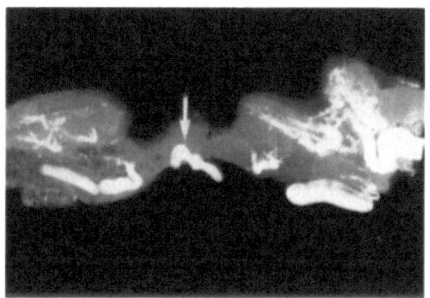

Plate 30

25. (Chapter 10) Chronic ulcer with non-bleeding visible vessel. The patient with severe UGI bleeding was included in a RCT of laser treatment.
26. (Chapter 10) Chronic ulcer with active spurting bleeding. This patient is the type randomized on CURE randomized trials.
27. (Chapter 11) Nd-YAG laser catheter and helium-neon aiming light.
28. (Chapter 11) Nd-YAG treatment of a spurting ulcer. Left is before, middle during, and right is after laser treatment.
29. (Chapter 11) Gastric ulcer (GU) with a non-bleeding visible vessel has a pseudoaneurysm on histopathology.
30. (Chapter 11) A GU whose artery was injected with barium. The artery courses below the ulcer surface.

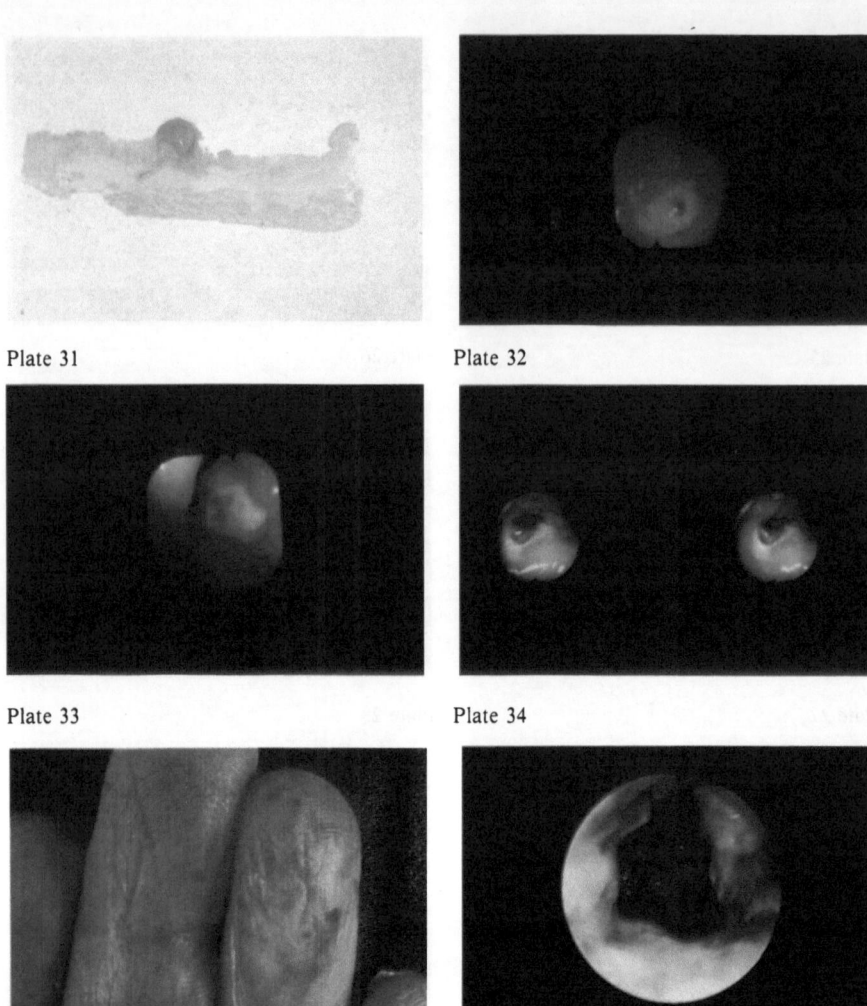

Plate 31

Plate 32

Plate 33

Plate 34

Plate 35

Plate 36

31. (Chapter 11) A GU with visible vessel. The artery loops away from the bleeding point.
32. (Chapter 11) A posterior GU with a non-bleeding visible vessel.
33. (Chapter 11) A flat red spot on a high lesser curvature GU.
34. (Chapter 11) A GU with an adherent, non-bleeding clot.
35. (Chapter 14) Endoscopic view of a mucosal, exophytic esophageal cancer before treatment.
36. (Chapter 14) Endoscopic view one week after YAG laser coagulation of an exophytic cancer.

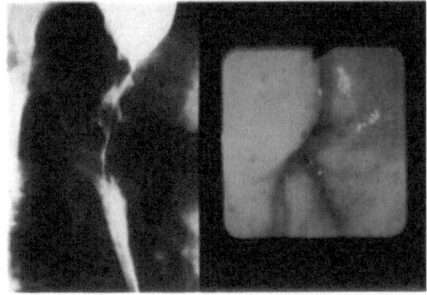

Plate 37

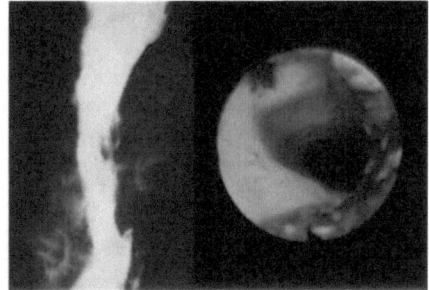

Plate 38

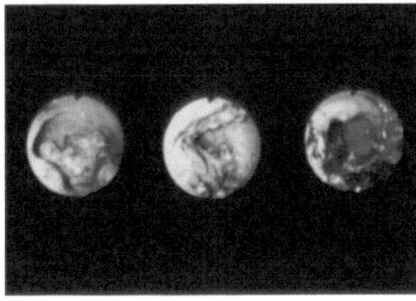

Plate 39

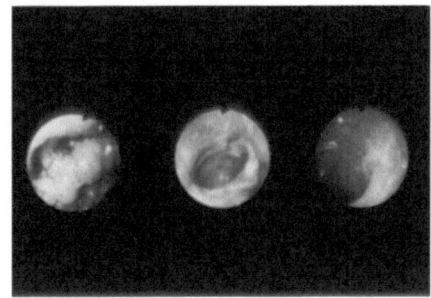

Plate 40

37. (Chapter 14) Endoscopy and esophogram of a submucosal esophageal cancer before YAG laser treatment.
38. (Chapter 14) Endoscopy and esophogram of a submucosal esophageal cancer one week after YAG laser treatment.
39. (Chapter 16) Serial photographs of an obstructing rectal adenocarcinoma. On the left, before laser; in the center, during laser treatment, on the right, at the end of the treatment. The lumen is patent.
40. (Chapter 16) Serial photographs of a villous adenoma receiving laser therapy. In the photo on the left a large villous adenoma can be seen prior to treatment. In the center photo is the central ulceration which occurs after laser treatment. In the photo on the right a pale white scar is the only remnant of the treated villous adenoma, three months after the last laser treatment.

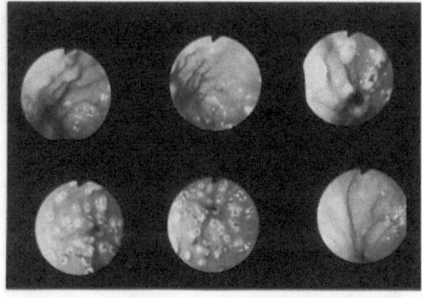

Plate 41

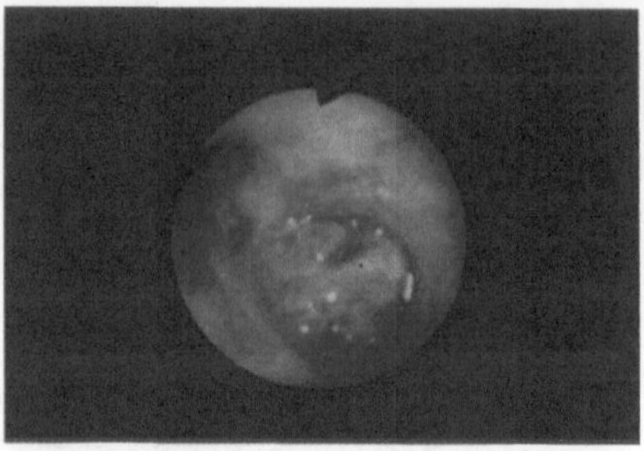

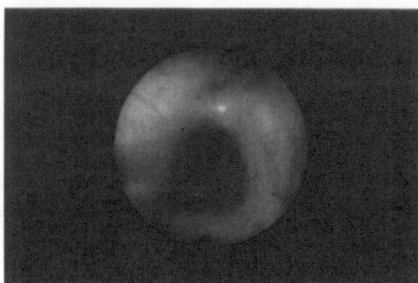

Plate 43

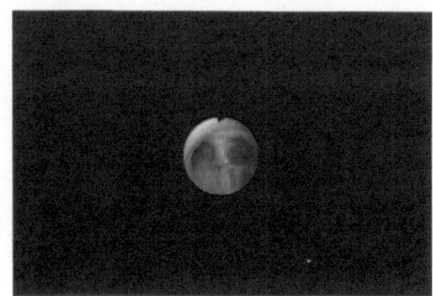

Plate 42

Plate 44

41. (Chapter 16) Serial photograph of a rectal polyposis. Upper left and middle: rectal polyposis before laser. Upper right, bottom left and middle: polyps coagulated or vaporized after argon laser. Bottom right: control one month after laser with complete healing of the mucosa.
42. (Chapter 18) Hamartoma of right mainstem bronchus before Nd-YAG treatment in a 19-year-old female.
43. (Chapter 18) Right mainstem bronchus hamartoma after Nd-YAG treatment.
44. (Chapter 18) Obstruction of right mainstem bronchus by squamous cell carcinoma in an 82-year-old male with respiratory failure.

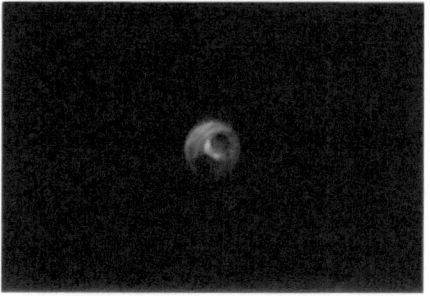

Plate 45

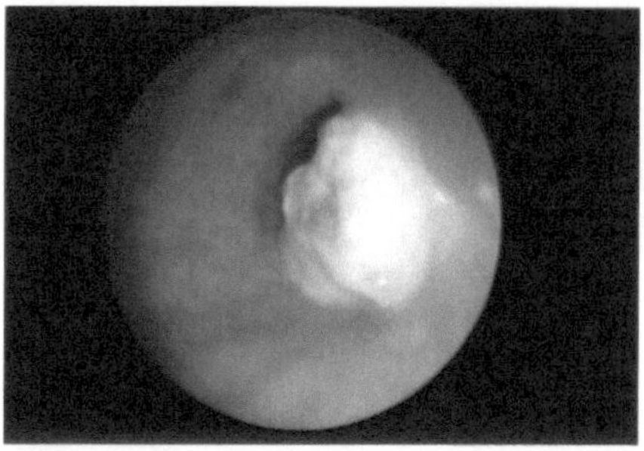

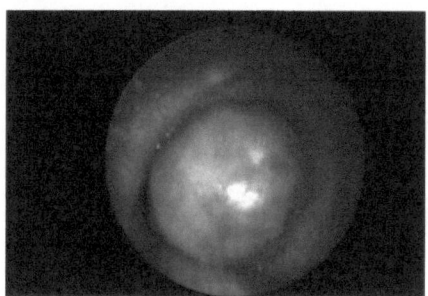

Plate 46

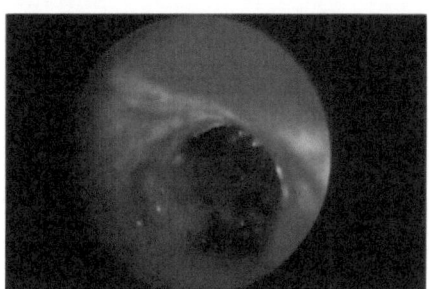

Plate 47

Plate 48

45. (Chapter 18) Patient of Plate 44 after Nd-YAG treatment of obstructing carcinoma of the right mainstem bronchus.
46. (Chapter 19) Leiomyoma: 72-year-old woman had repeated infections of the right lower lobe for 6 years. At bronchoscopy, there was total obstruction of the bronchus by a smooth and mobile tumor. The biopsy was leiomyoma.
47. (Chapter 19) We treated the patient of Plate 46 with the Cilas YAG laser at 50 W, delivering 1150 J to achieve total ablation of a thin pedicle. The resection was bloodless. There was no recurrence 5 years later.
48. (Chapter 19) Carcinoid: This 35-year-old man had fever from atelectasis of the entire left lung. Shows the initial endoscopic view. The biopsy revealed carcinoid.

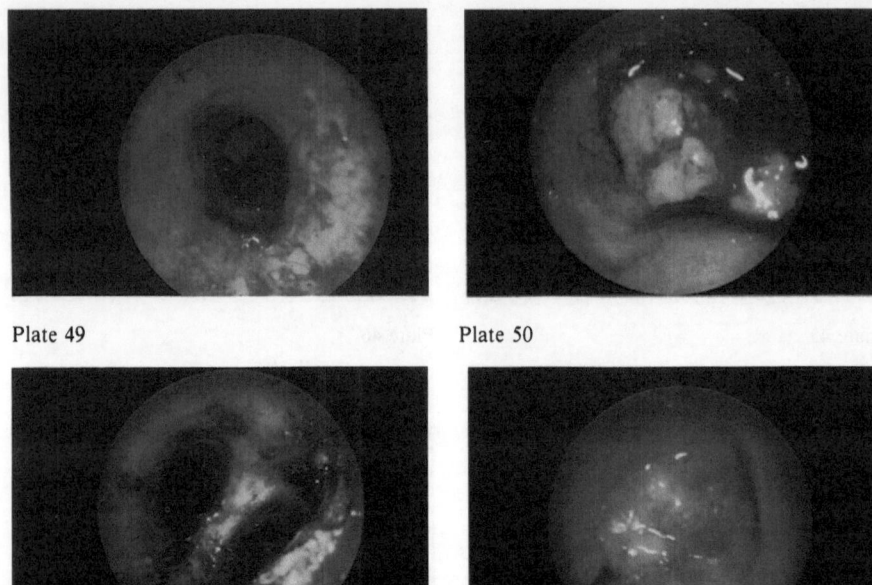

Plate 49

Plate 50

Plate 51

Plate 52

49. (Chapter 19) Endoscopic laser resection of the carcinoid of the patient of Plate 48 was done before a classical surgical sleeve resection to determine the exact insertion and extent of this obstructive tumor. Treatment was with Cilas YAG laser at 60 W for a total of 3000 J.

50. (Chapter 19) Squamous cell carcinoma: This is a 48-year-old man with a chronic bronchitis. For 4 months the dyspnea progressively increased. This man had acute asphyxia for 2 days from tracheal carcinoma. The biopsies revealed squamous cell carcinoma.

51. (Chapter 19) Treatment of the tracheal carcinoma of Plate 50 was with 60 W Cilas YAG laser and a total of 4000 J. After treatment, there was restoration of the bronchi to a nearly normal caliber. Radiotherapy was started 3 days after the laser session. Death occurred 14 months later from multiple metastases.

52. (Chapter 19) Carcinoma of the carina: This is a 67-year-old man previously treated with a left lower lobectomy 3 years ago for a carcinoma. Recurrence was treated by radio and chemotherapy for the last 6 months. This man arrived at the hospital comatose from anoxia. At bronchoscopy an obstructing carinal cancer was found.

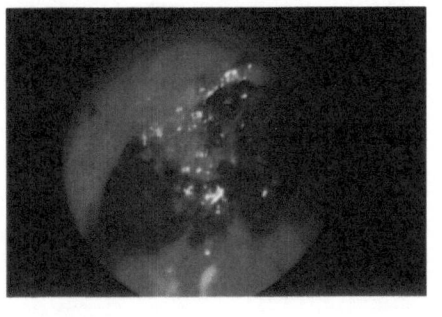

Plate 53

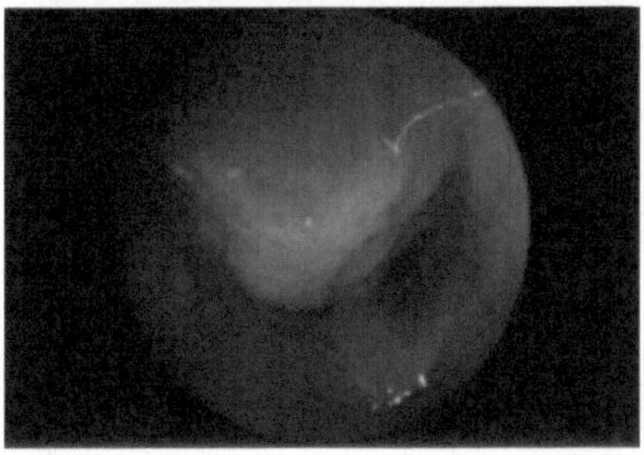

Plate 54

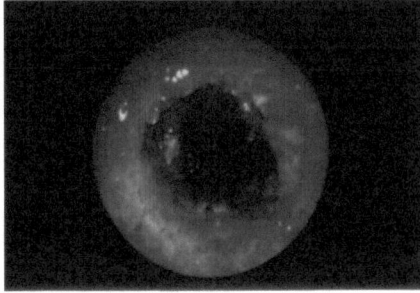

Plate 55

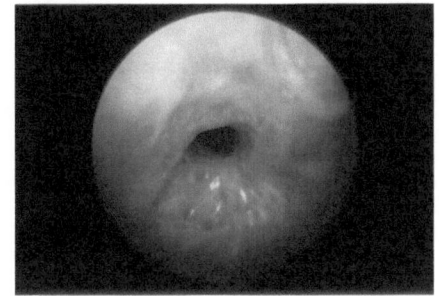

Plate 56

53. (Chapter 19) Using a Cilas YAG laser, 60 W and 8000 J total, there was restoration of a good caliber on both sides of the case of Plate 52. There was a little bleeding that was easily controlled. Three other laser resections were done during the follow-up period of 16 months after this first session. Death was caused by massive hemoptysis 27 days after the last laser resection.

54. (Chapter 19) Tracheal stenosis in a 48-year-old woman who had a tracheostomy after a traffic accident that caused rib fractures. After removing of the tracheostomy tube, the patient had severe dyspnea. Bronchoscopy revealed a diaphragm-like stenosis.

55. (Chapter 19) We used the Cilas YAG laser at 80 W and a total of 1050 J for vaporization of the tracheal stenosis of Plate 54. There was restoration of a good caliber of the trachea within a few minutes without blood loss. There was a good result with no recurrence in two years of follow-up.

56. (Chapter 19) Tracheal Granuloma in an 18-year-old boy with paraplegia from a T4 fracture. He had a tracheostomy for 1 month. After removing the tracheostomy tube, a granuloma was diagnosed by routine bronchoscopy. It was located above the tracheostomy ostium.

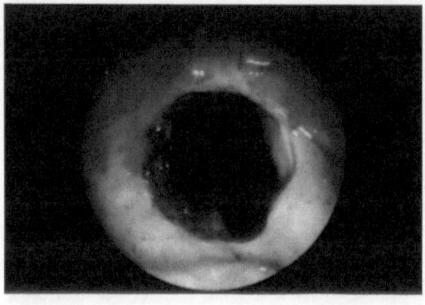

Plate 57

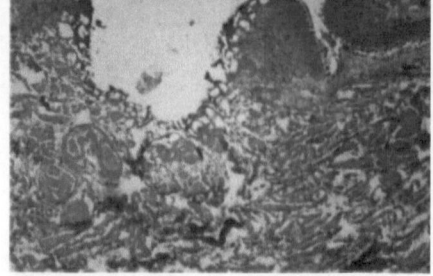

Plate 58

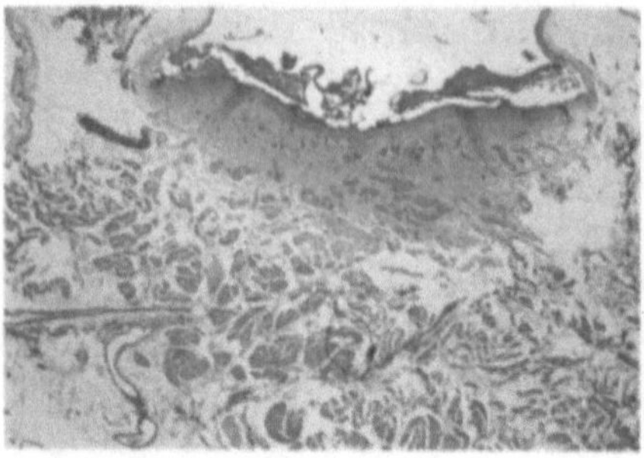

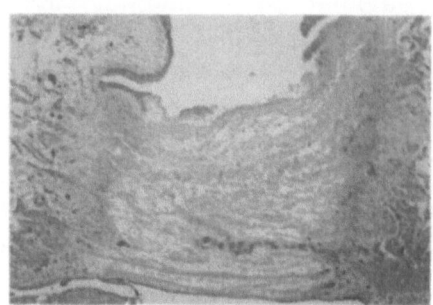

Plate 59

Plate 60

57. (Chapter 19) We vaporized the entire lesion of Plate 56 with the YAG laser, using 80 W and a total of 600 J. In 4 years of follow-up, there has been no recurrence.
58. (Chapter 20) Rabbit bladder. Histologic changes after CO_2 laser application.
59. (Chapter 20) Histologic changes after Argon laser application to rabbit bladder.
60. (Chapter 20) Transmural histologic changes after Nd:YAG application to rabbit bladder.

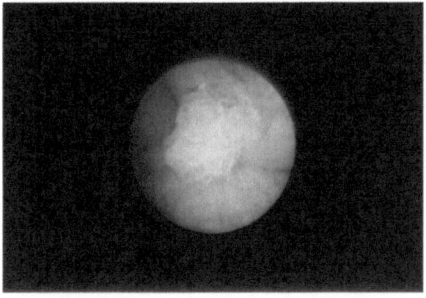

Plate 61

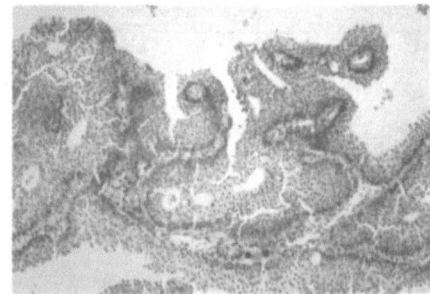

Plate 62

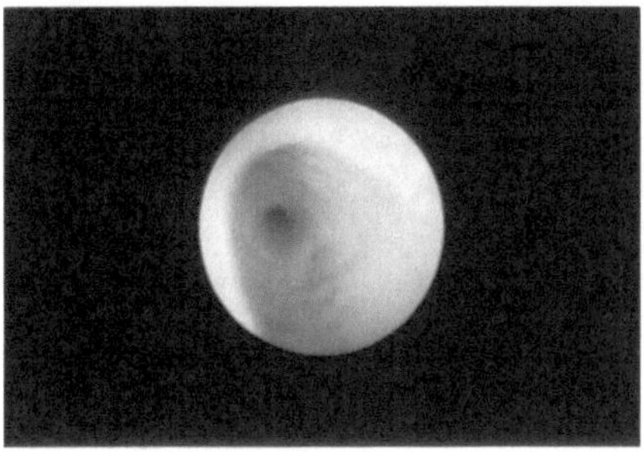

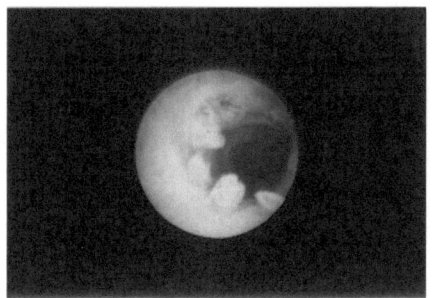

Plate 63

Plate 64

61. (Chapter 20) Papillary tumor, left ostium.
62. (Chapter 20) Grade I-II papillary tumor histopathology.
63. (Chapter 20) Urethral tumor three months after Nd:YAG laser irradiation.
64. (Chapter 20) Condylomata acumamata in the urethra.

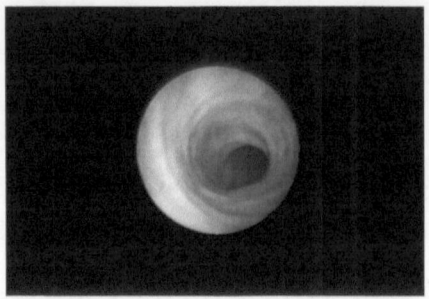

Plate 65

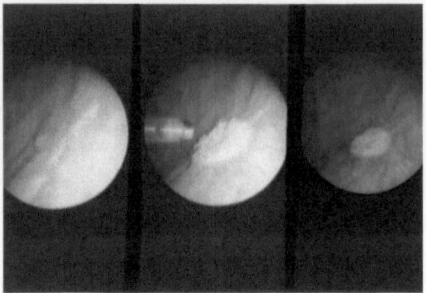

Plate 66

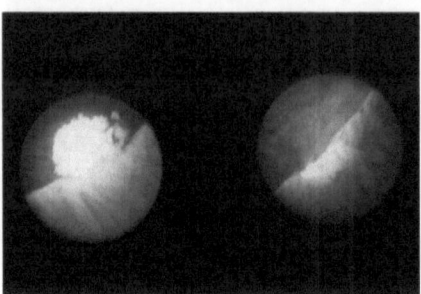

Plate 67

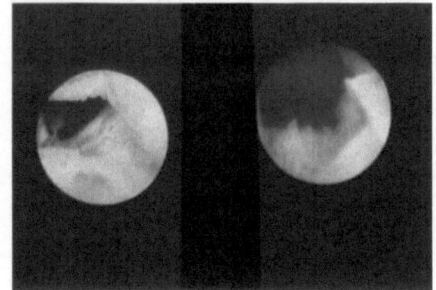

Plate 68

65. (Chapter 20) Condylomata acumamata one month after Nd:YAG laser irradiation.
66. (Chapter 22) Bladder tumor before (left), during (middle), and after (right) argon laser coagulation.
67. (Chapter 22) A papilloma of the bladder before (left) and after (right) argon laser photocoagulation.
68. (Chapter 22) Bladder neck stenosis before (left) and after (right) argon laser treatment.

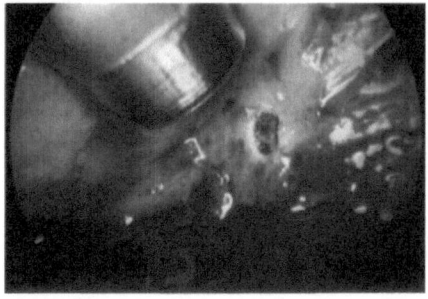

Plate 69

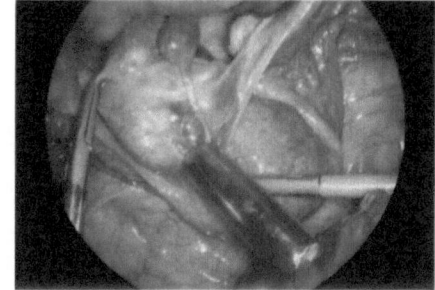

Plate 70

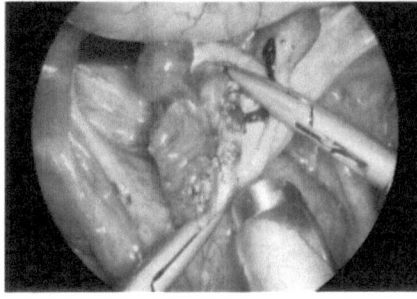

Plate 71

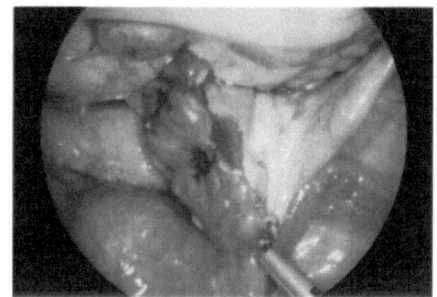

Plate 72

69. (Chapter 23) Endometriosis vaporization with a CO_2 laser.
70. (Chapter 23) Laparoscopic salpingostomy using a second puncture CO_2 laser probe. Initial appearance.
71. (Chapter 23) Laparoscopic salpingostomy with a CO_2 laser probe: radial incision of the fimbria – partial salpingotomy.
72. (Chapter 23) Laparoscopic salpingostomy with a CO_2 laser probe. Near completion of salpingotomy.

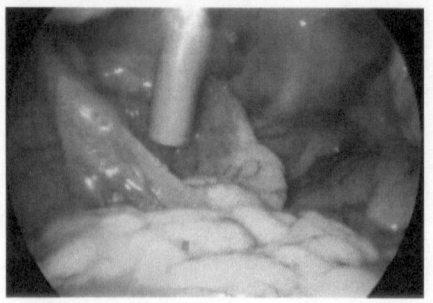

Plate 73

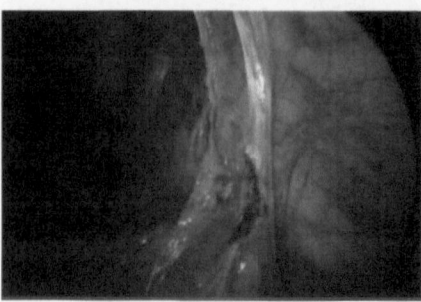

Plate 74

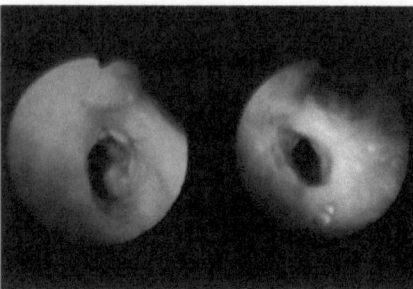

Plate 75

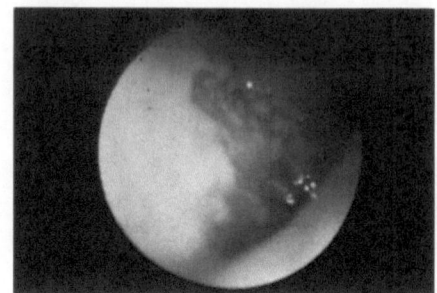

Plate 76

73. (Chapter 23) Lysis of an adhesion at laparoscopy with a CO_2 laser – initial appearance.
74. (Chapter 23) Adhesiolysis with the CO_2 laser laparoscope – appearance after lysis.
75. (Chapter 25) A nodular tumor (squamous cell carcinoma) 2.0 mm in diameter, in the right B2b before PDT (left). The tumor regressed after PDT (right), squamous cell carcinoma.
76. (Chapter 25) A superficially invading tumor in the cervical esophagus after reconstruction of the esophagus.

11. RESULTS, COMPLICATIONS AND TECHNIQUES OF LASER TREATMENT FOR BLEEDING PEPTIC ULCERS: CONCLUSIONS AND RECOMMENDATIONS AFTER TWO CONTROLLED TRIALS

PAUL SWAIN

In 1979, controlled trials were started at two hospitals in London, United Kingdom, in order to test the possible efficacy of laser photocoagulation in the endoscopic treatment of bleeding peptic ulcer. The study was undertaken because of promising accounts and observations of the efficacy of laser photocoagulation in models of experimental bleeding in animals (1-3) and because of enthusiastic but uncontrolled reports of efficacy in upper gastrointestinal hemorrhage in man (4, 5).

The trials had to be conducted between two hospitals in order to generate sufficient numbers of patients with UGI bleeding to test the hypothesis that laser photocoagulation might influence the incidence of rebleeding, need for urgent surgery and death following admission for bleeding peptic ulcer. Two controlled trials were carried out, the first testing the efficacy of the argon ion laser lasted fifteen months and the second, conducted according to the same protocol, tested the efficacy of the Nd-YAG laser and lasted for two years.

The argon laser was studied first (6). This laser was chosen because in 1979 animal studies of its efficacy and safety were more advanced than those of Nd-YAG laser and it seemed clear from comparative studies that the argon laser was safer than the Nd-YAG in terms of limited depth of penetration and seemed of similar if marginally lower efficacy in animal models of ulcer bleeding. The Nd-YAG laser was studied subsequently (7) because it was felt that this more deeply penetrating laser might offer greater efficacy since its energy could penetrate through overlying blood or clot to coagulate an underlying bleeding vessel and that greater efficacy might offset the increased theoretical hazard.

Setting up the trials

a) Materials

The argon lasers used in the first trial (Cooper Medical Devices 770 argon ion laser system; 12 Watts maximum output) were modified for endoscopic use with the beam focused onto the cleaved end of a 200 um single quartz fiber contained in a 1.7 mm plastic catheter. The endoscopy rooms at the two hospitals were altered to provide the necessary 3 phase electrical service and

D.M. Jensen and J.M. Brunetaud (eds), Medical Laser Endoscopy. 135-148.
© 1990 Kluwer Academic Publishers, Dordrecht

high flow water supply for laser cooling. Once the lasers were installed at both hospitals they were used for several months in uncontrolled studies before the trials were started. The Nd-YAG lasers were installed at both hospitals in 1981 (Barr and Stroud, Fiberlase 100 system; 100 Watts maximum output). The waveguide used with this laser was a 600 um single glass fiber contained in a 2.6 mm teflon catheter. A red helium neon laser beam, coupled into the light path of the invisible infra-red Nd-YAG laser output was used for targeting. (See Plate 27 in the atlas). The Nd-YAG lasers were used in uncontrolled studies for a four month period before embarking on the second controlled trial with this laser.

b) Funding

These controlled trials were funded by the British Government (Department of Health and Social Security, Clinical Trials Division and by the Research and Development Division). They supplied funds for the salary of a single gastroenterologist (honorary senior registrar grade) who was to be on call to endoscope all patients with gastrointestinal bleeding at both hospitals every day and night, using the lasers when appropriate. They bought 3 of the 4 lasers used in these studies as well as two operating endoscopes.

c) Ethical Approval and Consent

Ethical committee approval was sought for the trial and was readily granted. Careful attention was given to the wording of a patient consent form which read as follows. 'I consent to take part in a clinical trial of laser treatment for bleeding from the stomach. I understand that I shall receive all the usual treatment given to patients with this problem. I understand that it is part of modern treatment for bleeding from the stomach to be asked to swallow a flexible telescope ('endoscope') so that the nature and severity of the bleeding can be accurately determined. When that is being done, I may be given a new form of treatment in which an attempt is made to stop further bleeding by sealing the bleeding spot with a laser beam which can be passed down the endoscope.' It may be noted that potential complications such as perforation were not detailed in the consent form but were explained verbally to patients who inquired, nor was the nature of the randomization process spelled out in this form.

d) Uniformity of Conventional Management

It was necessary to seek the agreement of all the admitting physicians and surgeons at both hospitals that their patients should enter this trial and that they and their staff should be 'blind' to the endoscopic therapy. Furthermore, they should make day to day decisions on the conventional management of these patients and should also decide, independently of the endoscopist/laser therapist, whether rebleeding had occurred and when emergency surgery was needed.

A uniform policy of conventional management of patients with peptic ulcer was essential for the conduct of the trial and was agreed with the admitting physicians and surgeons based upon existing practices. Hypovolemia was reversed with transfused whole blood and central venous monitoring was used when possible.

Patients were considered for urgent surgery at the earliest sign of rebleeding in the hospital. All patients were treated with cimetidine (1g/24hrs, given intravenously for the first 24 hrs). This medication was given not because it was thought likely to influence outcome but to ensure uniformity of treatment in treated and placebo groups.

e) Technique of Endoscopic Laser Treatment

The patients were endoscoped as soon as possible after admission, preferably on their way from the emergency room to the ward. The laser was left running during the procedure, having been tuned to give appropriate power and pulse duration before the patient is intubated. During the endoscopy, particular attention was given to the identification and preparation of the bleeding site prior to randomization or treatment. Loose, overlying clot obscuring the view of the ulcer floor was removed by gentle endoscopic washing using a syringe full of water attached to the biopsy channel or to a washing catheter or pipe inserted through the biopsy channel. We did not observe that washing precipitated bleeding from ulcers. Clearing clot facilitated the recognition of the precise source of bleeding within an ulcer which was the target for endoscopic laser treatment. This was particularly helpful in deciding if active bleeding was present or not – often a difficult decision when there was oozing or intermittent bleeding. An overlying clot can absorb laser energy and prevent penetration to the bleeding vessel.

Once the bleeding point was identified, the laser waveguide was passed through the biopsy channel. The low power blue-green aiming beam of the argon laser or the red helium-neon aiming beam of the Nd-YAG laser was identified and was pointed at the target.

Ideally, the fiber was held a centimeter from the bleeding point but guessing distance at endoscopy was not easy. One technique which helped was to advance the waveguide until it almost touched the lesion and then withdraw the waveguide just under a centimeter at the biopsy channel port, holding the endoscope steady. The argon laser was fired in short bursts of 1-3 seconds until hemostasis was achieved; or in the case of non-bleeding lesions especially visible vessels until visible changes were seen which ranged from blanching to superficial charring. To avoid cell destruction and maintain maximum mechanical strength, no further laser treatment was applied once charring was observed. We attempted to treat circumferentially around the vessel. Sham endoscopic treatment consisted of only applying the aiming beam to the bleeding point but not applying laser power. The washing procedure was the same for controls as well as treated patients. Randomization only occurred when the aiming beam had shown that a bleeding point was accessible to laser treatment.

With the Nd-YAG laser animal studies have suggested that short (0.3–1 sec) pulses at high powers (70–90 Watts) are more effective and safer than longer or continuous laser treatment (8-10). This modifies the method of treatment somewhat. About 8 pulses of laser energy are fired to form a tight ring of spots around the bleeding vessel (See Plate 28 in the atlas). This technique may increase the chances of thermally damaging the bleeding artery distally and proximally to the bleeding point, and may diminish the chances of causing or increasing arterial hemorrhage which occasionally may occur if the laser is fired directly at an unstable plug of clot or pseudoaneurysm protruding from a bleeding point. This rationale is also based upon anatomical observations in resected gastric ulcers from control patients with rebleeding requiring emergency surgery from this series which revealed pseudoaneurysms (See Plate 29 in the atlas) in 54% and arteries of 0.1-1.8 mm sometimes coursing parallel to and immediately below the surface of the ulcer (See Plate 30 in the atlas) but more often looping up to and away from the bleeding point (See Plate 31 in the atlas). There are no animal studies to support this particular treatment technique and in practice it is often hard to place each pulse exactly, because the target moves, especially high in the stomach. Placebo treatment with the Nd-YAG laser involved aiming the low powered helium-neon aiming beam at the bleeding point without firing the Nd-YAG laser.

f) Definitions of Endoscopic Subgroups and Trial Endpoints

In the absence of spurting arterial bleeding (See Plate 28 in the atlas) or a pulsating pseudoaneurysm indicating the site of a vessel, a visible vessel (See Plate 32 in the atlas) was defined as an elevated red or black spot that protruded from the ulcer crater, was resistant to washing and was often associated with a fresh clot in the ulcer crater. When no vessel was visible, an ulcer was regarded as having stigmata of recent hemorrhage (SRH) if oozing was seen, if fresh blood or non-elevated black or red spots (See Plate 33 in the atlas) were seen in the crater.

Ulcers were stratified according to the type of endoscopically observed stigmata of recent hemorrhage and according to whether active bleeding was seen at any time during endoscopy even if it started or stopped spontaneously during the procedure. Six groups were defined: group 1 – visible vessel, active bleeding; group 2 – visible vessel, no active bleeding; group 3 – SRH other than a visible vessel, active bleeding; group 4 – SRH other than a visible vessel, no active bleeding; group 5 – clot obscuring part of the crater, active bleeding; group 6 – clot obscuring part of the crater, no active bleeding (See Plate 34 in the atlas). See Tables 11.1 and 11.2.

In group 1 there was active bleeding with pulsatile flow, in groups 3 and 5 oozing could be observed. In groups 5 and 6 the precise point of bleeding was not identified but these patients were included so that it might be possible to assess the effect of laser treatment through a small amount of clot.

Rebleeding in the hospital as judged by a clinician – blinded as to the nature of the endoscopic therapy – was taken as an indication of urgent surgery. Evidence of rebleeding was regarded as definitive if fresh hematemesis occurred, but as suggestive if there was fresh melena, a sudden rise in pulse rate, fall in blood pressure or central pressure, or unexplained drop in hemoglobin concentration following stabilization. In cases where rebleeding was uncertain it was confirmed by repeat endoscopy. All deaths or ulcer operations during the period of hospital admission were included in the analysis.

g) Trial Design

The trials were designed to test the null hypothesis that argon or Nd-YAG laser photocoagulation does not affect the rebleeding rate, need for urgent surgery or death following admission with bleeding peptic ulcer with a source of bleeding accessible to laser therapy.

Controlled trials of endoscopic therapy in gastrointestinal bleeding cannot be conducted in the same fashion as controlled trials of a pharmacological agent where it may be reasonable to give all patients a safe drug in the hope of helping a few. Treatment has to be applied selectively and trials have to be conducted using randomized high risk groups of patients. It would be pointless to fire the laser at all patients with gastrointestinal bleeding since 80% will do well with no treatment. It is crucial that the processes of selection are performed prospectively, prior to randomization. It is also important that the selection process is effective in identifying patients at risk of further bleeding or death. An ideal trial would only randomize patients at risk of further bleeding and death but would randomize all of them. These trials take advantage of two endoscopic findings valuable in the prediction of recurrent hemorrhage. The first of these is the identification of a visible vessel (bleeding or non-bleeding) at endoscopy which in our hands carries a high risk of further bleeding (58% of our controls with this finding have further bleeding and more than 90% of patients who died following admission with bleeding peptic ulcer had this finding). The second is the absence of stigmata of recent hemorrhage (SRH) i.e. blood or clot in an ulcer of a patient recently admitted because of gastrointestinal bleeding. Absence of SRH was effective in predicting that patients would not bleed again: no patients with no SRH in an ulcer had further bleeding or died during the period of these two trials. We included all patients with SRH accessible to laser therapy in our trials but expected most of the action to take place in the visible vessel subgroup, which had been randomized prospectively and separately, since the majority of the rebleeding and mortality was confined to this important subgroup.

Prospective randomization was carried out within our subgroups in blocks of ten patients. A sealed envelope which indicated laser or sham treatment was opened during endoscopy while the laser aiming beam pointed at the source of the bleeding within the ulcer. Prior to randomization the endoscopist had to decide whether there was a visible vessel, minor SRH, overlying clot and whether these subgroups were actively bleeding prior to randomization since he had to select a randomization envelope which indicated the subgroups in which the patient would remain.

Testing of endoscopic accessibility prior to randomization was an important feature of trial design. Our hypothesis was whether laser treatment was superior to no laser treatment for patients with bleeding peptic ulcer. To include patients who could not be treated with the laser for technical or endoscopic reasons would have only diluted and weakened the answer to this question. Other trials may have been weakened by failing to adhere to this design principle.

Argon laser trial: patients

During the 15 month period of this controlled trial, a consecutive series of 330 patients had urgent endoscopy following admission for acute upper gastrointestinal tract bleeding.

Table 11.1. Argon laser trial. Frequency of rebleeding in treated and control ulcers.

Category	Total	Laser		Control	
		Rebleed	No rebleed	Rebleed	No rebleed
Group 1 (visible vessel, bleeding)	11	4	3	4	0
Group 2 (visible vessel, not bleeding)	41	4	13	13	11
Group 3 (other SRH bleeding)	6	0	2	0	4
Group 4 (other SRH, not bleeding)	11	1	4	0	6
Group 5 (overlying clot, bleeding)	2	0	1	0	3
Group 6 (overlying clot, not bleeding)	5	2	2	0	1
Total	76	11	25	17	23

Ulcers were seen in 155 cases. One hundred-eight of these patients with ulcers had SRH and all 76 of those patients with SRH accessible to laser treatment were included in the trial. None of the 47 ulcers without SRH rebled. The reasons for initial exclusion from the trial of 32 patients who had ulcers with SRH were as follows: 17 were excluded because of endoscopic inaccessibility, 10 because of problems with a deformed or stenosed duodenal cap, 3 because of excessive bleeding, 2 with inaccessible high lesser curve ulcers. Seventeen were excluded because of other technical factors. The laser was not operating for 7 cases, the operator was unavailable for 4, patient intolerance excluded 4, a misdiagnosis of cancer and a closed perforation excluded one each. Of these 32 patients with SRH excluded from the trial, 10 rebled and 4 died.

The mean age of treated patients was 65 and of controls 67. There were 23 men and 13 women in the treated group and 22 men and 18 women in the control group. The mean admission hemoglobin was 8.6 g/dl in treated patients and 9.1 g/dl in controls. Thirteen of thirty-six patients in the treated group and 12/40 in the control group had an admission systolic blood pressure of less than 100 mm Hg. None of these differences are significant suggesting that the patients had been randomized without bias.

Thirty-nine gastric, 33 duodenal and 4 stomach ulcers were included in the trial. A vessel was visible bleeding and non-bleeding) in 52, other SRH only were present in 17, and in 7 the bleeding point was covered by overlying clot, not removed by washing. The incidence of rebleeding in treated and untreated ulcers is shown for each group in Table 11.1. Rebleeding in the treated ulcers was significantly less than in the controls in group 2 alone (visible vessel, not bleeding)($x^2 = 3.85$; $p < 0.05$) and in groups 1 and 2 combined ($x^2 = 3.88$; $p < 0.05$), although these results do not reach statistical significance in group 1 alone (visible vessel, bleeding). All the deaths and 25 of the 28 rebleeds occurred in groups 1 and 2, i.e. those patients with a visible vessel. No patient randomized to laser treatment died, although 7 in the control group did. All the deaths occurred in patients who had been diagnosed as having rebled, and in all but one case the deaths occurred after emergency surgery. Emergency surgery was carried out in all 8 patients with rebleeding in the treatment group and in 14 of 17 in the control group. Transfusion comparisons analyzed from 24 hours after admission showed that controls used more units of blood than laser treated patients (transfusion requirements in the first 24 hours relate mainly to blood lost in the period prior to admission and were not significantly different).

Complications were few. There were no perforations. On two occasions, firing the laser at visible but non-bleeding vessels (group 2) caused arterial bleeding which could not be stopped by further application of the laser. Both patients were taken to surgery immediately and did well afterwards.

In summary, this trial of argon laser photocoagulation suggests that argon laser photocoagulation can significantly reduce mortality from bleeding peptic ulcers accessible to this form of treatment. The trial also showed a significant reduction in rebleeding rate, at the lowest (5%) level of statistical significance, and all deaths occurred in patients in the control group who had rebled, suggesting that the reduction in mortality rate was at least in part due to the effect of the laser treatment.

There was a problem with one aspect of these results. It was difficult to explain why 7/19 control patients who rebled died while there were no deaths in 8 patients in the treatment group who rebled. Attempts to identify bias between the two groups suggested that they were well matched for other factors known to affect case fatality rate, such as age, hypotension on admission, low initial hemoglobin level and gastric ulcer to duodenal ulcer ratio. It seemed therefore reasonable to assume that the unequivocal improvement in mortality was due at least in part to laser treatment and the consequent reduction in rebleeding rate.

Some lessons were learned during the conduct of this trial and from some criticisms on its publication (11, 12). The first was that improvements in mortality rate required unequivocal reductions in rebleeding rate and need for emergency surgery in order to carry conviction that a therapy was influencing outcome in gastrointestinal bleeding. The second was that the benefits of prospective subgroup analysis of high risk groups (used for the first time in trials of gastrointestinal bleeding) could be mistaken for unwanted patients exclusion. The important lesson was that larger patient numbers were required for unequivocal demonstration of benefit, even though at the date of its publication 1981 it was amongst the largest controlled trial conducted in gastrointestinal bleeding drawing from 330 patients with upper gastrointestinal bleeding.

Table 11.2. Nd-YAG laser trial. Frequency of rebleeding in treated and control ulcers.

Category	Total	Laser		Control	
		Rebleed	No rebleed	Rebleed	No rebleed
Group 1 (visible vessel, bleeding)	19	2	8	7	2
Group 2 (visible vessel, not bleeding)	54	2	23	14	15
Group 3 (other SRH, bleeding)	9	0	4	1	4
Group 4 (other SRH, not bleeding)	19	0	12	0	7
Group 5 (overlying clot, bleeding)	6	0	2	1	3
Group 6 (overlying clot, not bleeding)	16	1	8	1	6
Total	123	5	57	24	37

Nd-Yag laser trial: patients

During the 24 month period of this controlled trial, 465 unselected patients admitted consecutively with upper gastrointestinal hemorrhage underwent urgent endoscopy (7). Peptic ulcers were seen in 232. All 123 ulcer patients with stigmata of recent hemorrhage (SRH) accessible to laser therapy were included in the trial (24 inaccessible, 85 had no SRH). None of the 85 ulcers without SRH rebled.

The reasons for exclusion from the trial of 24 patients who had ulcer with SRH are as follows. Eleven were excluded because of endoscopic inaccessibility, 9 because of duodenal stenosis or deformity, 2 because of inaccessible high lesser curve lesions. Thirteen were excluded because of other technical problems. The laser was not operating for 7 cases, the operator was unavailable for 4 cases. Patient intolerance prevented randomization of 1 and torrential bleeding in another one.

Matching of controls and treated patients suggested that the patients had been randomized without bias. The mean admission hemoglobin was 8.6 g/dl in treated patients and 9.3 g/dl in controls. Seventeen of the sixty-two treated patients vs. 19/61 of controls had a systolic blood pressure of less than 100 mm Hg on admission. The mean age of treated patients was 68 and of controls 71. GU/DU ratio was 34/28 in treated patients and 27/34 in controls.

Results

Sixty-one gastric and 62 duodenal ulcers with SRH were included in this trial of Nd-YAG laser photocoagulation. A vessel was visible vessel (bleeding or non-bleeding) in 73, other SRH were present in 28, and in 22 the bleeding point was covered by overlying clot not removed by washing. The incidence of rebleeding in treated and untreated ulcers is shown for each group in Table 11.2. Considering all patients in the trial 5/62 treated vs. 24/61 control patients rebled ($p<0.05$ Chi squared with Yates correction). The most important subgroup was the visible vessel group where most of the rebleeding took place (4/35 treated vs. 21/38 controls rebled, ps0.05). Rebleeding was reduced in patients with spurting from a visible vessel (2/10 treated vs. 7/9 controls, $p<0.05$). Visible vessels without bleeding were technically easier to treat than those with spurting. Results in this subgroup suggested that laser treatment reduced rebleeding (2/25 treated vs. 14/29 controls rebled, $p<0.05$). Considering patients with other SRH, few rebled on the control group and as expected no benefit was shown for the treatment group (0/16 treated vs. 1/12 controls rebled). In the group with overlying clot there were few rebleeds and consequently no evidence of benefit (1/11 treated vs. 2/11 controls rebled). As in the argon laser trial there was no overall reduction in transfusion requirement, but when transfusion requirements for 24 hours after admission was analyzed, there was a significant reduction in units of blood required by the treated group (the transfusion requirements after 24 hours relate to further bleeding in hospital).

No perforations occurred in laser treated patients but 4 patients with non-bleeding visible vessels bled during Nd:YAG laser treatment. All were stopped with further laser pulses but one rebled later.

The requirement for emergency surgery was significantly reduced in laser treated patients (5/62 laser treated but 19/61 controls required operations). Mortality also was reduced (1/62 laser treated patients died while 8/61 controls died, $p < 0.05$). All patients who died did so following an episode of rebleeding.

In summary, this controlled trial of laser photocoagulation suggests that the Nd-YAG laser significantly reduced the rebleeding rate, need for emergency surgery and mortality in patients with bleeding peptic ulcer with SRH accessible to laser treatment.

A comparison of the relative efficacy of the argon and Nd-YAG laser in two controlled trials

When the results of these two trials are compared, 11/36 (31%) argon laser patients rebled, compared with 5/62 (8%) Nd-YAG laser treated patients. Of the controls 17/40 (42%) rebled in the argon laser trial compared with 24/62 (39%) in the Nd-YAG laser trial. These results in the two trials carried out to the same protocol by the same staff suggest that the Nd-YAG laser, with its more penetrating beam, had a significantly ($p < 0.05$) greater effect on the rebleeding rate than the argon laser, whereas the rebleeding rate in the control group remained the same in the two trials. Greater operator experience gained in the course of these trials may have contributed to the superior results with the Nd-YAG laser.

Conclusion

The results of these two controlled trials of laser photocoagulation for bleeding peptic ulcer seem encouraging. Their results in general support trends reported in other controlled trials of endoscopic laser treatment in upper gastrointestinal bleeding (13-17) although further confirmatory reports would be valuable. The impact of lasers on the problem of gastrointestinal bleeding remains to be assessed and questions remain, as in any growing subject. It has to be admitted that some treated lesions rebleed, particularly when a large vessel is found in the crater of an ulcer (Plates 29-31 in the atlas). A proportion of patients have lesions that are inaccessible to treatment. Technical solutions to problems of large vessel bleeding and inaccessibility need to be found so that endoscopic therapy becomes less of a gamble. It is not clear that lasers are superior to probe type endoscopic thermal methods. Indeed animal studies suggest that they are of similar efficacy. The high capital cost of lasers raises the suspicion that even if they are highly effective clinically they may not be cost effective, and they are certainly less portable than electrocoagulation or heater probe devices. The results of controlled clinical trial for these cheaper devices have not been reported although such trial have been initiated. Prospects for advancement in the field of gastrointestinal bleeding depend crucially on the execution of properly conducted controlled trials. It is important that the freedom to conduct controlled trials is defended by gastroenterologists and ethical committees and that those involved in their design and practice should improve on these early trials. Through careful controlled trials the common goal of effective and reliable endoscopic hemostasis may evolve into a demonstrable clinical reality.

APPENDIX

Some tips on the endoscopy of patients with gastrointestinal bleeding

Patients requiring endoscopy following a gastrointestinal bleed are a little more difficult to endoscope that routine, non-bleeding patients. They are generally sicker and often more restless and frightened. Engaging their confidence is essential before starting endoscopy. I prefer to use minimal or no sedation in the elderly or ill patients who are bleeding. But I sometimes prefer opiate sedation in restless young patients with high alcohol intake who may become disinhibited with benzodiazepines. Since the stomach may not be empty, a lateral position with head down is even more essential than with conventional endoscopy. Gently seeking a succussion splash before starting can diminish the chance of unexpectedly encountering a stomach full of blood. I prefer not to lavage the stomach out before endoscopy since lavage tubes can cause erosions and diagnostic confusion.

If there is a large volume of blood in the stomach when the endoscope is passed it may be helpful to encourage the patients not to retch and to move the endoscope quickly but gently through the esophagus, inspecting it for varices and Mallory-Weiss tears, to enter the fundus where a finger is held on the air inflation button. As the upper stomach inflates, blood will fall away into the fundus and this maneuver will sometimes lift a posterior high lesser curve ulcer out of a pool of blood. It is less common to find significant bleeding ulcers in the fundus or high on the greater curve where this pool tends to collect.

If the blood is fresher in the fundus than in the duodenum this may hint at a high gastric lesion missed on the way down. Because of the head down position of the patient, blood will tend to run in a cephalad direction, fresh blood high in the stomach may have come from the duodenum. A clot prolapsing through the pylorus and obscuring it usually indicates duodenal ulceration. If there is partial duodenal stenosis and bleeding, the ulceration is usually distal to the stenosis. There are two common sites associated with severe bleeding from peptic ulcers: the first is high posterior position on the lesser curve, and the second is postero-inferior in the proximal duodenal bulb.

There are some catches in endoscoping bleeding patients. Antral ulcers can be mistaken for a major bleeding source when the true bleeding lesion is a duodenal ulcer. Small antral ulcers are common in the presence of duodenal ulceration. Multiple ulcers high on the lesser curve can cause problems, the most proximal, usually largest ulcer is the most likely to cause major bleeding.

There are problems diagnosing active bleeding. Spurting often stops spontaneously. A jet of blood can look like a string of blood clot. Pulsatile movement of blood can be caused by cardiac or respiratory movements moving pools of blood rhythmically. Bleeding can be caused by the endoscope touching mucosa or granulation tissue. Therefore, it is wise to under diagnose active bleeding in lesions which were missed or seen not to bleed as the endoscope passes them but appear to be bleeding on pull back. The diagnosis of oozing is subjective, requires careful washing and should only be diagnosed in ulcers that were not touched by the endoscope.

The diagnosis of non-bleeding visible vessels can cause difficulty. If I am in doubt about a possible vessel, (See Plate 32 in the atlas) I ask myself whether the spot in question within the ulcer crater is the only point from which the bleeding is likely to have come and I move the endoscope to check that the spot is raised. Gentle washing, trying to clear loose debris from the ulcer is particularly helpful. Endoscopic features which increase the chance of rebleeding when a visible vessel is observed include: spurting, visible pulsation, loud arterial doppler signal, large ulcer size, low hemoglobin or shock on admission.

Although fresh blood can sometimes be effectively aspirated through a large channel endoscope, if there are lumps of clot it is usually unwise to try suction which can block the endoscope and cause loss of vision.

Blood absorbs light. It is easier to see erosions with a large diameter endoscope and a bright light source. Severely anemic patients have very pale mucosa and color contrast between normal mucosa and ulcer may be lost. Changing to a large diameter instrument, waiting until the stomach has been emptied of blood and transfusing the patient can bring out lesions missed at a first endoscopy.

The following tips may be helpful to those beginning to practice therapeutic endoscopy for gastrointestinal bleeding. It is hard to place each pulse precisely, especially high on the lesser curve because the target moves. Movement can be controlled to some degree by giving buscopan or glucagon judiciously if peristalsis is a problem. Asking the patient to hold his breath while the laser is fired may assist if respiration is interfering with the aim. Major bleeding from ulcers is common in two sites, the posterior aspect of the high lesser curve and the postero-inferior aspect of the duodenal bulb. Both these sites can be difficult to treat and are usually approached at acute angles of between 45° and 0° using forward viewing endoscopes. On the high lesser curve, access can be improved by curving the endoscope with a J maneuver, and rotation of the endoscope with its eccentrically placed biopsy channel sometimes may give a different and more useful angle of approach. If the laser aiming beam disappears or cannot be seen, it is usually wise to withdraw the fiber without firing it and cleaning any blood or adherent mucus from the tip. The laser tip can be destroyed by firing it when it is contaminated. The use of an initial 'sighter' spot on the edge of the ulcer may be helpful in allowing a biological test of the laser's function. At effective coagulation powers, a single pulse should produce a ring of blanched mucosa but should not break the surface of the mucosa. Blackening due to the oxidation of hemoglobin pigment can be mistaken for charring or vaporization of tissue.

Acknowledgements

I wish to express my gratitude to my colleagues, David Storey, Paul Salmon, Steve Bown, John Kirkham and Tim Northfield for their assistance during the four year period of these trials, and also to the many patients with gastrointestinal bleeding who gave their consent to participate in these controlled trials.

References

1. Silverstein FE, Protell RL, Gilbert DA et al. Argon vs. Neodymium-YAG laser photocoagulation of experimental canine gastric ulcers. Gastroenterology 1979;77:491-496.
2. Bown SG, Salmon PR, Kelly DF et al. Argon laser photocoagulation in the dog stomach. Gut 1979;20:680-687.
3. Dixon JA, Berenson MMN, McCloskey DW. Neodymium-YAG laser treatment of experimental canine gastric bleeding. Acute and chronic studies of photocoagulation, penetration and perforation. Gastroenterology 1979;77:647-651.
4. Fruhmorgen P, Bodem F, Feidenbach HD. Endoscopic photocoagulation by laser irradiation in the gastrointestinal tract of man. Acta Hepatogastroenterologica 1978;25:1-5.
5. Kiefhaber P, Nath G, Moritz K. Endoscopic control of massive gastrointestinal hemorrhage by irradiation with a high-power Neodymium-YAG laser. Progr Surg 1977;15:140-155.
6. Swain CP, Bown SG, Storey DW et al. Controlled trial of argon laser photocoagulation in BICAP peptic ulcers. Lancet 1981;11:1313- 16.
7. Swain CP, Bown SG, Salmon PR et al. Gastrointest Endosc 1984;30:137A.
8. Johnston JH, Jensen DM, Mautner W and Elashoff J. YAG laser treatment of experimental bleeding canine gastric ulcers. Gastroenterology 1980;79:1256-61.
9. Bown SG, Salmon PR, Storey DW. Nd-YAG laser photocoagulation in the dog stomach. Gut 1980;21:818-25.
10. Rutgeerts P, Vantrappen G, Geboes K, Broeckaert L. Safety and efficacy of Neodymium-YAG laser photocoagulation: an Experimental study in dogs. Gut 1981;22:38-44.
11. Bateson MC, Henry DA, Langman MJS, Cotton PB, Vallon AG, Piper DW, Northfield TC et al. Letters. Lancet 1982;1:99, 172, 230,231,402,508.
12. Peterson WL. Laser therapy for bleeding peptic ulcer. A burning issue? Gastroenterology 1982;83:485-6.
13. Vallon AG, Cotton PB, Laurence BH et al. Randomized trial of endoscopic argon laser

photocoagulation in bleeding peptic ulcers. Gut 1981;22:228-30.

14. Jensen DM, Machicado GA, Tapia JI, Elashoff J. Controlled trial of endoscopic argon laser for severe ulcer hemorrhage. Gastroenterology 1984;86:1125A.

15. Ihre T, Johansson C, Seligson U, Torregren S. Endoscopic YAG laser treatment in massive upper gastrointestinal bleeding. Report of a randomized controlled study. Scand J Gastroenterol 1981;16:633-40.

16. Rutgeerts P, Vantrappen G, Broeckhaert L et al. Controlled trial of Nd-YAG laser treatment of upper digestive hemorrhage. Gastroenterology 1982;83:410-16.

17. MacLeod IA, Mills PR, Mackenzie JF et al. Neodymium-yttrium- aluminum-garnet laser photocoagulation for major hemorrhage from peptic ulcers and single vessels: A single blind controlled study. Br Med J 1983;286:345-48.

12. ENDOSCOPIC Nd:YAG LASER THERAPY FOR ACUTE UPPER GASTROINTESTINAL BLEEDING

DAVID FLEISCHER AND STEPHAN G. BOWN

Introduction

There are more published data about Nd:YAG laser therapy for acute upper gastrointestinal bleeding (UGIB) than for any other endoscopic modality. A far greater number of controlled studies have been recorded than with all other laser devices combined. Initially there were many investigators who argued that the argon laser was better suited for treating acute UGIB. A major concern existed that the Nd:YAG laser penetrated too deeply and the risk of perforation would be too great. Although there is no controlled scientific information which demonstrates one laser superior to another, the fact that greater than 90% of the GI lasers in use today for endoscopic hemostasis are Nd:YAG, certainly is a testimony to the fact that most endoscopists prefer it to the argon laser. This chapter summarizes the results of the controlled trials from around the world which assess the efficacy and safety of endoscopic Nd:YAG laser therapy for acute UGIB and summarizes the American experience.

Equipment

Lasers

Commercially-produced lasers from several companies are available in the United States. Power outputs at the tip of the fiber range from 80 to 110 watts. Although all are potentially movable, none is portable in the most specific sense of the term.

The price range is between $80,000 and $100,000 (U.S.).

Endoscopes

Any endoscope can be used to treat UGIB but most American endoscopists prefer the larger therapeutic instruments. There is divided opinion as to whether the endoscope with a single large (>3.5 mm) biopsy channel is preferable to a two channel (one 2.8 mm and the other 3.5 mm or both 3.7 mm) scope. An additional wash channel is also present. Video-endoscopes are also

D.M. Jensen and J.M. Brunetaud (eds), Medical Laser Endoscopy. 149-162.
© 1990 Kluwer Academic Publishers, Dordrecht

being adapted with a protective distal filter so that they may be used with lasers.

Fibers

Flexible quartz or glass fibers convey the beam from the laser to the target organ. The unsheathed fiber is approximately 1 mm in diameter. Generally a plastic sheath encircles the fiber with a space between for the delivery of coaxial gas or water. The outside diameter varies, but most are 1.8 to 2.4 mm. The beam usually exits straight ahead (180°). Although the results that will be given were accrued using these conventional fibers, two new developments bear close scrutiny in the near future. Hashimoto et al. (1) have developed a lateral prismatic tip wherein the beam exits at 60 to 90° offering the endoscopist the option of delivering the beam perpendicularly even when the endoscope cannot be placed in the en face position. Joffe (2) has championed the use of the contact endoprobe wherein a sapphire tip is attached to the distal end of a standard quartz fiber. This may allow coaptive coagulation with a 'touch' technique as opposed to the conventional 'no-touch' method. Results are too preliminary at this juncture to speculate on its efficacy and safety compared to the standard method.

Accessories

In addition to routine endoscopic equipment some accessories may be of value. A forceful water pump may be attached to the extra wash channel and it will provide a good cleansing source. An overtube is employed in selected circumstances if reintroduction of the endoscope will be required repeatedly. It is seldom used. There is no good way to remove a large gelatinous clot. Occasionally a sphincterotomy/stone retrieval basket or a polyp grasper is of some use for removing clot from the area of the bleeding site.

Results

Controlled or Prospective Trials

To date 8 (3 9, 11) controlled and one other prospective YAG trial (10) have been done to assess the efficacy and safety of Nd:YAG laser therapy for acute UGIB (3-11). In all of the trials except one by Fleischer (11), the majority of patients have non-variceal bleeding, and most look at patients with peptic ulcer bleeding only.

The published trials can be divided into 3 groups, according to the nature of the lesion treated and the precision used to define the bleeding point and the target for treatment. These are:

a) Hemorrhage from peptic ulcers – endoscopic stigmata of recent hemorrhage and treatment target not fully defined.

b) Hemorrhage from peptic ulcers – bleeding point defined prior to treatment.

c) Hemorrhage from esophageal varices.

No controlled studies have been reported for endoscopic laser treatment of any other lesions causing upper gastrointestinal hemorrhage (such as esophageal gastric or duodenal erosions; Mallory-Weiss tears; vascular lesions or tumors).

Group (a)

The 3 trials in this group were the first to be reported, and used a protocol similar to that developed in 1979 by the American Society for Gastrointestinal Endoscopy (ASGE). They limited inclusion of patients who had a massive bleed (more than 3 units of blood required to restore the circulating blood volume) and who were actively bleeding at the time of initial endoscopy. No further details were given on the nature of the bleeding point for the individual cases in the laser treated and control groups.

Trial 1 (3) was carried out by Ihre et al. in Stockholm, Sweden, and the results for peptic ulcers are shown in Table 12.1. Forty-two patients fulfilled their entry criteria (including ulcers and varices). Twenty-three were randomized to receive laser treatment, but in 8 this was not possible, due to poor access or other technical reasons.

Table 12.1. Results of trial 1 (peptic ulcers only) – Ihre et al.

	Total	Rebleed	Emergency surgery	Died
Laser	12	5	5	2
Control	13	5	5	2

No significant difference.

Trial 2 (4) was carried out by Escourrou et al. in Toulouse, France. Seventy-one ulcers were randomized. Patients were randomized before accessibility to treatment was determined, i.e. whether the laser could be aimed at the bleeding lesion. Full details have not yet been published. Refer to Table 12.2. There was no significant difference between control and laser treated patients with regard to mortality and the need for emergency surgery.

Trial 3 (5) was carried out by Rohde et al. in Marburg, West Germany. One hundred and five patients with active bleeding were randomized. Refer to Table 12.3. There was no difference between the laser and the control groups with

Table 12.2. Results of trial 2 (ulcers) – Escourrou et al.

	Total	Rebleed	Emergency surgery	Died
Gastric ulcers				
Laser	22	7	6	5
Control	23	3	3	4
Duodenal ulcers				
Laser	20	5	5	1
Control	18	4	3	2

No significant difference.

regard to the incidence of recurrent bleeding or mortality. A significantly smaller number in the laser treated group required emergency surgery.

Table 12.3. Results of trial 3 – Rohde et al.

	Total	Rebleed	Emergency surgery	Died
Laser	62	35	13*	24
Control	43	25	41	27

* Significant difference only in rate of emergency surgery.

Group (b)

The 5 trials in this group provide the most precise data currently available both on the importance of the identification of a visible vessel in the crater of an ulcer that has recently bled and on the efficacy of the Nd:YAG lasers in reducing both the need for emergency surgery and the mortality. Trials 4-7 were randomized, double-blind controlled trials and Trial 8 was another type of prospective trial (See Trial 8 below).

Trial 4 (6)

This trial is from Rutgeerts et al. in Belgium. From an unselected series of 338 patients presenting with upper GI hemorrhage, 152 patients with stigmata of recent hemorrhage were included in the trial of which 129 were peptic ulcers (the rest were mostly erosions or Mallory-Weiss tears). Stratification was in 3 groups: spurting arterial hemorrhage, active bleeding (non-spurting) and non-bleeding (red clot or visible vessel). The results (for ulcers only) are shown in Table 12.4.

Table 12.4 Results of trial 4 (peptic ulcers only) – Rutgeerts et al.

		LASER				CONTROL		
	Total	Rebleed	Emergency Surgery	Died	Total	Rebleed (spurting)	Emergency Surgery	Died
Group 1	23	14	14	7(7*)	NIL (ethical reasons)			
Group 2 (active bleeding)	38	2	1	6(1*)	32	12	4	5(4*)
Group 3 (non-bleeding)	14	3	2	2(2*)	22	7	5	3(2*)

* post-rebleed
Rebleeding:
  Group 2 – p <0.001
  Group 3 – no significant difference
  Emergency Surgery – no significant difference

Trial 5 (7)

This trial from MacLeod et al. in Glasgow was limited to patients with major blood loss from peptic ulcers (shock or Hb less than 10 g/dl) and identifiable visible vessels or red or black spots in the ulcer crater at endoscopy (bleeding or not bleeding). From 657 unselected patients, 184 had peptic ulcers. Forty-one fulfilled all the criteria for inclusion and had lesions accessible to laser therapy. None of the 25 with red or black spots rebled (treated or untreated). The results for those with visible vessels are shown in Table 12.5.

Table 12.5. Results of trial 5 (peptic ulcers) – MacLeod et al.

	Total	Rebleed	Emergency surgery	Died
Laser	8	1	1	–
Control	8	8	8	2

Rebleeding: p<0.02.
Emergency surgery: p<0.02.
Mortality: no significant difference.

Trial 6 (8)

In this trial from Swain, Bown et al., patients were stratified into 4 groups: spurting arterial hemorrhage, non-bleeding visible vessels, oozing, and stigmata other than a visible vessel without active bleeding. From 465 unselected admissions for upper gastrointestinal hemorrhage, peptic ulcers were seen in 232. All 101 with stigmata of recent hemorrhage (SRH) accessible to laser therapy were included in the trial (85 had no SRH, 46 were inaccessible or could not be cleaned of overlying clot). The results are shown in Table 12.6.

Table 12.6 Results of trial 6 (peptic ulcers only) – Swain, Bown et al.

	Laser				Control			
	Total	Rebleed	Emergency Surgery	Died	Total	Rebleed	Emergency Surgery	Died
Spurting	10	2	2	1	9	7	6	2
Visible Vessel (not bleeding)	25	2	2	0	29	14	11	5
Oozing or other minor SR H	16	0	0	0	12	1	1	1
Total	51	4	4	1	50	22	18	8

Rebleeding: whole trial p $<$0.001
     spurting and visible vessel
       combined p$<$0.001
     visible vessel alone p$<$0.001
     other SRH: no significant difference

emergency surgery p$<$0.005
mortality p$<$0.05

Trial 7 (9)

In this study by Krejs et al. from Dallas, Texas, patients were divided into two groups – those with active bleeding and those with stigmata of recent hemorrhage. Patients who were so severely ill that they could not be transported to the laser (e.g., on respirators or in intensive care units) were excluded. Patients with active bleeding or SRH who received laser therapy fared no better than controls. Results are shown in Table 12.7.

Table 12.7. Results of trial 7 (peptic ulcers) – Krejs et al.

Active bleeding	Total	Rebleed	Emergency surgery	Died
Laser	20	3	4	1
Control	16	5	4	0
Stigmata recent hemorrhage	*Total*	*Rebleed*	*Emergency surgery*	*Died*
Laser	66	13	9	0
Control	74	13	10	1

No significant differences.

Trial 8 (10)

Trudeau et al., in Sacramento, California, assessed the efficacy of Nd:YAG laser therapy for non- bleeding ulcers with visible vessels in a non-randomized trial. Thirty-three patients were included. Consecutive patients managed by standard treatment (seen by non-laser physicians) were prospectively compared with YAG laser treatment (seen by laser physicians). The incidence of rebleeding and emergency surgery was less in the laser group. The results are shown in Table 12.8.

Table 12.8. Results of trial 8 (non-bleeding visible vessels) – Trudeau et al.

	Total	Rebleed*	Emergency surgery*	Died*
Laser	18	2	1	2
Control	15	6	4	5

*Differences are significant.

Group (c)

Only 2 controlled studies have been reported on laser treatment for hemorrhage from esophageal varices. Both used the Nd:YAG laser and both were small studies. Ihre's results were published with his results for peptic ulcers (3) and are shown in Table 12.9.

Table 12.9. Results of trial 1 (varices only) – Ihre et al.

	Total	Rebleed	Died
Laser	3	3	2
Control	5	3	3

No significant differences.

The other trial, Trial 9, was carried out by Fleischer in Washington (11) and the results are shown in Table 12.10.

Table 12.10. Results of trial 9 (varices) – Fleischer.

	Laser	Control
Total	10	10
Endoscopic hemostasis*	7	0
Rebleed or ongoing bleed	7	7
Died	4	7

* Endoscopic hemostasis significantly different.

For the treatment of hemorrhage from peptic ulcers, the different results obtained in these trials reflect the slightly different questions asked in each. The most convincing results come from the trials that identify which ulcers are at highest risk of further hemorrhage (those with a visible vessel – bleeding or non- bleeding) and limit inclusion to cases in which it is technically possible to apply laser therapy to the precise bleeding point. In the first 3 trials, Group (a), the main criteria for inclusion were a large initial bleed and active bleeding (arterial or diffuse oozing) seen at endoscopy. Arterial hemorrhage was seen

155

in some cases in all trials, but it is not clear how often this occurred in laser treated or control patients or how often the ulcer crater was fully visualized and therapy applied to the precise bleeding point. It is unlikely that shots aimed at fresh blood or clot in an ulcer crater will influence hemorrhage from an underlying artery whose exact position is not known. Even if a spurting artery can be identified, it is technically more difficult to treat than the other larger group of high risk cases: ulcers with a non-bleeding visible vessel, which were included in the later trials. These factors may explain the negative results in these 3 early trials. In addition, in Trial 1, the Nd:YAG laser was used at 50W power, a level found less effective in experimental studies (12). The other 8 Nd:YAG trials used 70-90W. Trial 4 grouped ulcers by the endoscopic findings although the precise bleeding point was not always defined. Their Group 1 consisted of those with spurting arterial hemorrhage. Following a decision of the local ethical committee, there were no control cases in this group. For laser treated cases with spurting, 61% had further bleeding or rebleeding and required urgent surgery. The authors commented that the laser treated cases did better than similar patients treated in the same hospital before a laser was available. Their Group 2 ulcers with active bleeding other than arterial hemorrhage included those oozing from diffuse areas or bleeding around a clot. Some that rebled were found to have an obvious artery under the clot when submitted to surgery, so this group included some high and some low risk lesions, but significant benefit was shown for the treated cases. Although the mortality did not differ, 5% of laser cases rebled vs. 37.5% of controls. Their Group 3 also contained high and low risk lesions as it included non-bleeding visible vessels and lesions in which adherent clot was not cleared. There was a trend towards benefit in the treated cases not quite reaching statistical significance: 21% of laser cases rebled vs. 33% of controls. The mixture of endoscopic stigmata of hemorrhage in Groups 2 and 3 of this trial makes comparisons with other results difficult, but the numbers included were large and the results encouraging.

The other 5 non-variceal trials all tried to identify the exact bleeding point in every case and all stratified ulcers with spurting arteries or non-bleeding visible vessels separately from those with other SRH (oozing from a diffuse area or flecks of red or black clot). Four of these five studies (studies 4, 5, 6, and 8) suggested that endoscopic laser therapy was beneficial. The largest study, the one by Krejs, is the only one of these 5 in which the laser group fared no better than the control. One possible explanation is that the laser is not effective. However, it should be noted that the sickest patients – those too sick to be transported to the laser area – were excluded. It may be in this subgroup that the laser is of most value. In the four other studies the laser was beneficial.

The combined results of all ulcer studies are shown in Table 12.11.

The results of the only controlled study assessing Nd:YAG laser therapy for varices (11) suggest that treatment is reasonably effective for achieving initial hemostasis. However, the benefit is frequently temporary and rebleeding is a problem. It is interesting that Jensen (13) also found the Nd:YAG laser to be

Table 12.11. Combined trial results for Nd:YAG laser (peptic ulcers only).

	# of pts randomized	Major bleed only	Active bleeding + other SRH	Bleeding point defined	Benefit from laser
Ihre	25	+	+	–	NO
Escourrou	83	+	+	–	NO
Rohde	105	+	+	–	NO
Rutgeerts	129	–	–	±	YES
MacLeod	41	+	+	+	YES
Swain	101	–	+	+	YES
Krejs	176	–	+	+	NO
Trudeau	33	–	–	+	YES

effective for initial hemostasis in his variceal model in canines. However, on follow-up endoscopies of Nd:YAG treated varices, esophageal varices were often patent after one week. This suggests that YAG laser treatment alone is not a definitive means for variceal obliteration.

There is no registry in the United States in which the results of endoscopic laser therapy for the treatment of gastrointestinal diseases are collated. Therefore, firm data are lacking. However, some information is available. By mid-1985, there were approximately 300 medical centers using lasers for GI purposes. This represents an astonishing growth. As recently as 1982, less than 30 centers were using lasers. More than 95% of the units have Nd:YAG lasers. A few have only argon lasers and some use both.

It is impossible to know how many patients have been treated with the laser for GI bleeding. Several endoscopists have treated greater than 100 patients. The largest series is that of Dwyer (14). He has utilized the laser for hemorrhage in more than 400 patients. In his unselected series, initial hemostasis was achieved more than 90% of the time. Johnston (15) achieved permanent hemostasis in 68% of patients.

It is encouraging that the complication rate has been acceptably low. Perforations occur with a frequency of 1-2%. Induced bleeding, caused by vaporization of vessel, occurs in about 10% of patients. This has been seen most commonly with the non-bleeding visible vessel in ulcers.

Technique (Fleischer)

Ulcers

Treatment is most likely to be successful when the bleeding site is well-visualized. It is technically easier if the lesion is viewed en face, although this is not always possible. Lesions high in the fundus of the stomach or in the duodenal bulb can be particularly difficult. It may be impossible to locate the source of bleeding on the greater curve of the fundus if the blood cannot be evacuated.

157

If an ulcer with a clear base or a small black or red spot is seen, I do not consider laser treatment. In these situations the incidence of further bleeding with endoscopic treatment is minimal. I consider treatment if a) there is active bleeding; if b) there is a fresh clot on the surface; or if c) there is a non-bleeding visible vessel on the surface.

Controversy exists as to what a visible vessel actually represents and about rates of rebleeding. I believe it may either be an actual vessel protruding through the ulcer crater or a sentinel clot on top of a vessel or a pseudo-aneurysm. These are endoscopically indistinguishable. I also believe that the incidence of rebleeding is high so I treat them if I encounter them. An attempt is made to view the ulcer en face. I aim the beam close to, but not at the vessel. I rim the vessel. Some experienced endoscopists choose to rim the ulcer first and then the vessel, but I do not. After I have rimmed the vessel, I will aim at the vessel. It has been shown that relatively high powers (70–90 watts) and short pulse durations (0.3–0.5 seconds) are most effective. After treatment edema and a white coagulum is seen around the vessel. Induced bleeding occurs in 10–15% of cases, although usually this can be controlled with further treatment. Presumably the energy density is too great and the vessel is vaporized and ruptured prior to successful coagulation.

If the lesion cannot be viewed en face, treatment will be more difficult and less successful. The same principles apply, but with tangential direction of the beam, circumferential therapy is usually not possible and the risk of induced bleeding increases.

The same technique is used when a spurting vessel is encountered, except it is more difficult. In these instances, a catheter with a water jet is particularly useful to tamponade the spurt and to cleanse the area. Often aiming the beam is not as precise and the vessel itself may be treated sooner rather than later.

Some modification occurs if there is a fresh clot sitting on the ulcer. In this situation, I very much prefer a two channel endoscope. After I have secured the best position, I will put the laser fiber down one channel and the second channel will be loaded with an endoscopic accessory used to remove the clot (e.g., a polyp grasper or sphincterotomy basket). I extend the polyp grasper toward the clot and I am poised to fire the laser the second the clot is pulled free. If clot removal leads to active bleeding, I know I will have only 15–60 seconds to clearly see the area where the blood is emanating. If there is a visible vessel, I treat as described above. If the ulcer base is clean under the clot, I don't treat.

Rutgeerts (16) has modified the standard method by pre-treating the ulcer with injection therapy. He uses a sclerotherapy needle to inject a vasoconstrictive agent (e.g. norepinephrine) around the bleeding site prior to laser treatment. He believes this enhances the efficacy of the therapy.

The techniques I discussed are those that I use when I work with the standard non-contact laser fiber. The newly developed sapphire probes may be attached to the end of a modified fiber. They employ laser energy plus coaptation, a technique similar to the heater probe. With these probes, laser energies of 15–20 watts are used and the treated area is actually touched by the sapphire tip. No clinical series using these tips for ulcer bleeding has been reported.

Varices

Although I believe that Nd:YAG laser therapy effectively coagulates many acutely bleeding varices, I do not feel it is definitive therapy. Those who use the laser to treat variceal bleeding often follow it with sclerotherapy.

Treatment is often difficult because an en face view cannot be obtained in the esophagus. With torrential bleeding, clear visualization and aiming at the precise bleeding point is difficult and the risk of aspiration is great. Therefore many, including myself, recommend medical intubation prior to laser therapy. Concomitant intravenous vasopressin may be useful if the bleeding is marked. Some have used a Linton tube to balloon tamponade the inflowing blood stream so the bleeding site can be localized.

Once a site is seen the beam is aimed either directly at it or distal to the bleeding site. Dwyer (14) has advocated the Z-technique, in which he treats the varix as well as surrounding normal tissue to create edema. Powers of 70–90 watts and pulse durations of 0.3–0.5 seconds are used. Hashimoto (1) has reported that the lateral prismatic fiber is particularly effective for treating varices. At the present time it is not commercially available.

UGI Angioma

See the Chapter 6 and 7.

Other Lesions

Mallory-Weiss tears are handled like ulcers. If they have stopped bleeding at the time of endoscopy, I do not treat them since recurrent bleeding is uncommon. Because they are located at the esophagogastric junction, it is usually not possible to obtain an en face view, so usually they are treated tangentially as if one were treating an ulcer. Isolated gastric erosions are handled like small ulcers. I think it is of limited value to treat diffuse erosive gastritis endoscopically. I prefer pharmacologic therapy with prostaglandins. Some advocate treating the largest eroded sites as if one were treating an ulcer. Others feel that a spray technique has merit. In the latter situation, the beam is 4-8 cm away from the tissue. Large spot sizes (e.g., 4-6 cm diameter) are used so that the beam sprays a large area. Stalks of gastric polyps that bleed post-polypectomy may not abate spontaneously. The laser may be aimed at the tip of the stalk remnant or at the base to achieve coagulation.

Discussion

Endoscopic Nd:YAG laser therapy for upper gastrointestinal bleeding is safe. The overall incidence of perforation in a high-risk population is about 1%, an acceptable rate. It also appears to be effective in many instances. The advantage of endoscopic therapy is that it can be piggy-backed to the diagnostic endoscopy, the preferred investigational study of UGI bleeding.

Where endoscopic laser therapy fits into the overall endoscopic armamentarium for patients with UGI bleeding is unknown. Its merits when compared to other modalities are still being debated and defined. So far, no prospective controlled studies have been reported which compare Nd:YAG laser therapy to other endoscopic therapies (e.g., heater probe, BICAP, injection treatment). More scientific information supports the efficacy of the laser than the other modalities, but comparative studies are needed. The main disadvantage of the laser is that it is not portable. Therefore if a bleeding lesion is encountered during an endoscopy in an intensive care unit, a second procedure must be done. If the endoscopist wishes to use another portable modality, he can perform the treatment at once. Laser advocates argue that a patient who is having major hemorrhage should not be handled at a bedside setting, but rather in a specialized area (e.g., endoscopy suite or operating room). In real life, portability is important. On the other hand, the Nd:YAG laser is more versatile than these other instruments and that may be an important feature.

A question that is still unanswered related to the relative merits of contact vs. non-contact for therapy of acute bleeding. One of the initial appeals of laser treatment was that it represented a non-contact technique. The advantages are that it is easier to aim at the bleeding site and there is no chance that the coagulum will be dislodged or pulled off. However, since investigators report that the ability to tamponade the bleeding site as is done with contact methods (e.g., heater probe) is extremely valuable for control of arterial hemorrhage (17). Coaptation decreases blood flow during the thermal delivery, thereby reducing the heat sink effect and also welding the vessel walls more efficiently. The contact probe tips which were discussed above allow the laser to be used for coaptive coagulation and also utilize less power. Whether contact laser tips will be practical and effective for tamponade of active ulcer bleeding and whether they will improve laser hemostasis of such lesions is unknown. The answers to these important questions are awaited with excitement.

Technologic advances are being made so rapidly that treatment methods in the future may be vastly different than those used today. The evolution in the lasers themselves, fibers, endoscopes, and accessories could further revolutionize the field. Perhaps a laser of another wavelength is better-suited for this purpose. In the past few years new delivery systems (contact laser probes, lateral prismatic fibers) have been introduced which offer great promise. Endoscopes will get smaller and undoubtedly give better access to difficult-to-reach areas. The application of accessories could also change the equation. An endoscopic doppler or ultrasound that defined the path and size of feeding vessels would be extremely useful. An effective tool to remove overlying gelatinous clots would also be welcomed.

The endoscopic therapy of UGI bleeding is an exciting area. Laser therapy has been an important step in moving toward a solution. Most complex clinical problems do not have a single solution, but solutions for defined subsets of the problem. It seems likely that laser therapy will be one of the methods used to treat acute UGI bleeding in the future. Technologic advances will undoubtedly affect the equation.

References

1. Hashimoto D. Takami M, and Idezuki Y. Prismatic tip lateral radiation probe in YAG laser endoscopy. Gastrointest Endosc 1985;31:153.
2. Joffe SN, Sankar MY, Salzer D, and Daikuzono N. Preliminary clinical applications of the contact surgical rod and endoscopic microprobes with the Nd:YAG laser. Gastrointest Endosc 1985;31:155.
3. Ihre T, Johansson C, Seligson U et al. Endoscopic YAG laser treatment in massive upper gastrointestinal bleeding. Scand J Gastroenterol 1981;16:633-40.
4. Escourrou J, Frexinos J, Bommelaer G et al. Prospective randomized study of YAG photocoagulation in gastrointestinal bleeding. Proceedings of Laser Tokyo '81. Ed. K Atsumi and N. Nimsakul 1981;5-30.
5. Rohde M, Thon K, Fischer M et al. Results of a defined therapeutic concept of endoscopic neodymium-YAG laser therapy in patients with upper gastrointestinal bleeding. Brit J Surg 1980;67:360.
6. Rutgeerts P, Vantrappen G, Broeckhaert L et al. Controlled trial of YAG laser treatment of upper digestive hemorrhage. Gastroenterology 1982;83:410-416.
7. MacLeod I, Mills PR, Mackenzie JF et al. Neodymium YAG laser photocoagulation for major haemorrhage from peptic ulcers and single vessels. Br Med J 1983;286:345-348.
8. Swain CP, Bown SG, Salmon PR et al. Controlled trial of Nd:YAG laser photocoagulation in bleeding peptic ulcers. Gastrointest Endosc 1984;30:2,137.
9. Krejs GJ, Little KH, Westergaard H, Hamilton JK, and Polter DE. Laser photocoagulation for the treatment of acute peptic ulcer bleeding: A randomized controlled clinical trial. N Engl J Med 1987;316:1618-1622.
10. Trudeau W, Siepler JK, Ross K, Cornish D, and Prindiville T. Endoscopic Nd:YAG laser photocoagulation of bleeding ulcers with visible vessels. Gastrointest Endosc 1985;31:138.
11. Fleischer DE. Endoscopic Nd:YAG laser therapy for active esophageal variceal bleeding. Gastrointest Endosc 1985;31:138.
12. Bown SG, Salmon PR, Storey DW et al. Nd:YAG laser photocoagulation in the dog stomach. GUT 1980;21:818-825.
13. Jensen DM, Silpa MC, Tapia JI, Beilin DB, Machicado GA. Comparison of methods for endoscopic hemostasis of bleeding canine esophageal varices. Gastroenterology 1983;84:1455-1461.
14. Dwyer R. Treatment of upper gastrointestinal bleeding. Washington Laser Symposium. Washington, D.C. April 18, 1985.
15. Johnston J, Sones J, Long B, Posey EL. Comparison of heater probe and YAG laser in endoscopic treatment of major bleeding from peptic ulcers. Gastrointest Endosc 1985;31:175-180.
16. Rutgeerts P, Van Trappen G, Broeckart L, Coremans G, Janssens J, and Geboes K. A new and effective technique of YAG laser photocoagulation for severe upper gastrointestinal bleeding.

Endoscopy 1984;16:115-117.

17. Johnston JJ, Jensen DM, Auth D. Experimental comparison of endoscopic neodymium-yttrium-aluminum-garnet laser, electrosurgery, and heater probe for coagulation of canine gut arteries: Importance of compression and avoidance of erosion. Gastroenterology 1987;92:1101-1108.

13. CANCER IN THE ESOPHAGUS: PRINCIPLES OF LASER TREATMENT

RENE LAMBERT

The 5 year survival rate for esophageal cancer is very low in cancer registries. The crude data (around 3 percent) are not significantly improved when multicentric surveys collect cases either in the surgical, or in the radiation therapy departments, reaching respectively 4 and 6 percent (1, 2). Figures improve when restricted to cases effectively receiving radical treatment. However, the current therapy available in the period 1960-1970 does not significantly alter the natural history of the disease. Radical curative resection of the tumor is the best procedure available, with a 5 year survival rate reaching 20 percent in occidental countries and 50 percent in China or Japan (3, 4, 5). However, curative surgery is only feasible for a small percentage of cases. During the last 10 years, a tendency to improved efficacy of therapy has been observed with a drastic reduction in the post-operative mortality and morbidity, a higher ratio of 'effectiveness to side effects' in radiation therapy (linear accelerator, computerized dose assessment...) and now chemotherapy with new agents (of which the main is cisplatin). An increased survival rate at 1 and 2 years is obtained while long term data are not yet available.

Laser photodestruction of the tumor, introduced in 1982 as a palliative procedure to relieve dysphagia in patients with esophageal cancer, was proposed as an alternative to the endoscopic stent. Now we suggest its application in association with other agents in a combined modality protocol (6, 7), as an approach to a radical non-surgical treatment.

Methodology

Histology of the tumor

Under the term 'cancer in the esophagus', two different tumors have been described: squamous cell carcinoma and adenocarcinoma. However, a clear cut distinction should be made as they differ in etiology, natural history, and susceptibility to treatment.

Squamous cell carcinoma is the main type and is intra- mucosal (in situ) at the early stage. It is often multicentric or associated with cancer in other sites of the upper digestive and respiratory tracts. Rapid mediastinal and abdominal lymphatic spread follows extension to the submucosa. In occidental countries,

D.M. Jensen and J.M. Brunetaud (eds), Medical Laser Endoscopy. 163-176.

the etiology is related to alcohol and tobacco consumption.

Adenocarcinoma in the esophagus is a rare disease when restricted to tumors arising from the Barrett's epithelium (above the esophagogastric junction). It should be distinguished from stomach adenocarcinoma at the cardia arising from the gastric side of the junction and progressing to the lower esophagus. An esophageal obstruction with dysphagia is observed in both situations. Histologic distinction between squamous cell cancer and adenocarcinoma is usually easy but may require repeated biopsies and specific staining when the grade of tumor differentiation is low.

Morphology of the Tumor

In squamous cell cancer the TNM staging is based preoperatively upon radiology, endoscopy, bronchoscopy, CT scan, and ultrasound of the liver, The following characters should be determined:

1) *Location*: In the upper, mid and lower third of the esophagus. The upper third includes tumors of the cervical esophagus at the upper esophageal sphincter (the distance from the incisors is 16-18 cm in fibroscopy). These have poor prognosis. The mid third includes tumors which require a careful analysis of their extension to the bronchial tree.

2) *Length*: Tumors over 10 cm in length, covering more than one third of the esophagus, have an unfavorable prognosis.

3) *Form and degree of parietal invasion*: The pre-1987 TNM classification of esophagal tumors was used in this study. *T1 tumors* are non-circumferential and less than 5 cm in length. Two types should be distinguished, the flat superficial cancer and the exophytic tumors. In the latter condition the presence of an ulceration with parietal infiltration is a factor of poor prognosis as compared to polypoid tumors. *T2 tumors* are either circumferential or more than 5 cm in length. Again two types should be distinguished. Flat superficial tumors may still be classified as early cancer even when circumferential. On the other hand, circumferential tumors obstructing the esophagus may be classified according to their severity into three groups: exophytic or elevated non-stenotic tumors, exophytic ulcerative and stenotic tumors, infiltrative submucosal stenotic tumors. *T3 tumors* have a transparietal extension, including mediastinal invasion; bronchial compression, invasion or fistula; or laryngeal paralysis. In this stage, one should also be included tumors with transparietal lymphatic spread and nodular infiltration of the mucosa at a distance from the primary lesion.

The same TNM stage list will be proposed for adenocarcinoma in the esophagus. However, most tumors are of the T2 or T3 type with circumferential invasion of the full thickness of the esophageal wall. Stage 1 tumors with a superficial and non-circumferential tumor are very unusual.

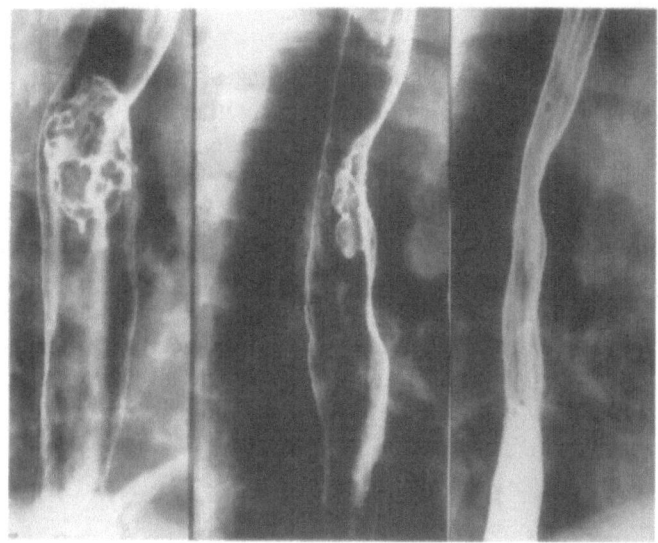

Fig. 13.1. Male patient aged 58. Squamous cell cancer. TNM stage I. Left – before treatment. Middle – at 3 weeks after 1 chemotherapy session and laser photodestruction. Right – at 3 months after radiotherapy (curative protocol). Normal esophageal wall. Biopsies negative.

The patients

Symptoms

Dysphagia should be staged at the first examination of the patient as proposed by Fleischer (8): no dysphagia, restriction to ground foods, restriction to liquids, or total dysphagia. The body weight before symptoms started, weight loss and nutritional status should be recorded, as a basis for the follow-up.

General Condition

Assessment of the health condition of the patient is usually adapted to test the patient for surgery. Three operative contra- indications are designated. 1) Contra-indication due to *old age* is very subjective. However, over the age range 75-80, most cases are not accepted by the surgeon in spite of a good health status. 2) Contra-indication due to *other diseases* is common in patients with a squamous cell cancer such as cirrhosis, respiratory insufficiency, or cardiac failure and 3) contra-indication due to *advanced cancer* (large regional extension, distant metastases) is also common. Extension to the bronchial tree has the worst prognosis.

Case History

New cases include tumors at various TNM stages and the surgical alternative should always be considered before adopting the non- surgical solution. *Previously treated cases* include *persisting evolution* after a non-surgical protocol (radiation therapy, chemotherapy, and esophageal stent). Inflammatory fibrosis is usually associated with cancer infiltration at the site of esophageal obstruction. *Recurrence at the level of anastomosis* after total esophagectomy and an esophago-gastric anastomosis occurs commonly. The neoplastic lesions usually involve both sides of the anastomosis. *Recurrent cancer* at the same site as the primary tumor sometimes follows complete destruction by a non- surgical protocol. *New cancer* at a different site in the esophagus may follow complete destruction of the primary tumor.

Objective of Therapy

Therapy should be designed carefully, often by a multidisciplinary team, taking in account all the parameters previously described.

Palliative Therapy

The objective of palliative therapy has been often questioned and analyzed (9-13). The purpose is symptomatic, i.e. relieving dysphagia. There is no concern as to a prolonged survival. Palliative therapy should be proposed when the patient cannot be submitted to any form of aggressive therapy. If symptomatic relief is not achieved, the palliation should be considered a failure.

Curative or Radical Therapy

The main objective is eradication of the disease and therefore improved survival. If this is not achieved, there is failure. In a surgical protocol, curative surgery means that the resection of any tumoral tissue (primary tumor, lymph nodes, even metastases) is complete. In a non-surgical protocol an assumption of radical treatment is obtained only through the follow-up. As for esophageal cancer, the mucosal surface should return to normal or scar (with negative biopsies) while there is no evidence for lymph nodes mediastinal extension and/or metastases.

The YAG laser session

Relief of esophageal obstruction

Photodestruction of the exophytic part of the tumor in the esophagus is performed with a YAG source. The first step in the presence of a tumoral stenosis is dilation. This is achieved by catheterizing the tumor with an angiographic (rather than metallic) guide wire and passing smooth Savary bougies until the diameter is at least 12.8 mm. The fiberscope is then introduced and a complete examination of the entire tumor stricture is performed including the aboral pole. Laser photodestruction is conducted under visual control while the scope is progressively withdrawn (aboral to oral). The power of the laser source is selected between 70 and 90 Watts, distributing an amount of 3000 to 12000 Joules per session. The use of an unprotected quartz fiber, without coaxial gas insufflation improves the tolerance as well as the technical approach of the tumor by the tip of the fiber. Operation under video control with a camera is convenient because filters can be eliminated from the ocular. The laser session is usually carried out under light premedication. Hospitalization is not required if the preliminary step of bougiennage has not been associated with a complication. Relief of dysphagia is immediate after laser treatment and eating is possible after recovery from the premedication. The initial stage of relief of the obstruction requires 1 to 3 laser sessions at 2 to 3 day intervals but varies with the size of the tumor.

Maintenance Therapy

A palliative protocol requires repeated sessions at 4 to 8 week intervals to maintain a patent lumen in the esophagus. Development of inflammatory fibrosis plays a role in the recurrent stenosis. Therefore sessions often combine dilation and laser photodestruction. YAG laser photodestruction is proposed as a sole procedure when there is contra-indication to the use of radiotherapy or chemotherapy. Such patients are very old (over 80), have an advanced cancer, or very poor health. The objective of the treatment is limited to the relief of dysphagia for a short life span.

Photodynamic Therapy (P.D.T.)

While still under investigation, this procedure is based upon photobiology and the use of a photosensitizing agent (4, 15-20). The main studies were conducted by Lipson (21), Dougherty (16) and Hayata (17). Application to esophageal cancer is limited to squamous cell cancer in a curative protocol. Its use in palliation is not recommended. The patient selected for a PDT treatment is injected with a photosensitizing agent (Photofrin II), which has been proposed for therapeutic and also diagnostic (21, 22) purposes. In the therapeutic protocol, a delay of 48 to 72 hours allows clearance of this agent from the non-tumor tissue. Laser photoradiation is used to activate the hematoporphyrin derivative which in turn is thought to activate tissue oxygen to the 'singlet' status which is cytotoxic. The laser beam (630nm) is usually obtained through a dye laser circulating Rhodamine B and pumped by an argon laser. The tumor should receive between 100 and 200 J/cm2. Prompt necrosis of tumor tissue follows irradiation. Its duration varies according to the depth of the tumor: one week if the cancer is superficial to more than one month if it is implanted in the muscular layer. The patient must completely avoid direct sun exposure for one month to prevent severe sunburn.

This procedure is proposed with a curative objective. Therefore, it is restricted to small or flat tumors. These include superficial cancers as a new case or small recurrence in a patient previously treated and cured by radiotherapy. In these cases, PDT is often proposed as a sole procedure without association of radiotherapy or chemotherapy. In such cases, the management of the patient is simple and there is not risk of cumulative toxicity.

Laser Photodestruction in a Combined Modality Protocol

This protocol is based upon addition of destructive effects from 3 different agents. Radiation is considered as the main agent in the therapeutic course (23, 24). Potentiation rather than addition characterizes the action of adjuvant chemotherapy. The basic principle of the combined modality protocol is the reduction of the tumor mass prior to radiotherapy and/or surgical excision (25-30). According to Steiger (29), complete destruction of the tumor tissue is achieved by the association of chemotherapy-radiotherapy in one case out of three submitted to radical resection after this adjuvant therapy. Laser photodestruction will help to reduce the tumor mass but its role is not a principal one.

We propose a *protocol course of 13 weeks*:

Week 1: Requires hospital admission. Screening of the tumor and first chemotherapy course during 4 days of continuous venous infusion as proposed by Steiger (29): 5 FU 1 g/m² per day – 4 days, Cisplatin 80 mg/m² – 1 day. In patients over the age of 70, half the dose is prescribed. For patients over age 80, indications are limited to patients in very good health. A contra-indication to the use of the cisplatin is significant renal insufficiency. An objective response to chemotherapy is detected in 80% of cases, either at endoscopy (partial necrosis and ischemia of the tumor) or at radiology (reduction in the volume). YAG laser photodestruction is performed at the end of the chemotherapy course, requiring 1 or 2 sessions.

Weeks 2 and 3: The patients is at home and receives no therapy. This is a period of elimination of the necrotic tissue and reduction of inflammation.

Weeks 4 to 8: As an outpatient, the patients receives radiation therapy to the mediastinal and sub-clavicular areas (linear accelerator 18 to 24 MeV). The curative protocol includes 25 x 2 gy sessions in 5 weeks. It is adopted in patients in good health to minimize the side effects compared to the efficacy. In patients in poor health (or advance cancer disease), the dosimetry is concentrated: 10 x 3 gy sessions on weeks 4 and 5. During this period 1 to 2 sessions of chemotherapy are performed (weeks 4 and 8) as an adjuvant to radiation efficacy. This period requires admission to the hospital.

Weeks 9 to 12: The patient is at home on no treatment.

Week 13: Further dose of radiotherapy is given as 5 x 12 gy sessions, resulting in a full dose of 60 gy in the curative protocol. In patients submitted to the concentrated palliative protocol (split), 5 x 3 gy sessions are performed on week 10.

Late follow-up: During the following months, 1 to 3 further chemotherapy sessions may be prescribed according to the patient's status.

Personal experience with YAG laser photodestruction of esophageal cancer

In the first four years of treatment, we treated 355 patients:

Cases

Squamous cell cancer: For 266 patients, 70% were new cases and 30% were previously treated with other therapy. YAG laser was the only therapy in 35%, and YAG laser was used in a combined protocol in 65%. The tumor stages were: T1 = 20%, T2 = 40%, and T3 = 40%.

Adenocarcinoma in the esophagus (tumor in Barrett's epithelium): 14 cases

Adenocarcinoma in the esophagus (tumor extension from the cardia): 61 cases

Adenocarcinoma in the esophagus (tumor recurrence after gastrectomy for cancer): 14 cases located at the anastomosis.

Method

In most patients (338 cases) laser photodestruction was obtained through the YAG source. PDT was given to 31 patients, of which 23 had squamous cell carcinoma and 8 had adenocarcinoma (14 of these patients had also received YAG laser).

Results

Symptoms

Laser destruction of tumor

Relief of dysphagia is obtained in most cases when an exophytic tumor is the cause (6, 7, 31-37). Patients with moderate dysphagia (eating of ground food prior to treatment) return to normal. Patients with total or severe dysphagia return to moderate dysphagia. Complete failure is rare (less than 10%). Failure occurs in the following conditions: 1) failure to catheterize the tumor channel, 2) tumor with a bronchial fistula, 3) infiltrative submucosal tumor with a very narrow lumen, and 4) tumor located at the upper esophageal sphincter altering the mechanism of swallowing. On the other hand, the best results are obtained in exophytic non-circumferential tumors. If a combined modality protocol is adopted, relief of the dysphagia may be long lasting. Therefore, the weight loss is corrected and the patient is asymptomatic during the follow-up.

Maintenance therapy

Repeated laser sessions in a palliative protocol are required at intervals of 4-8 weeks to maintain luminal patency at an acceptable level and prevent dysphagia. Indeed, recurrence is observed after a few weeks. The limiting factors are the growth of the tumor and the progression of inflammation with fibrosis.

Therefore, sessions require combined dilation and photodestruction. On average, the patient is maintained with a moderate dysphagia and a stable weight without recovering normal predisease weight. The indication for an esophageal stent or a gastrostomy is delayed or postponed until the terminal period (death from advanced cancer or other disease). Best results are obtained in exophytic, non-circumferential tumors located at a distance from the bronchial tree and the upper esophageal sphincter.

Survival

Survival in the palliative protocol

The average life span of the patient is very short. In *squamous cell carcinoma*, most patients die during the first 6 months from advanced cancer or other disease. The median survival varies from 3 to 4 months (6, 7, 8, 10, 31-36) with a small group (less than 10% living at least 1 year). The endoscopic stent has been extensively analyzed in relation to the survival period (9, 11, 38, 39). It should not be proposed as an alternative to laser palliation but rather as a second stage treatment when fibrosis plus transparietal infiltration are the

170

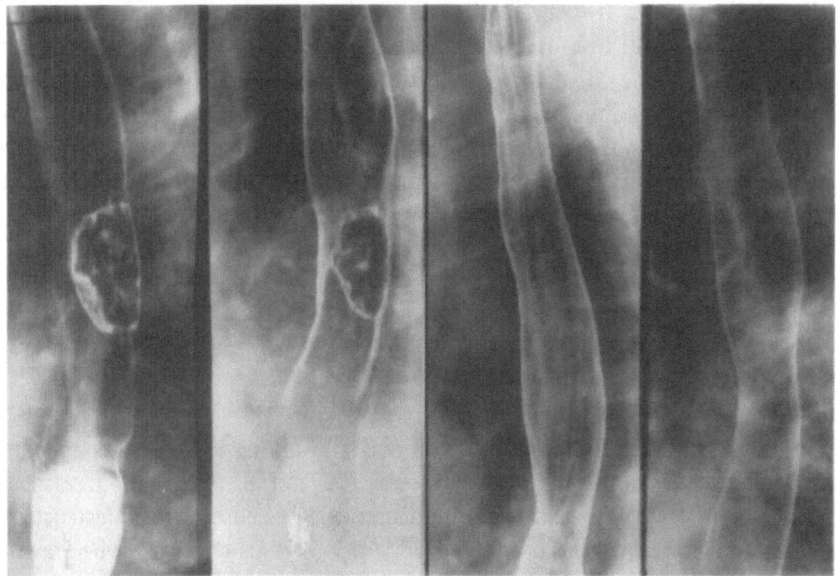

Fig. 13.2. Male patient aged 63. Squamous cell cancer. TNM stage I. Left – before treatment. Second left – at 1 week after 1 chemotherapy session. Second right – at 3 months after laser photodestruction. Right – at 3 weeks (esophageal mucosa returns to normal).

major problems. In *adenocarcinoma*, similar figures are obtained. For example, in our experience, the median survival is limited to 2.6 months while the mean survival reaches 3.9 months. A small percentage of patients in this group have a longer life span. About 30% survive at least 6 months and nearly 10% survive at least one year. An esophageal stent is the only alternative. It should be remembered that the distal pole of the stent has to be inserted in the stomach. This situation requires prevention of reflux.

Survival in the combined modality protocol

This protocol is proposed for patients with squamous cell carcinoma in different condition. Extremes might include young patients in good health with a small superficial T1 cancer (prolonged radiation therapy protocol) as one condition and a patient still in good health with an advanced inextirpable cancer with bronchial invasion and/or metastases (split radiation therapy) on the opposite extreme. Therefore, external factors such as age, associated diseases, or the presence of metastases must be taken into account when one is interpreting data concerning the primary tumor. Very preliminary results are available. In our experience, the global rate of survival at one year reaches 80% in T1 tumors, decreases to 40% in T2 tumors and is only 20% in T3 tumors. In the latter group, some patients survive in good health for more than 1 year. Cancer evolution in patients submitted to the combined modality protocol include: 1) persisting local evolution with fibrosis and/or necrosis with fistula in the mediastinum, 2) recurring cancer at the same location after complete healing of the initial lesion, 3) distant metastases (liver and lung) while the esophageal wall is negative for cancer, or 4) development of a new cancer at another site in the esophagus or in the upper pulmonary or digestive tract. As for adenocarcinoma, a combined protocol treatment with laser photodestruction and radiotherapy is proposed to some inoperable patients when the tumor is at an early stage.

Complications

Perforation

This is the main complication. It will occur in about 1% of cases and may result in severe symptoms or death. At the initial phase of treatment, perforation may be correlated with excessive YAG laser photodestruction. However, previous dilation combined with photodestruction on withdrawing the scope substantially reduces risk. Perforation can be induced at the stage of dilation prior to laser irradiation. Risk factors include very infiltrative tumors, location near the bronchial bifurcation and previous radiation therapy. Perforation into the mediastinum is treated by intubation, positioning of a nasogastric tube, antibiotics and parenteral nutrition. Recovery without sepsis is frequent. There is no need for surgical management in such patients. The combined protocol (laser sessions, chemotherapy, and radiotherapy) is postponed for 1 to 3 weeks if a perforation occurs. Later, at the stage of maintenance therapy or during the follow-up of a combined therapy protocol, perforation may occur into the mediastinum or bronchial tree. It is not usually induced by laser radiation. Factors involved include dilation, natural progression of the disease, and radiation therapy. The management is similar to the initial stage.

Complications of chemotherapy

If the exclusion criteria concerning renal insufficiency are followed, the tolerance to 1-5 sessions of chemotherapy is excellent. In a few patients (about 5%), transient medullary aplasia results. Further sessions of chemotherapy are not recommended in such cases.

Complications of PDT

If the principles concerning sun exposure are followed, skin tolerance is excellent and reactions are limited to a suntan. We observed edema and burns in 2 patients who had exposed themselves to direct sunlight. On the other hand, a cumulative toxicity for the skin may be observed if radiation therapy is performed with too short a delay (less than 6 weeks) after Photofrin injection.

In such conditions we observed 2 cases of severe radiation epithelitis.

Indications in squamous cell cancer

Laser photodestruction in monotherapy (palliative protocol)

Relief of esophageal obstruction is proposed in presence of severe dysphagia when there is a simultaneous contra-indication for surgical resection and for aggressive non-surgical procedures (radiation therapy or chemotherapy). This concerns patients in poor health, at a late stage of the disease, or when all other procedures have been rejected. Effective symptomatic relief may be obtained when the tumor is exophytic and non-circumferential. The limitations of the laser method should be recalled: presence of a bronchial-esophageal fistula or infiltrative submucosal tumor. A stent should be placed in such patients. When the tumor is located at the upper esophageal sphincter, the only possibility is often a gastrostomy (performed by the percutaneous route). In patients with persisting symptoms and tumor in the esophagus after radiation therapy, laser photodestruction is proposed and may eventually be combined with chemotherapy. Similar indications for laser photodestruction are found when recurrent cancer obstructs the esophageal lumen near the anastomosis after gastrectomy for stomach cancer.

Laser photodestruction in the combined modality protocol

Surgical versus non-surgical treatment

Adoption of a non-surgical protocol requires a cautious analysis of the surgical alternative in patients who could be submitted to a radical procedure. Of course, small resectable tumors detected in 'poor risk' patients are excellent indications for a non- surgical protocol. When it is assumed from preliminary exploration that surgical extirpation of the tumor tissue would be incomplete, a non-surgical treatment is usually preferred to palliative surgery. The indications for surgical palliation are now quite limited. However, surgery should still be proposed to a young patient with a circumferential, infiltrative tumor invading the mediastinum. Surgical bypass followed by radiation therapy will give a better symptomatic relief than the endoscopic treatment of obstruction. Taking into account the present status of the disease, its detection, and its treatment in occidental countries, most cases can be managed without surgery. In a small percentage of patients, radical surgery is still proposed but this occurs in less than 10% of cases. Such an approach is for patients with tumors at the T1 or T2 stage.

TNM staging and the non-surgical protocol

T1 tumors: Best results are obtained in superficial and in exophytic, non-ulcerated cancers. The protocol can be proposed to patients in a good health even if they are young. When the morphology of the tumor includes elevation and ulceration, surgery should be recommended for young patients.

T2 tumors: Results are not as good as in the T1 stage, especially if the tumor is circumferential and infiltrative. Therefore, surgery should be proposed to young patients in good health.

T3 tumors are an elective indication for the non-surgical protocol. When there is invasion (but no fistula) of the bronchial tree, adjuvant chemotherapy is a fundamental approach. Radiation therapy should be proposed only if there is regression of the bronchial lesion. This prevents perforation. When there is no regression, positioning of a stent is recommended prior to radiation.

Photodynamic therapy

The method is proposed only for patients with a squamous cell carcinoma in the following conditions. 1) Superficial cancer, small or extensive, detected in a patient at a very old age, or with a very high operative risk or 2) recurrent cancer after a previous treatment (radiation therapy or esophagectomy) when the lesion is small (less than 3 cm) and of slight elevation. When these criteria are used, a complete destruction of the tumor is usual with return of normal mucosa.

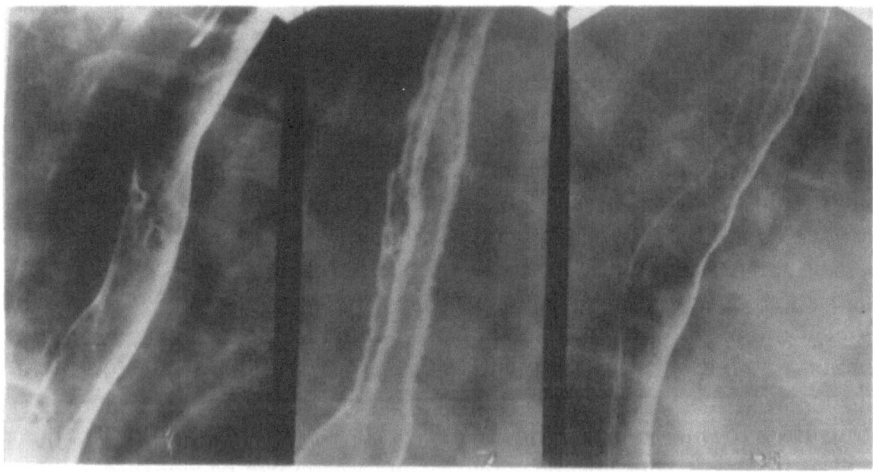

Fig. 13.3. Female patient aged 83. Squamous cell cancer. TNM stage I. Left – before treatment. Middle – after photodynamic therapy at one week (extensive mucosal necrosis). Right – at 3 weeks (esophageal mucosa returns to normal). From left to right.

PDT alone is prescribed in patients previously treated or in 'new cases' at a very old age. PDT is included in a combined modality protocol in 'new patients' with good health.

References

1. Cunha Melo Jr. Oesophageal squamous cell carcinoma: I. A critical review of surgery. Brit J Surg 1980;67:381-390.
2. Cunha Melo Jr. Oesophageal squamous cell carcinoma: II. A critical review of radiology. Brit J Surg 1980;67:457-461.
3. Tsurumaru M, Kawamura T et al. Principles of surgical treatment for carcinoma of the esophagus. Analysis of lymph node involvement. Ann Surg 1981:194;438-446.
4. Launois B, Paul JL, Lygidakis NJ et al. Results of the surgical treatment of carcinoma of the esophagus. Surg Gynecol Obstet 1983;156:753-760.
5. Wu Yink D'Ai, Huang Kuo Chun. Chinese experience in the surgical treatment of carcinoma of the esophagus. Ann Surg 1979;190:361-365.
6. Lambert R, Sabben G, Chavaillon A et al. Nd-YAG laser treatment in epidermoid esophageal cancer. Lasers Surg Med 1984;3:340.
7. Lambert R, Sabben G, Chavaillon A et al. Nd-YAG laser therapy for epidermoid cancer of the esophagus. Gastroenterology 1984;86:1151.
8. Fleischer D, Kessler F. endocopic Nd-YAG laser therapy for carcinoma of the esophagus: a new form of palliative treatment. Gastroenterology 1983:85:600-606.
9. Den Hartog Jager FCA, Bartelsman JF et al. Palliative treatment of obstructing esophago-gastric malignancy by endoscopic positioning of a plastic prothesis. Gastroenterology 1979;77:1008-1014.
10. Fleischer D, Kessler F, Haye O. Endoscopic Nd-YAG laser therapy for carcinoma of the esophagus: A new palliative approach. Am J Surg 1982;143:280-283.
11. Graham DY, Dobbs SM, Zubler M. What is the role of prosthesis insertion in esophageal carcinoma? Gastrointest Endosc 1983;29:15.
12. Hankins JR, Cole FN, Attar S, McLaughlin JS. Carcinoma of the esophagus: Twelve year's experience with a philosophy for palliation. Ann Thorac Surg 1982;33:464.
13. Orringer MB. Palliative procedures for esophageal cancer. Surg Clin North Am 1982;63:941-950.
14. Diamond I, Granelli S, McDonagh AF et al. Photodynamic therapy of malignant tumors. Lancet 1972;2:1175.
15. Dougherty TJ, Grindey GB, Fiel R, Weishaupt KR et al. Photoradiation therapy: II. Cure of animal tumors with hematoporphyrin and light. J Natl Cancer Inst 1974;55:115.
16. Dougherty TJ, Kaufman JH, Goldfard A et al. Photoradiation therapy for the treatment of malignant tumors. cancer Res 1978;38:2628.
17. Hayata Y, Kato H, Aida H et al. Laser photoradiation therapy for early stage esophagus and stomach cancer. Scand J Gastroenterol 1982;17:128.
18. Hematopophyrin derivative radiation therpy. In Lasers Surg Med – Special issue – 1984;4:1-131.
19. Lambert R, Sabben G. Cancer in the esophagus: treatment by photoradiation therapy. Lasers Surg Med 1964;3:341.
20. McCaughan JS, Hicks W, Laufman L et al. Palliation of esophageal malignancy with photoradiation therapy. Cancer 1984;54:2905-2910.
21. Lipson RL, Blades EJ, Olsen AM. Hematopophyrin derivative: A new aid of endoscopic detection of malignant disease. J Thoracic Cardiovasc 1961;42:623.
22. Gregorie HB Jr, Jorger EO, Ward JL et al. Hematopophyrin derivative fluorescence in malignant neoplasms. Ann Surg 1968;167:829.
23. Pearson JG. The present status and future potential of radiothreapy in the management of

oesophageal cancer. Cancer 1977;39:882-886.

24. Zong YIY, Gu XZ, Zhoo S et al. Long term survival of radiotherapy for esophageal cancer: analysis of 1136 patients surviving for more than 5 years. Int J Radiat Oncol Biol Phys 1983;9:1769-1773.

25. Advani SH, Saikia TK, Swaroop S et al. Anterior chemotherapy in esophageal cancer. Cancer 1985;56:1502-1506.

26. Bains MS, Kelsen DP, Beattie EJ et al. Treatment of esophageal carcinoma by combined preoperative chemotherapy. Ann Thorac Surg 1982;34:521.

27. Franklin R, Steiger Z, Vaishampayan G et al. Combined modality therapy for esophageal squamous cell carcinoma. Cancer 1983;51:1062-1071.

28. Kelsen DP, Bains A, Hilaris B et al. Combination chemotherapy of esophageal carcinoma using cisplatin, vindesine and bleomycin. Cancer 1982;49:1174-1177.

29. Steiger A, Francklin R, Wilson RF et al. Eradication and palliation of squamous cell carcinoma of the esophagus with chemotherapy, radiotherapy and surgical therapy. J Thorac Cardivasc Surg 1981;82:713-719.

30. Resbent M, Le Prise Fleury E, Benhassel M et al. Squamous cell carcinoma of the esophagus: treatment by combined vincristine – methotrexate plus folinic acid rescue and cisplatin before radiotherapy. Cancer 1985;1246-1250.

31. Fleischer D. Endoscopic laser therapy for gastrointestinal disease. Arch Intern Med 1984;144:1225-1230.

32. Fleischer D. Endoscopic laser therapy for upper gastrointestinal tract disease. Surv Dig Dis 1983;1:42-53.

33. Fleischer DE, Sivak MV. Selection of patients with esophagogastric cancer for endoscopic laser therapy: factors affecting outcome. Lasers Surg Med 1984;3:340.

34. Buset M, Dunham F, Baize M et al. Nd-YAG laser, a new palliative alternative in the management of esophageal cancer. Endoscopy 1983;15:353-356.

35. Mellow MH, Pinkas H. Endoscopic laser therapy for malignancies affecting the esophagus and gastroesophageal junction. Lasers Surg Med 1983;3:342.

36. Sabben G, Lambert R. Les Lasers en gastroenterologie. Gastroenterol Clin Biol 1984;8;165-176.

37. Groisser VW. YAG laser therapy of gastrointestinal tumors. Gastro Intest Endosc 1984;30:311-312.

38. Ogilvie AL, Dronfield MW, Ferguson R, Atkinson M. Palliative intubation of oesophago-gastric neoplasms at fiberoptic endoscopy. Gut 1982;23:1060-1067.

39. Rose JDR, Smith PM. Fibre endoscopic insertion of palliative oesophageal tube with the Nottingham introducer. JR Soc Med 1983;76:266-268.

14. ENDOSCOPIC TREATMENT OF UPPER GASTROINTESTINAL TUMORS

DAVID FLEISCHER

Introduction

When esophageal cancer is diagnosed, cure is seldom possible and palliation is the usual goal. Of the several forms of palliative treatment, all have limitations. Although potentially the most definitive, surgery has the highest morbidity and mortality. Often patients are designated as 'not surgical candidates.' Radiation therapy has several limitations.

Relief of symptoms may not occur until weeks after the treatment has begun. Additionally, if the patient has recurrence after a previous attempt at curative radiation therapy, he cannot be given a second course. Chemotherapy is seldom the only therapy chosen and the most effective agents have significant toxicity. Dilatation has the distinct advantages of being simple and inexpensive, but generally the benefit becomes short-lived as the disease progresses and eventually the patient and the doctor decide that it is not productive. The placement endoscopically of an esophageal prosthesis is valuable in some patients. This is the treatment of choice for patients who have tracheo-esophageal fistulae. Stent dislodgment and obstruction are recognized complications. Gastrostomy or jejunostomy are viewed by most as last resorts. Although they provide a conduit for nutrition, they eliminate the pleasure of eating.

Into this milieu of palliative therapies, came endoscopy laser therapy (ELT). Since my initial description in 1982 (1), more than 2000 patients have been treated in the United States, Europe and Japan. ELT has the appeal of being performed under direct vision and without general anesthesia. Unlike radiation therapy, there is no limitation to the number of sessions a patient may undergo. Initial results have been encouraging, but it is impossible to know how it should fit into the overall therapy of esophageal cancer since there are no comparative data. No randomized studies of laser versus other therapies have been reported. In most medical centers, conventional wisdom and local politics dictate what treatment is given, rather than conclusive scientific information. The purpose of this chapter is to review the techniques and results of ELT for tumors of the esophagus and gastric cardia.

D.M. Jensen and J.M. Brunetaud (eds), Medical Laser Endoscopy. 177-188.
© 1990 Kluwer Academic Publishers, Dordrecht

Evaluation

Not all patients are candidates of ELT. If there is any possibility of cure, surgery should be advised. If the patient is anorectic, markedly debilitated, or close to death, the physician must ask if an open lumen will benefit the patient. In many cases, the answer is no.

It is also important that the physician and the patient define the goals of therapy. The patient must understand that treatment will not be curative but palliative in most cases. The physician is best equipped to proceed if he defines his endpoint in advance of therapy. Before ELT begins, the physician should consider whether ancillary treatment is planned. We do not know the best sequence of combined modality therapy. If more than one therapy will be used, the endoscopist should plan the combinations in advance.

It is useful for each patient to have three diagnostic studies before beginning ELT – a barium swallow, a screening endoscopy, and an imaging study (CT, NMR or EUS). The barium swallow is the best test to look for a tracheo-esophageal fistula and helps to define the extraluminal anatomy. The endoscopy allows the physician to plan therapy and answer several specific questions: will dilatation be required? which endoscope will be used? how many treatments will be needed? Either a thoracic/abdominal computerized tomogram (CT) or nuclear magnetic resonance (NMR) study will provide important information. Endoscopic ultrusonography, a newer technology, shows promise for localizing extent J. tumor penetration and local nodal involvement. These may help determine the extent of the tumor, the thickness of the esophageal wall, and the proximity of the neoplasm to other critical structures (e.g., trachea, bronchi, aorta, left ventricle, etc.).

Equipment

My experience is with a Nd:YAG laser at a power output of 90-120 watts I have a wide variety of endoscopes available. Single channel instruments ranging from 7 to 13 mm have been employed as well as two channel instruments. Often only the smaller gastrointestinal endoscopes or bronchoscopes can maneuver through the tumor and they must be used. Most commonly I employ a 9 mm endoscope with a single 2.8 mm channel. The endoscope should have the tip modified. A white heat resistant material should be exchanged for the routine black plastic. Ideally a protective eye filter will be built into the endoscope. Adaptors can be attached to the proximal entry port of the biopsy channel to exhaust gas.

The YAG laser waveguide has a quartz fiber of 400-600 microns with a cladding that increases the fiber diameter to 1 millimeter. A plastic sheath brings the outer diameter to 2 mm (Fig. 14.1). Coaxial gas flow protects the fiber. My experience has been accumulated with these conventional fibers. I sometimes prefer to use the naked (1 mm) fiber without the surrounding

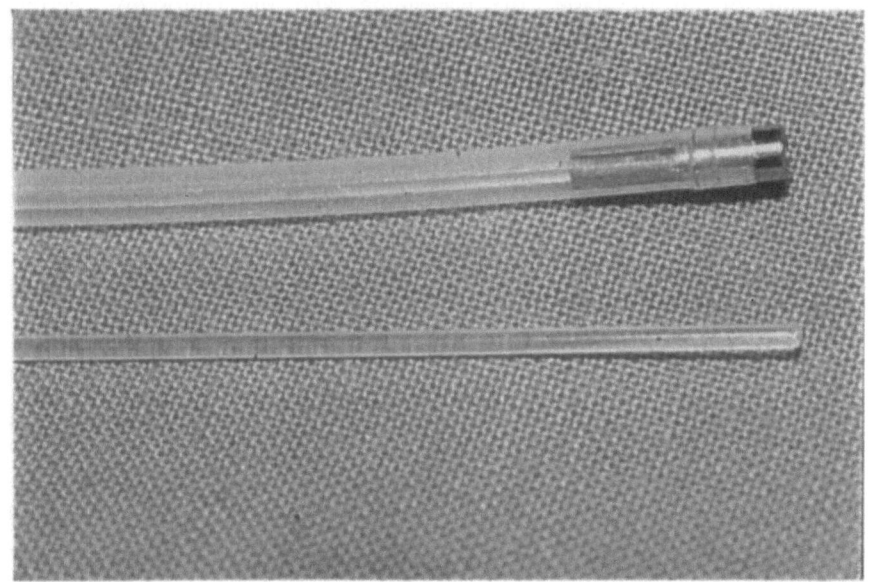

Fig. 14.1. Quartz fibers of Nd:YAG lasers. Sheathed (top) and unsheathed /naked (bottom).

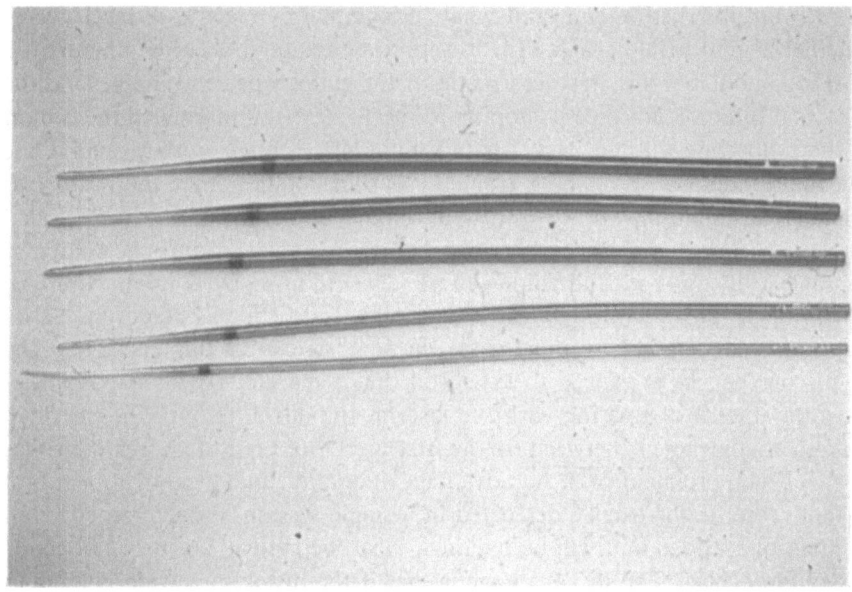

Fig. 14.2. Savary dilators. Tapered polyvinyl dilators which fit over specially made guidewire.

sheath. It provides 2 major advantages. Gaseous overdistention is avoided and it can be used with smaller diameter endoscopes. However, the risk of contaminating and melting the fiber tip is increased without the gas flow to protect it. With conventional fibers the laser beam exits straight ahead with a beam divergence of 8-10°.

In addition to the laser, the waveguide, and the endoscope, certain accessories are necessary. Dilation is often part of the procedure. A guidewire delivery system of dilators first described by Savary (2) have been extremely valuable. They represent a modification of and advance over the Eder-Puestow dilators (Fig. 14.2). Additionally, a variety of accessories to remove necrotic tissue or to debride tumor must be at hand. These include biopsy and grasping forceps, sphincterotomy baskets, water pumps and brushes.

Preparation and technique

(Refer also to Plates 35-38 in the Atlas.)

General anesthesia is not required. Intravenous sedation with meperidine (Demerol®) or sublimaze and midazolam (Versed®) is given. If there is complete esophageal obstruction or if the tumor is high in the esophagus, an anticholinergic agent is given to decrease salivary secretions. At least two health personnel should accompany the physician, one to care for the patient and one to work with the physician and/or the laser.

The procedure begins with the introduction of a small diameter endoscope. It is advanced to the superior margin of the tumor and the topography is surveyed. I note whether the tumor is exophytic or submucosal, whether or not there is an obstruction rim, and what the luminal diameter will be. I decide whether a stent would seat well if it were to be required. At this juncture, no decision about stenting has been made. If the endoscope can pass beyond the proximal tumor, I advance it, hoping to reach the distal margin to the tumor. If the endoscope will not pass, I pass a guidewire through so that I can dilate the tumor stenosis. If I know from the barium swallow that the passage is relatively straight I may proceed without fluoroscopy. If the X-Ray had revealed a tortuous course or if I encounter the slightest resistance during the guidewire passage, I do not pass the guidewire blindly. Fluoroscopy is used. After the guidewire is passed through the tumor, the endoscope is removed. Serial dilation is carried out. In most cases the stenosis can be dilated so that the endoscope can be advanced to the distal tumor margin. If this is possible, I have the option of treating with the laser at the distal margin, the proximal margin or anywhere in between. In the first cases that I reported, treatment was always begun proximally (1). An advantage of dilation and distal treatment first is that more tumor can be destroyed in a single session, reducing the overall number of sessions that will be required. Also the patient can be suctioned if distention occurs. The disadvantage is that if the distal narrowing is tight, it is technically difficult to aim the beam when the endoscope is wedged into the tumor. Often the fiber has to be turned directly toward the esophageal wall which will increase the possibility of perforation. Also the treatment site is very close to the tip of the endoscope and heat and carbon debris from the tissue vaporization may damage the instrument.

If treatment is begun distally, the endoscope is withdrawn and ELT continues during the withdrawal. Every attempt is made to keep the endoscope and the beam in the axis of the lumen. This minimizes the risk of perforation.

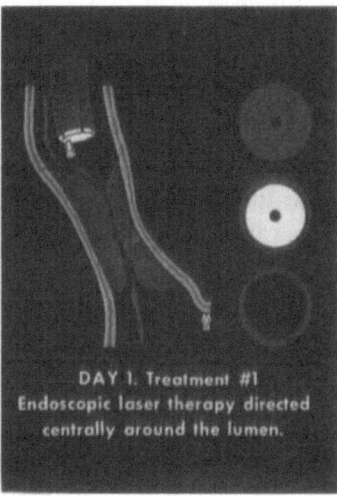

Fig. 14.3. Technique – En face treatment of proximal margin. The laser beam is aimed centrally around the lumen. Circumferential treatment proceeds toward but not to esophageal wall. Initially tumor tissues whiten with coagulation and then blacken with vaporization.

When the scope is in position to treat the superior margin of the tumor, certain principles are applied. This position may have been reached by the withdrawal or a decision may have been made to start the treatment proximally. Technically this is the easiest position from which to treat. The beam is aimed circumferentially around the lumen, beginning centrally and advancing toward but not to normal esophageal wall. Initially a coagulative effect will be seen. The endoscopic correlate is whitening. If further energy is delivered the tissue heats even more, and vaporization is noted. The endoscopic correlate is black charring, the formation of divots, or actual evaporation of tissue. Smoke is present. the endpoint is reached when the entire superior margin has been vaporized.

The physician just beginning to use the laser is anxious to know how much energy should be used. What are the laser settings for power and duration? What is the total energy that should be applied for each session? An experienced endoscopist chuckles to himself, because he knows that no such answers exist, but remembers he asked the same questions before he began to use the laser.

Because the beam exits from the fiber tip at a divergent angle, the energy density (energy/unit area) varies considerable with distance. If the tip is 1 centimeter from the tumor, the energy will be considerably greater than if it is 3 cm away. Yet the recorder on the laser would register the same total energy, since it does not factor distance into the equation. Therefore, it is the tissue effect that the experienced endoscopist uses as his guideline. A setting of 50 watts for 1 second at a distance of 0.5 cm from the tissue may cause vaporization just as 100 watts x 1 second from 2 cm may cause vaporization.

Having said that, I set the laser at a power of 90-100 watts with pulse durations of 2.5 seconds. I attempt to place the tip of the fiber one centimeter from the tissue. But it is the tissue effect, the signs of vaporization, that I care about, not the readings on the machine.

If the treatment session was done on Day #1, a second session is planned on Day #3. The 48-hour interval serves two purposes. Maximal tissue necrosis will occur at this juncture so that it will be easier to debride and the patient is usually grateful for the rest between procedures.

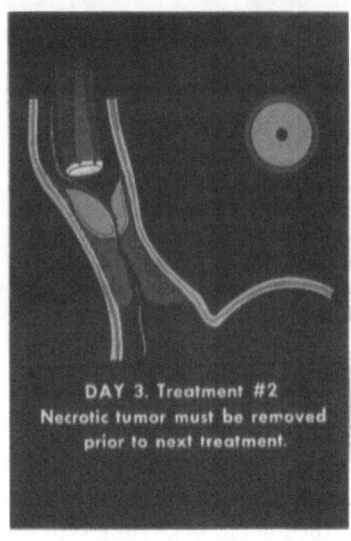

Fig. 14.4. Illustration of the antegrade approach. On Day 3 necrotic cancer must be removed with a suction tube or debrided by dilatation before further therapy.

Attention must be given to nutrition in the interim. If there is some luminal opening, full liquids with nutritional supplements can be used. If the lumen is obstructed or if several sessions will be required, parenteral nutrition must be considered. Additionally, the patient must be warned that after a laser session dysphagia may actually increase temporarily because of tissue edema.

At the beginning of the second session on Day #3, a screening endoscopy is performed with a small diameter endoscope. This allows me to determine the efficacy of the previous therapy and to plan ELT for that day. Usually the session begins with guidewire dilation. The logic is similar to its use on Day #1 and it has the additional benefit of debriding necrotic tissue.

Serial treatments are carried out until the endpoint is reached. I often document lumen size with repeat barium swallow. Refer to Fig. 14.4 for an example of barium swallow before and after treatment. Although the clinical and endoscopic goals must be individualized, I prefer to obtain passage of an 11 mm endoscope if possible. Consideration should be given to additional treatment that may be required (e.g., chemotherapy, radiation, stent).

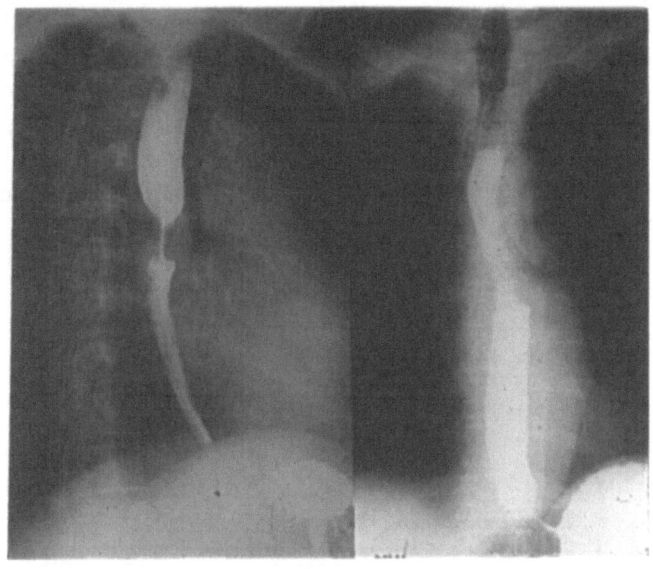

Fig. 14.5. Barium swallow showing esophageal cancer before and after laser therapy.

Results

My series is the largest American series, with 120 patients in Washington (Veterans Administration Medical Center, Washington Hospital Center, Georgetown University Hospital) and Cleveland (Cleveland Clinic Foundation) by July, 1985. Seventy percent had primary squamous cell carcinoma of the esophagus and most of the remaining patients had adenocarcinoma involving the distal esophagus and proximal stomach. Refer to Table 14.1. The majority of patients had prior non-laser therapy. The mean number of laser sessions to achieve luminal patency was 3.6 for squamous cell carcinoma and 2.8 for adenocarcinoma of the GE junction.

Table 14.1. Palliation of esophagogastric cancer (clinical – endoscopic aspects).

	Squamous cell	*Adenocarcinoma*	*Total*
Patients	81	39	120
Prior RX			
Radiation	39	0	39
Surgery	9	20	29
Both	7	3	10
Dilatation	67	30	97
Mean YAG laser RXs	3.6	2.8	3.3

From our experience, Sivak and I (3) identified parameters which predicted good or poor initial outcomes (Figs. 14.6 and 14.7). The endoscopic appearance was extremely important. If the tumor was exophytic and predominantly mucosal, treatment was technically much easier and clinical improvement was better than when the tumor was extrinsic or primarily submucosal. The location in the esophagus was another useful parameter. Tumors in the cervical esophagus generally had the poorest outcome. Treatment was often difficult or impossible if the tumor abutted upon the cricopharyngeus.

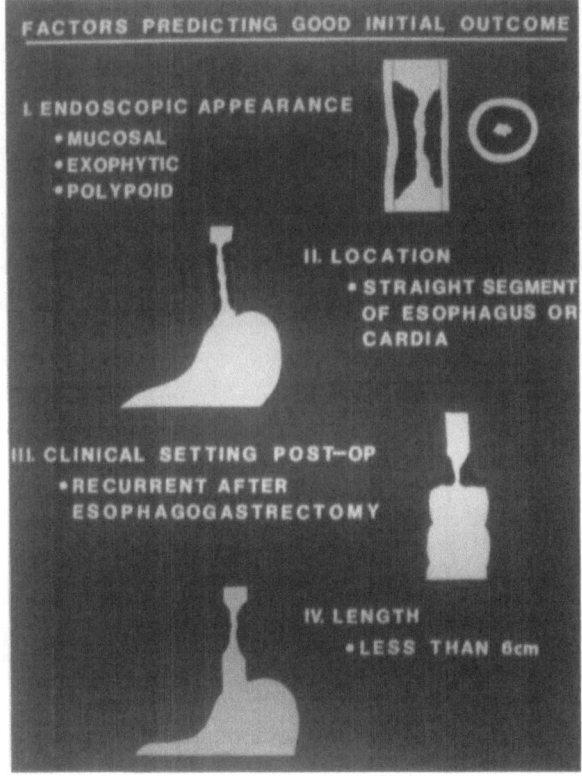

Fig. 14.6. Parameters which predict good initial outcome after endoscopic laser therapy.

In some of these cases, even if luminal patency was achieved, swallowing did not get better. Presumably this relates to the neuromuscular debility secondary to extra-esophageal involvement or radiation toxicity. Tumors in a straight segment of the esophagus were easiest and safest to treat. Those lying in a horizontal segment at the gastroesophageal junction were problematic.

It was more difficult to safely aim the laser beam and even after the lumen was opened, food would lodge in their horizontal, aperistaltic segment. The longer and more advanced the malignant process, the greater the number of sessions required to relieve the obstruction and the poorer the overall prognosis.

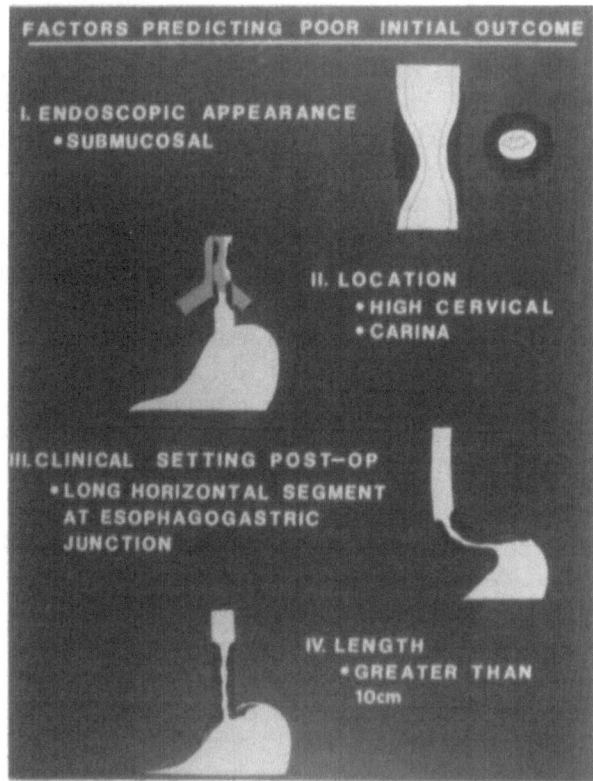

Fig. 14.7. Parameters which predict poor initial outcome after endoscopic laser therapy.

Table 14.2 summarizes our results for overall patient outcome. It should be noted that about 95% of tumor strictures could be technically opened, but not all were (73%) functionally improved.

Table 14.2. Endoscopic ND:YAG laser. Palliation of esophagogastric cancer (outcome).

	Squamous cell	*Adenocarcinoma*	*Total*
Patients	81	39	120
Technical success	77 (95%)	37 (94%)	114 (95%)
Functional success	61 (75%)	25 (64%)	88 (73%)
Major complications	5 (6%)	2 (5%)	7 (5%)
Minor complications	19 (24%)	6 (15%)	25 (21%)
Mortality 2° to Laser	0	0	0

Definitions:

Technical success – Luminal patency achieved and documented by objective criteria with no major complication at time of the procedure.

Functional success – Luminal patency achieved and oral intake improved.

Major complication – Death, perforation.

Minor complication – Overdistention, suspected aspiration, clinical sepsis, uncontrolled bleeding, severe pain during procedure (fever, WBC, pain after procedure, initial increased dysphagia – not included).

Discussion

More than 2000 patients with esophagogastric cancer have been treated in the United States by ELT. The rate of technical success (the ability to relieve the esophageal obstruction) is about 90%. However, the functional success (the ability to maintain adequate nutrition by peroral ingestion) is less – about 70%. The discrepancy is related to the fact that although luminal patency can be achieved, nutrition cannot be maintained either because of anorexia; painful metastases; or complication of therapy, tumor or treatment associated esophageal motility disturbances. These data relate to the initial results. It is extremely difficult to interpret long-term results of laser palliation. On one hand, many patients who are referred for ELT have already undergone other therapy and are only given laser treatment as a 'last resort.' Since ELT is only designed to open the lumen, it is often combined with other adjuvant therapy such as chemotherapy. When the obstruction recurs it may relate to rate of tumor growth or effectiveness or lack of efficacy of the adjuvant therapy. Some studies are underway in the United States to try to determine how ELT can best fit into the overall treatment schema.

Table 14.3. Complications of laser RX esophagogastric cancer.

	Squamous cell	Adenocarcinoma	Total
Total patients	81	39	120
MAJOR			
Perforation	5 (6%)	2 (5%)	7 (5%)
Procedure-related death	0	0	0
Totals – Major	5 (6%)	2 (5%)	7 (5%)
MINOR			
Overdistention	8	6	14
Suspected aspiration	5	0	5
Clinical sepsis	0	0	0
Uncontrolled bleeding	0	0	0
Severe pain during procedure	5	1	6
Totals – Minor	18	7	25 (20%)

The major complication has been perforation. The incidence is 5-10%. Minor complications include gaseous overdistention, transient bacteremia, fever, and pain during and after the procedure.

Most laser fibers incorporate a coaxial flow of gas into their design. When ELT is performed proximal to the obstructing tumor, this gas may pass into the stomach and beyond. Neither instrument suction or belching prevents the overdistention in 10-20% of patients, if the gas is used. Wolf et al. (4) described a 40% incidence of bacteremia in patients undergoing ELT for esophageal cancer. They established that the bacteremia is related to the passage of the endoscope through the necrotic tumor and was not specifically related to firing the laser. Bacteremia is related to the passage of the endoscope through the necrotic tumor and was not specifically related to firing the laser. Bacteremia was transient and prophylactic antibiotic treatment was not indicated unless the underlying medical condition dictated endocarditis prophylaxis. Low-grade temperature elevations occur in some patients. When the temperature of the treated tissue is high, the patient experiences pain during the laser treatment. If the endoscopist senses this and withholds therapy until the tissue has cooled, discomfort abates. The pain is much more apt to occur if submucosal tumor is being treated. Pain after treatment is related to irritation of raw ulcerated tissue by ingestion or acid reflux. Mortality related to laser therapy of UGI tumors per se is approximately 1%.

There are two new laser catheter developments which are potentially very important. Hashimoto (5) has used a fiber with a lateral prismatic tip. The beam exits laterally at an angle of 90°. This allows the endoscopist to aim the laser beam perpendicularly if he so desires. A second development has been championed by Joffe (6). He describes a variety of sapphire endo probes which can be fitted onto the distal tip of the fiber. With this method, laser energy is delivered with the tip in contact with the tumor tissue. Because energy is concentrated, lower energy settings (10-15 watts) are used with the Nd:YAG laser than with conventional tips.

Limitations and future expectations

Endoscopic laser therapy for esophageal cancer is currently bound by both clinical and technological limitations.

The clinical efficacy and safety of opening an esophageal lumen are reasonably well defined and we are just beginning to define parameters that help us decide in which patients technical success is most likely, but we certainly do not begin to understand where ELT fits into the overall schema for treatment of esophageal cancer. The role of the laser is to maintain luminal patency. This can be achieved by other methods (surgery, radiation therapy, dilatation, peroral prosthesis). We do not know which is best. We do not know if a combination of treatments is superior. The laser, likely has little role in the second aspect of therapy of esophageal cancer, retarding tumor growth. For this we depend on surgery, radiation therapy, or chemotherapy. Does pretreatment with the laser increase or decrease the efficacy and toxicity of these modalities? Further studies are needed to answer these questions.

Technologically, ELT is in its infancy. The technique I described uses high power lasers, with fibers, endoscopes, and accessories that are far from ideal. Refer to the chapters by Lambert (Chapter 13) and Brunetaud (Chapter 15) for a description of other techniques of laser palliation of UGI tumors. It is likely that when appropriate modifications are made in these three areas, ELT will be safer, more effective, and more efficient. I believe that in the years ahead we will regard the current methodology as primitive.

References

1. Fleischer D, Kessler F, Haye O. Endoscopic Nd:YAG laser therapy for carcinoma of the esophagus: A new palliative approach. Am J Surg 1982;143:280-283.
2. Savary M. Cours d'endoscopie de la clinique O.R.L. de Lausanne du 15 au 18 settembre 1980.
3. Fleischer DE, Sivak MV Jr. Endoscopic Nd:YAG laser therapy as palliative treatment for advanced adenocarcinoma of the gastric cardia. Gastroenterology 1984;87:815-820.
4. Wolf D, Fleischer D, Sivak MV Jr. Incidence of bacteremia with elective upper gastrointestinal endoscopic laser therapy. Gastrointest Endosc 1985;31:247-250.
5. Hashimoto D, Takami M, Idezuki Y. Prismatic tip lateral radiation probe in YAG laser endoscopy. Gastrointest Endosc 1985;31:153.
6. Joffe S, Sankar MY, Salzer D, Dalkuzono N. Preliminary clinical applications of the contact surgical rod and endoscopic microprobes with the Nd:YAG laser. Gastrointest Endosc 1985;31:155.

15. PALLIATIVE TREATMENT FOR ESOPHAGOGASTRIC CANCER BY LASER PHOTOABLATION

J.M. BRUNETAUD, V. MAUNOURY, D. COCHELARD,
A. CORTOT AND J.C. PARIS

Esophagogastric cancers have a poor prognosis (5). Progressive dysphagia is responsible for the poor quality of life during the short survival length of non-surgical patients (4, 5). Different methods have been used to avoid the gastrostomy, but they have limitations and complications (5). Laser photoablation has proved to be safe and effective in preliminary studies (3, 4, 8). Our purpose is to analyze the results of laser treatment of 115 non- surgical patients and the factors influencing immediate and long-term successful palliation.

Patients and methods

Patients

For palliation of biopsy documented esophagogastric carcinoma one hundred and fifteen patients (23 females and 92 males) were treated at the Lille Laser Center from December 1979 to November 1986. The mean age was 69 years (range 40-92). They were divided into 2 groups. The 99 patients of group I had dysphagia. The 16 patients of group II had a small lesion. A small lesion was defined as exophytic without gross evidence of ulceration or submucosal infiltration of the wall, less than 3 cm in length, involving less than one third of the circumference of the lumen, and without sign of regional or general dissemination.

The reasons for treatment are given in Table 15.1. The localization and the circumferential extension are given on Table 15.2. The circumferential extension was graded from C1 to C3 as a function of the tumor base extension: less than 1/3 of the circumference was C1, between 1/3 and 2/3 was C2, and more than 2/3 was C3. The histology is given on Table 15.3 as a function of the tumor localization.

Methods

An 80 W Nd:YAG 100 or 101 (Cilas, Marcoussis, France) was used at 40 W in 1 sec pulses. Spot size was approximately 2 mm which resulted in

D.M. Jensen and J.M. Brunetaud (eds), Medical Laser Endoscopy. 189-194.
© 1990 Kluwer Academic Publishers, Dordrecht

Table 15.1 Reasons for treatment in the 115 patients.

	# of patients	% of total
Laser as a first treatment:		
Non-surgical patient	56	49
Metastasis	13	11
Regional extension	10	9
Recurrence after a non-laser treatment:		
Radiation	12	10
Surgery	12	10
Laser as an additional treatment after:		
Radiation	8	7
Chemotherapy	1	0.5
Endoprothesis	1	0.5
Gastrotomy	2	2

Table 15.2. Localization and circumferential extension of the tumors in the 115 patients.

99 GROUP I PATIENTS WITH DYSPHAGIA

Localization			Circumferential extension		
	#	% of total		#	% of total
upper 1/3	19	19	C1	6	6
middle 1/3	27	27	C2	26	26
lower 1/3	11	11	C3	12	12
cardia	30	30			

16 GROUP II PATIENTS WITH A SMALL TUMOR

Localization			Circumferential extension		
	#	% of total		#	% of total
upper 1/3	6	37	C1	16	100
middle 1/3	5	31			
lower 1/3	2	12			
cardia	3	19			

approximately a 1200 J/cm^2 fluence for each pulse. Exophytic tumors were coagulated to a whitish appearance without vaporization.

A 10 W argon laser (Cooper Lasersonics, Santa Clara, Calif.) was used to supplement Nd:YAG laser in 3 patients with a small tumor. An 8W continuous beam (spot size 1 mm, irradiance 1000 W/cm2) was used for vaporization of the tumor when it was small and nearly flat with the mucosal surface.

Olympus GIF Q and P3 endoscopes (Olympus Corp. Tokyo, Japan) were used for the laser treatment. The core diameters of the laser optic fiber was 200 um for the argon laser and 400 um for the Nd:YAG laser. The fiber was inserted in a 1.6 mm external diameter catheter. Nitrogen was used to protect the fiber tip. The small diameter of the catheter allowed the gas to escape through the

Table 15.3. Localization and histology of the tumors in the 115 patients.

99 GROUP I PATIENTS WITH DYSPHAGIA

Localization	Adenocarcinoma #	% of total	Squamous #	% of total
upper 1/3	0	0	19	19
middle 1/3	1	1	26	26
lower 1/3	11	11	12	12
cardia	30	30	0	0
total	44	44	57	57

16 GROUP II PATIENTS WITH A SMALL TUMOR

Localization	Adenocarcinoma #	% of total	Squamous #	% of total
upper 1/3	0	0	6	38
middle 1/3	0	0	5	31
lower 1/3	1	6	1	6
cardia	3	19	0	0
total	4	25	12	75

biopsy channel of the GIF Q endoscope during the laser treatment. In 8 patients the tumor could be reached by the fiber only tangentially, and a special contact sapphire was used at the tip of the fiber (SLT, Tokyo, Japan). Cooling of the sapphire was obtained by water circulation.

Patients were treated as outpatients, without sedation. Laser photoablation was performed from the distal to the proximal part of the lesion, after endoscopic dilatation when the endoscope was unable to pass through the tumor. During initial treatment, patients were treated once or twice a week until disappearance of the dysphagia or complete destruction of the tumor. During follow-up, patients were re-endoscoped every month and eventually retreated.

Four types of non-laser treatments were combined with laser photoablation: endoscopic dilatation prior to the laser in 21 patients in group I, radiation therapy in 7 patients in group I and 5 patients in group II, chemotherapy in 1 group I patient, and BICAP in 4 group I patients.

Evaluation

A nutrition scale was used for evaluation of the patient's stage: 5 = aphagia, 4 = liquid diet only, 3 = soft diet, 2 = difficulties with some hard solids, and 1 = normal diet. The initial success in group I patients was defined as reaching grade 3 or better during a minimum period of 15 days without retreatment. The treatment was judged successful in group II patients when a total tumor

191

destruction was obtained with repeatedly negative biopsies.

Results

Group I Patients: Initial Treatment

The initial treatment was successful in 76 of 99 patients (83%). The initial treatment required 2 treatment sessions and lasted 12 days on the average. The mean nutrition score before treatment was 3.9 ± 0.1. It was 2.0 ± 0.1 after initial treatment. Among the 16 unsuccessfully treated patients, five of them were treated only once. Three had only one treatment because the lesion was too advanced for any possible benefit, one patient because an acute gastric distention occurred after the first treatment which required a gastrostomy and one because the patient did not come back after the first treatment. In eleven patients the treatment was judged unsuccessful after two to four treatment sessions. All of them had a very advanced lesion with regional extension. The localization, and the circumferential extension of the 16 tumors with unsuccessful treatment are given on Table 15.4. Extrinsic compression by lymph nodes was the reason for the two failures in the C1 subgroup. The failure rate was also effected by the reason for treatment. It was 32% in patients treated for a recurrence after a non-laser treatment versus 12% in the other patients (p=0.05).

Table 15.4. Localization and circumferential extension of the 13 unsuccessfully treated group I patients.

Localization				Circumferential extension		
upper 1/3	7/19	(37%)		C1	2/6	(33%)
others	9/80	(11%)		C2	0/22	(0%)
				C3	14/71	(20%)
total	16/99	(16%)			16/99	(16%)
p=0.02				C2/C3: p=0.02		

Group I Patients: Long-Term Results in the 76 Successfully Treated Patients

Eight patients were still under treatment. The treatment was stopped in 68 patients and the Average Duration of Improvement (ADI) was 130 days ± 16 (range 17-886). The reasons for treatment, the localization, and the histology did not influence the ADI. The ADI was 172 days (range 20-500) in the patients with a C1 and C2 tumor and 112 days (range 10-886) in the patients with a C3 tumor. This difference was nearly statistically significant (p<0.1).

Group II Patients

Among the 16 patients with a small tumor, one was still under treatment, one was unsuccessfully treated by laser and was referred for radiation therapy. The other fourteen patients had total destruction with negative biopsies after an average of 2.5 treatments. Two patients had a local recurrence after 5.5 months, and were referred for radiation therapy. Four patients were lost to follow-up after an 18 month average follow-up, 5 deceased from other causes, and 3 had negative biopsies with a 12 month average follow-up (range 3-29).

Tolerance and complications

All the patients tolerated the treatment well except 4 who interrupted the laser treatment after initial success. Two of them were over 90 years old and one had severe a major pulmonary insufficiency. Four complications (4%) occurred, all in group I patients: two esophagotracheal fistulae treated with a prosthesis, an acute gastric dilatation requiring a gastrostomy, and one fatal hemorrhage.

Discussion

In a large survey (2), the overall survival rate at four years for patients with an esophageal cancer was 5%. 'Curative' surgery was possible in 10% and the survival rate of that subgroup at 4 years was 13%. Therefore, the treatment of esophageal cancers is mainly palliative. The aim of the treatment is to palliate the dysphagia, with a minimum of discomfort and morbidity for the patient.

Our 83% success rate in patients presenting initial dysphagia (group I) is comparable to the 80% of Fleischer (4). In our experience, localization at the upper 1/3, C3 extension and referral for a recurrence after a non-laser treatment were factors of poor prognosis. Extrinsic compression by lymph nodes was the reason for the failure in two of our patients despite total destruction of a C1 tumor. Furthermore, cancer anorexia can be the cause of the lack of improvement. Only about 70% of the patients with satisfactory destruction of intraluminal tumor will have a normal alimentation after laser palliation of advanced esophagogastric cancers (3, 4, 5).

The duration of improvement after laser photoablation has not often been reported. The ADI of our patients was short (130 days) despite new laser treatments. But the improvement lasted as long as the patient survived. A gastrostomy was required in only 14% of our patients. A C3 extension was the only factor of poor prognosis concerning the ADI.

Our 4% complication rate in group I patients was slightly lower than the 8% of Fleischer (4) or the 7% of Naveau (7). Perforation of the esophagus is the main complication. Its rate was 5% in Fleischer experience (4) and in a large

European survey of 326 patients and 2000 treatments (1). Our two tracheal-esophageal fistula occurred at the beginning of our experience when narrow stenoses were not dilatated before laser photoablation. Our acute gastric distention was secondary to the nitrogen gas in the stomach which could not escape through a spastic pylorus nor through an incompletely destroyed tumor of the GE junction. Now we dilate esophageal or GE junction tumor strictures prior to laser treatment and systematically suck the gas from the stomach at the end of the treatment. Our single fatal accident was secondary to a massive digestive hemorrhage occurring the day after the treatment.

Even small esophageal cancers invade the lymph nodes early and often spread to several sites in the esophagus. Therefore, local destruction by laser photoablation should be limited to non-surgical patients. Fourteen of our 16 patients had negative biopsies, but two recurrences occurred after a 5.5 month follow- up. The treatment of these non-surgical patients with small squamous tumors is not well established. Patrice (8) reported disappearance of all 8 tumors using laser and radiation. Lambert (6) combined chemotherapy, laser and radiation and reports an 83% survival rate at 12 months in 13 patients.

In our experience laser photoablation was able to improve 83% of patients with dysphagia. The improvement lasted as long as the patient survived and the complication rate was acceptable. Twelve of our 16 patients with small lesions have negative biopsies without local recurrence. Laser photoablation is an effective technique with a low rate of severe complications. The exact role of the laser photoablation has to be established by further controlled or comparative studies.

References

1. Delvaux M, Escourrou J. Complications observées au cours du traitement par laser des tumeurs du tractus digestif supérieur. Acta Endoscopica 1985 15;1:13-17.
2. Faivre J, Millan C, Hillon MC, Klepping C. Incidence du cancer de L'oesophage dans le départment de la Côte d'Or. Gastroentérol Clin Biol 1981;5:251-256.
3. Fleischer D, Kessler F, Haye O. Endoscopic Nd:YAG laser therapy for carcinoma of the oesophagus. A new palliative approach. Am J Surg 1982;143:280-283.
4. Fleischer D, Siwak M. Endoscopic Nd:YAG laser therapy as palliation for oesophagogastric cancer. Gastroenterology 1985;89:827-831.
5. Jensen DM. Lasers in the GI cancer war and on other fronts. Gastroenterology 1984;87:974-976.
6. Lambert R, Sabben G, Chevaillon A, Gerard J, Descos F. Traitement non chirurgical du cancer épidermoïde de l'oesophage: approche combinée. Gastroenterolo Clin Biol, 1985;2bis:204A (abstract).
7. Naveau S, Poitrine A, Poynard T, Thuvignon E, Chaput JC. Traitement palliatif des cancers de l'oesophage et du cardia par le laser YAG neodyme (essai préliminaire non contrôlé). Gastroenterol Clin Biol 1984;8:545-550.
8. Patrice T, Jutel P, Le Bodic L. Traitement par laser des cancers intra-muqueux de l'oesophage chez des patients inopérables. Gastroenterol Clin Biol, 1985;4:374.

16. LASERS IN RECTOSIGMOID TUMORS

J.M. BRUNETAUD, V. MAUNOURY, D. COCHELARD,
A. CORTOT AND J.C. PARIS

Lasers were developed in GI endoscopy for their hemostatic properties. They are now used more commonly for tumor destruction (1-2). At the Lille Laser center, three types of sessile rectosigmoid tumors are treated by laser photo-ablation: cancers (advanced and small tumors), villous adenomas and small rectal polyps in familial polyposis syndrome after total colectomy and ileorectal anastomosis.

Material and methods

Patient Preparation

Patients were treated on an outpatient basis, without anesthesia or premedication. Patients were prepared with a small enema at the Laser Center and no special diet was required before the treatment. Patients were treated once or twice a week until functional improvement (advanced cancers) or until complete destruction of the tumor. Then they were followed up every two weeks until complete re-epithelialization. Subsequently, patients with an advanced cancer were retreated every month, and the other patients were followed up and retreated if a recurrence or new lesions occurred.

Material for histology

The main disadvantage of laser photo-ablation is the lack of material available for a total histologic study of the tumor. Before the treatment multiple biopsies have to be performed. For large tumors, a partial snare electroresection is performed when feasible. Snare resection debulks the tumor and decreases the laser treatment time. More biopsies are performed during follow-up examinations.

Laser treatment modalities

Laser photo-ablation can be performed in two different ways: coagulation necrosis of the tumor with a delayed slough, or vaporization with immediate

D.M. Jensen and J.M. Brunetaud (eds), Medical Laser Endoscopy. 195-206.
© 1990 Kluwer Academic Publishers, Dordrecht

destruction. Coagulation necrosis occurs also at the border of the vaporized area but the amount depends upon the laser wavelength used.

Two types of lasers are used for GI endoscopic treatment at Lille: the argon laser and the Nd:YAG laser. See Fig. 16.1. The argon laser is a 770 Lasersonics (Santa Clara, California) with 10 Watts maximum power output. Its wavelength is well absorbed by the tissue. The argon laser was used for vaporization of superficial tumor (until a flat surface was obtained) at a power of 8 Watts and a spot size of 1 mm (power density: 1,000 Watts/cm²) with a continuous beam. Delayed necrosis is negligible after argon laser vaporization.

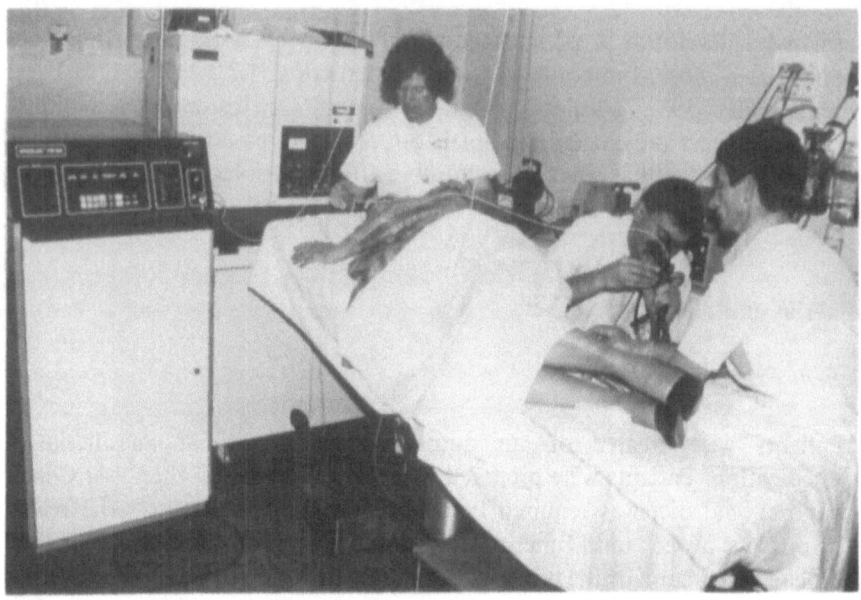

Fig. 16.1. The endoscopic laser room. The two lasers are ready for use: on the left the Cilas Nd:YAG laser and on the right the Cooper Lasersonics argon laser. A rectal neoplasm is being treated via endoscopy.

The Nd:YAG laser is the YM 101 CILAS (Marcoussis, France) with an 80 Watt maximum power output. The Nd:YAG laser wavelength is less absorbed by the tissue than the argon wavelength. The volume of delayed necrosis occurring after Nd:YAG vaporization can be difficult to predict from the macroscopic aspect of the tissue during the treatment (3, 4). Therefore, the Nd:YAG laser was used at Lille only for coagulation (blanching) of the tumor and an interval of 2 to 3 days between two treatments allows the coagulated parts of the tumor to slough off. Reproducible effects without unexpected necrosis were obtained at 70 Watts, 2 mm spot size (2,000 Watts/cm²), and 0.7 s exposure time.

A 200 um core optic fiber is used for argon laser transmission and a 600 um is used for Nd:YAG. In both cases the fiber is protected by a teflon catheter. Nitrogen gas flows at a rate of 2 liters/minute to protect the fiber tip. It also gives a neutral gas atmosphere in the rectum and avoids possible explosion when high temperature occurs with treatment. During endoscopy, care must be taken to avoid rectosigmoid overdistension because it is painful and it reduces the thickness of the rectosigmoid wall, thus increasing the risk of perforation. To evacuate the gas, a cannula is introduced in the rectum along side the endoscope. See Fig. 16.2. The fiber tip is maintained at a distance of 5 to 10 mm from the tissue during the treatment.

For lesions in the lower third of the rectum, rigid anoscopy is preferred to flexible endoscopy, if the patient can tolerate the knee-chest position. A suction

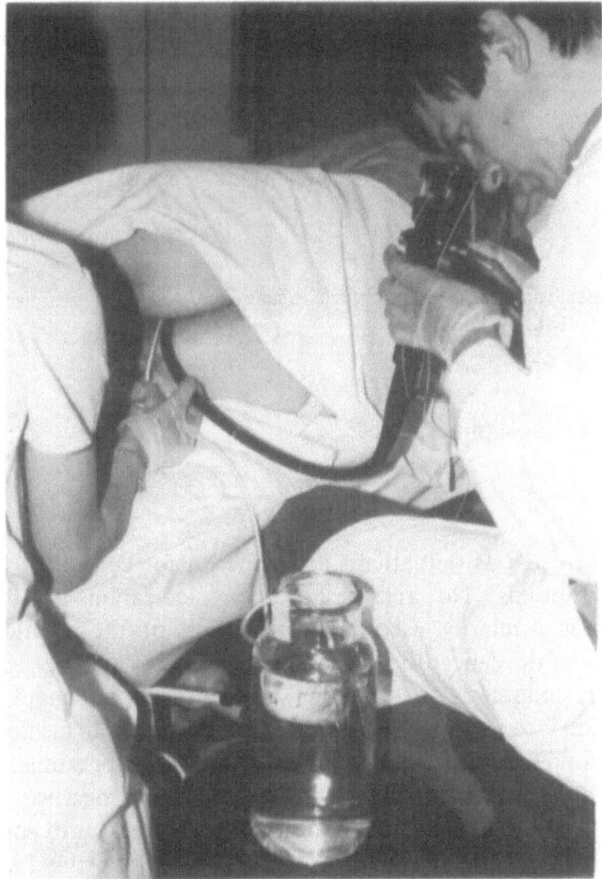

Fig. 16.2. Gas evacuation method. An 18 French Levine tube is passed beside the sigmoidoscope with the free end submerged in 20 cm of water. This maintains a constant luminal distention.

cannula evacuates necrotic tissue and blood with this technique. In this case the fiber is coupled to a rigid handpiece where a lens refocuses the laser beam to an 0.6 mm spot for argon laser and 1.2 mm spot for Nd:YAG laser. Refer to Fig. 16.3.

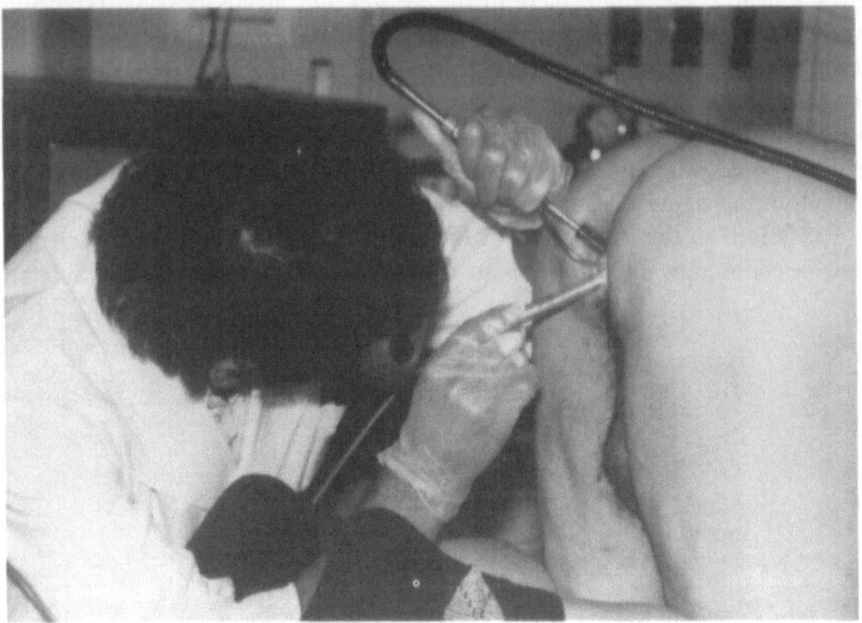

Fig. 16.3. The laser handpiece as used through an anoscope. Anoscopic treatment allows good visualization of the base of the rectum.

Patients with a rectosigmoid cancer

Techniques

Patients are treated as outpatients after referral for control of bleeding or obstructive symptoms. No anesthesia or premedication is administered. Nd:YAG laser is primarily used for coagulation of the intraluminal and exophytic parts of the cancer that cannot be removed by snare resection. After examination via endoscopy of the cancer size and location, coagulation of the whole cancer surface is performed from proximal to distal fashion. A rectal cannula decompresses the area and suctioning more proximally with the endoscope is done at the end of the treatment. Tumor necrosis and slough occur in 3–5 days so treatments are performed every week until control of the tumor mass and/or re-epithelization occurs (4). Refer to Atlas Plate 39.

Patients

One hundred and sixty-one patients with rectosigmoid cancer were treated from December 1979 to August 1987. The mean age of the patients was 78 years (range 47-94). One hundred forty-two patients were treated for an *advanced tumor*. Reasons for treatment, localization and circumferential extension are given on Tables 16.1, 16.2, and 16.3. The circumferential extension (annular size of the tumor base) was estimated by comparing the circumferential portion of the bowel lumen occupied by the tumor base to the complete luminal circumference. The main symptom at the beginning of the treatment was

Table 16.1. Reasons for treatment in patients with advanced and small rectosigmoid cancers.

Reasons for treatment	Advanced lesions		Small lesions	
	#	(%)	#	(%)
Non-surgical*				
without metastases	85	(60)	14	(74)
with metastases	22	(15)	1	(6)
Colostomy & abnormal discharge	20	(14)	0	(0)
Recurrence after surgery	11	(8)	2	(10)
Refusal of surgery	4	(3)	2	(10)
Total	142	(100)	19	(100)

* Non-surgical candidate because of severe medical or surgical problem making the risk of surgical resection unacceptably high in the opinion of the consulting surgeons and internists.

Table 16.2. Localization of advanced and small rectosigmoid cancers.

Localization	Advanced lesions		Small lesion	
	#	(%)	#	(%)
Rectum	96	(68)	12	(63)
Rectosigmoid junction	26	(18)	2	(11)
Sigmoid	20	(14)	5	(26)
Total	142	(100)	19	(100)

Table 16.3. Circumferential extension of the advanced rectosigmoid cancers.

	#	(%)
C1:	25	(18)
C2:	56	(39)
C3:	61	(43)
Total	142	(100)

C1 indicates <1/3 circumference, C2 indicates between 1/3 and 2/3 circumference, C3 indicates >2/3 circumference.

abnormal rectal discharge in 125 patients and obstructive symptoms in 17. Nineteen patients had a *small lesion*. Small lesions were defined as a tumor less than 3 cm in length, with a circumferential extension of the base less than one-third of the circumference, without signs of infiltration, and purely exophytic configuration without ulceration. The reasons for treatment and localization of the small lesions are given in Tables 16.1 and 16.2.

Results

Ninety percent of the patients with an advanced cancer improved after an average duration of 15 days for the initial treatment (average treatment member 2.5). The treatment was completed in 96 and the average duration of improvement (ADI) was 9.3 months (0.2-50.3). By life table analysis 48% of patients survived one year, and 92% of them had continued improvement. The improvement rate was higher in surviving patients with initial abnormal rectal discharges (97% at 6 months) than in those with obstructive symptoms (58%). Patients with a C1 tumor did much better than the others.

Ten percent of the patients with an advanced cancer failed to improve. This was more frequent in C2 and C3 patients (11.5% of failures) than in C1 patients (4%). Patients with initial obstructive symptoms improved less often (18% of failures) than patients with initial abnormal discharge (9%).

Negative biopsies were obtained without local recurrence in 6 of the 25 (24%) patients with a C1 tumor and in all the 19 patients with a small rectal cancer after an average treatment duration of 5.0 months. Among the C1 patients, one died from liver metastases 3 months after the end of the treatment, and 1 deceased from another etiology after 28 months of follow-up. The average follow-up of the 4 patients who are still followed is 4.6 months (range 1-12.3). Among the patients with a small cancer, one patient who had a metastasis before the treatment died 8 months later, 2 patients deceased from cause etiology and one was lost to follow- up. The average follow-up of the 15 patients who are still followed is 17.3 months (range 1-51.8).

Five complications occurred in the group of patients with an advanced rectosigmoid carcinoma (3.7% of these patients) after 1664 laser treatment sessions. There were two perforations at the rectosigmoid junction (fatal), one perirectal abscess and two recto-vaginal fistulae.

Lasers in rectosigmoid villous adenoma

Techniques

Patients with villous adenoma are treated almost the same way as patients with cancer. However, the argon laser is preferably used to vaporize the superficial parts of the tumors and patients are treated twice a week until complete tumor destruction (3). Refer to Atlas – Plate 40.

Patients

Two hundred and forty-seven patients were treated at Lille from December 1979 to August 1987 for a rectosigmoid villous adenoma. The mean age was 72 years (range 32-92). The indications for laser treatment were 1) non-surgical patients (89 patients, 36% of total), 2) surgical resection appearing to be too drastic for a tumor found benign on biopsy (98 patients, 40% of total), 3) recurrent tumor after a previous non-laser treatment (57 patients, 23% of total) and 4) patient's refusal of surgery (3 patients, 1% of total).

Localization, circumferential extension of the tumor base (from C1 to C3), and histology are given on Tables 16.4 and 16.5.

*Table 16.4.*Localization and circumferential extension of 247 villous tumors.

Localization			Circumferential extension		
	#	(%)		#	(%)
Lower rectum	62	(25)	C1	109	(44)
Middle rectum	89	(36)	C2	107	(43)
Rectosigm. jn	54	(22)	C3	31	(13)
Sigmoid	42	(17)			
Total	247	(100)		247	(100)

C1 indicates <1/3 circumference, C2 indicates between 1/3 and 2/3 circumference, C3 indicates >2/3 circumference.

Table 16.5. Histology of the 247 villous adenomas at the beginning of treatment.

	#	(%)
Mild dysplasia	117	(47)
Moderate dysplasia	83	(34)
Severe dysplasia	27	(11)
Carcinoma in situ	20	(8)
Total	247	(100)

A partial snare electroresection was performed in 71 patients, and forcep biopsies alone in 176.

Results

The treatment was not completed in 33 patients because 12 patients were lost to follow-up, 14 died from another cause during the treatment, and 7 are still under treatment. Results are available in the 214 remaining patients. Thirteen patients (6.1%) had positive biopsies during the treatment. However, only 9 of this latter group of 13 patients had a true adenocarcinoma (4.2%). The other 4 had no invasive cancer upon surgical resection.

Two patients (1%) could not be successfully treated. Both had a circumferential lesion previously treated by a non-laser procedure. The previous treatment was electrocoagulation in one which resulted in a very tight stenosis making any endoscopic treatment impossible. Therefore, only a diverting colostomy could be performed. The second patient had been treated by surgical transanal resection. He developed a stenosis after Nd:YAG laser treatment. The stenosis was not tight enough to require a colostomy but made the endoscopic treatment impossible.

One hundred ninety-nine patients were successfully treated. This represents 93% of the patients whose treatment was completed. Among these 199 patients, 46 were lost to follow-up after a mean follow-up post-laser treatment of 12.4 months (range 0.4-61.2), 6 died from another cause after a follow-up of 14.2 months (range 1.2-37.8) and 147 are still followed-up post treatment for an average of 24.4 months (range 0.9-66.6). Among the 199 successfully treated patients, 24 had a recurrence after an average of 11.6 months. All of them were easily retreated except one. The reason for laser treatment in this patient was a recurrence 6 months after surgical transanal surgery. No malignancy was found on the resection specimen nor on the biopsies performed on the first recurrence. The second recurrence of villous adenoma occurred 16 months after laser treatment and was found to be malignant.

During treatment with Nd:YAG, some patients experienced warmth in the rectum when the tumor was close to the anus. For 2 or 3 days after a laser session, patients often had spotting with blood and evacuation of necrotic tissue. Two patients experienced fever to 38°C for 2 days unassociated with pain. This spontaneously abated. Ten developed a stenosis but only 3 stenoses were symptomatic and required endoscopic dilatations (1.5% of the patients with completed treatment). No perforations or massive hemorrhages were observed.

The circumferential extension was the main predictive factor which influenced the frequency of cancer during initial treatment, the treatment duration until re-epithelialization, stenosis development requiring dilatation, and recurrence rate (Table 16.6).

Table 16.6. Influence of circumferential extension on outcomes.

Extension	Cancer	Rx duration	Stenosis	Recurrence
C1	1.0%	2.7 mo	0.0%	10.45
C2	2.2%	4.6 mo	0.0%	10.65
C3	24.0%	8.5 mo	18.8%	31.3%
Total	4.2%	4.0 mo	1.5%	12.2%

The effect of circumferential extension upon incidence of cancer during initial treatment, treatment duration, stenosis development requiring dilatation and recurrence rate.

The effect of circumferential extension upon incidence of cancer during initial treatment, treatment duration, stenosis development requiring dilatation and recurrence rate.

Lasers in rectal polyposis

Technique

Our technique was to vaporize small polyps which could not be removed by snare electrosurgery. Argon was primarily used. All polyps were treated in the same session. During subsequent examination, biopsies were performed for new polyps before laser ablation. Refer to Atlas – Plate 41.

Patients

Seventeen patients were treated for rectal polyposis. The mean age was 29 years (range 11-48). Twelve had familial polyposis and five Gardner's Syndrome. All of them had surgery with an ileorectal anastomosis prior to rectal treatment with the lasers.

Results

No rectal carcinoma was observed in the 12 patients with familial polyposis. Eleven were regularly treated at the Laser Center with an average follow-up of 8.5 years (range 1-15) after the colectomy. One patient was lost to follow-up 10 years after the colectomy. Among the 5 patients with Gardner's Syndrome, 2 were lost to follow-up 1 and 1.5 years after colectomy. Two are regularly followed for 2 years, and the last patient required a rectal amputation 5 years after the colectomy for an adenocarcinoma. No complications occurred in this group of patients.

Discussion

Our technique of using both argon and Nd:YAG lasers is rather original. The use of argon laser in GI endoscopy is not widespread, probably because the purchase of a second laser is found too expensive by most gastroenterologists. The multidisciplinary use of lasers (5) is a good solution to share the expenses with other specialities and to have the appropriate laser wavelength for each particular lesion. In fact, those who have access to an argon laser (6), prefer the absence of delayed effects, risk of perforation and thermal stenosis for treatment of some tumors compared with higher risks with Nd:YAG laser treatment.

The best technique for endoscopic use of Nd:YAG laser is also controversial. Some investigators vaporize the tissue with a very high power density (over 10,000 Watts/cm^2) (7) with Nd:YAG, or they coagulate small lesions and vaporize the larger ones (8-9). We prefer to coagulate with a lower power density (between 1,500 and 2,000 Watts/cm^2) and wait until the coagulated areas slough off (3-4). Others have stressed the increased safety of coagulation compared to vaporization treatment of cancer strictures (10).

Our treatment of ambulatory patients without a special diet beforehand or premedication is well adapted to our elderly population. Our treatment technique of using both argon and Nd:YAG lasers and limiting the Nd:YAG laser effects to coagulation is also safe. No complications occurred in the patients with small cancers or rectal polyposis. Our complication rate for advanced rectosigmoid cancers (3.7%) or villous adenomas (1.5%) is significantly lower than the 10% of Mathus-Vliegen (8-9) who uses high power Nd:YAG for vaporization and coagulation.

Our immediate success rate in palliation of advanced rectosigmoid cancers was 90%. At 6 months, 95% of our surviving patients whose presenting symptoms were abnormal rectal discharge and 60% of those with obstructive symptoms remained improved. Mathus-Vliegen (8) and Escourrou (11) have respective immediate success rates of 93% and 100% for hematochezia and 83% and 67% for obstructive symptoms. The benefit from laser treatment appears to be better for patients with hematochezia than with obstructive symptoms.

Complete local destruction of C1 cancers or small rectosigmoid cancers with negative biopsies can be achieved by endoscopic laser treatment. This result was obtained by us in 24% of the patients with C1 tumors and all 19 patients with small tumors. Similar results were reported by others (7, 11). However, possible local or regional spread of these tumors can not be detected and their endoscopic treatment has to be limited to non-surgical patients, in our opinion.

A large proportion of our patients with villous adenoma were difficult cases. Fifty-six percent of our patients with villous adenoma had a large lesion (C2 and C3) and 23% had a recurrence after a previous non-laser treatment. However, 198 of the 214 patients (93%) who completed treatment were cured by the laser treatment. These results are better than those of Mathus-Vliegen who has only a 40% cure rate in almost the same type of lesion (9). Our recurrence rate after laser treatment is 12.2%. This is much lower than other treatments such as transanal surgery where recurrence rates are greater than 20% in most series. In our series recurrences occurred a mean of 12.4 months after the end of the laser treatment. Therefore, our patients are followed up every 3 months during the first 18 months post-laser treatment and then every 6 months.

The treatment of C3 villous adenomas takes longer than C1 and C2. C3 tumors also have higher rates of recurrence and stenosis. However, laser photo-ablation is probably the only conservative treatment available at present for these tumors.

Nine malignancies (4.2%) occurred in our series of villous adenoma patients during the initial laser treatment. The malignancy rate was higher in C3 lesions (24.0%) than in C1 (1.0%) and C2 (2.2%). This is in accordance with the natural history of the villous adenoma where the malignancy rate increases with the tumor size. Mathus-Vliegen reported a 20% of malignant degeneration (9). Therefore, we think that it is very important to get the best histology possible from the tumor before the treatment with large snare resections when feasible. We also select our patients and we limit the indications to non-surgical, previously operated patients or those with small tumors which would require drastic surgery.

The management of patients with an ileorectal anastomosis for familial polyposis is not easy. The risk of malignancy, even in patients regularly treated, is not negligible. One of our patients developed a carcinoma 5 years after the colectomy. Therefore, the laser treatment has the same limitations as electrocoagulation in this type of palliation. But its main advantages over electrocoagulation are the rapidity (6) and the good healing quality without scarring, as demonstrated by Mathus-Vliegen (9).

In conclusion, endoscopic laser treatment is a safe and effective technique for the treatment of benign sessile rectosigmoid tumors and for palliation of symptoms from malignant tumors. The two main disadvantages of the lasers are their high purchase price and the lack of total histology, particularly with villous adenoma and familial polyposis. The first problem can be solved by a multidisciplinary use (5). The solution for the second problem is a very careful histologic investigation before, during, and after the treatment, and a good selection of the patients where the risk of malignancy has to be balanced with the risk of surgery. Patients with biopsy proven adenocarcinoma should be selected for palliation only if they are not candidates for surgery.

References

1. Fleischer D. Lasers and colon polyps. Technology and pathology the courtship continues. Gastroenterology 1986;90:2024-2025.
2. Jensen DM. Lasers in the GI cancer war and on other fronts. Gastroenterology 1984;87:974-976.
3. Brunetaud JM, Mosquet L, Houcke M et al. Villous adenomas of the rectum: Results of endoscopic treatment with argon and Nd:YAG lasers. Gastroenterology 1985;89:832-837.
4. Brunetaud JM, Maunoury V, Ducrote P, Cochelard D, Cortot A, Paris JC. Palliative treatment of rectosigmoid carcinoma by endoscopic laser photoablation. Gastroenterology 1987;92: 663- 668.
5. Brunetaud JM, Mosquet L, Bourez J et al. Organization of a multidisciplinary laser center, in Fleischer D, Jensen D, Bright- Asare P (eds): Therapeutic laser endoscopy in gastrointestinal disease, Boston, Martinus Nijhoff, 1983, pp 167-72.
6. Dixon JA, Burt RW, Roetering RH, McCloskey DW. Endoscopic argon laser photocoagulation of sessile polyps. Gastrointest Endosc 1982;28:162-165.
7. Lambert R, Sabben G. Photodestruction par laser des tumeurs colorectales: Résultats précoces

(Abstract). Gastroenterol Clin Biol 1983;7:59A.

8. Mathus-Vliegen EM, Tytgat GN. Nd:YAG laser photocoagulation in gastroenterology: Its role in palliation of colorectal cancer. Laser Med Sci 1986;1:75-80.

9. Mathus-Vliegen EM, Tytgat GN. Nd:YAG laser photocoagulation in colorectal adenoma. Evaluation of its safety, usefulness, and efficacy. Gastroenterology 1986;90:1865-1873.

10. Jensen DM. Palliation of esophagogastric cancer via endoscopy. Gastroenterol Clin Biol 1987;11:361-363.

11. Escourrou J, Delvaux M, Frexinos J et al. Traitement du cancer du rectum par le laser neodyme YAG. Gastroenterol Clin Biol 1986;10:152-157.

17. COMPLICATIONS OF GASTROINTESTINAL LASER ENDOSCOPY

JAMES H. JOHNSTON

Complications following endoscopic laser therapy may be divided into hazards related to the endoscopy itself, thermal injury, or the coaxial gas jet (Table 17.1).

Table 17.1. Complications of endoscopic laser therapy.

1. *Endoscopic*
   Aspiration
   Medication reaction
   Hypotension
   Arrhythmia
   Mallory-Weiss tear
   Induced hemorrhage
   Perforation
2. *Thermal*
   Acute – tissue erosion
     induced hemorrhage
     acute perforation
   Subacute – tissue necrosis
     ulceration
     delayed hemorrhage
     delayed perforation
     fistula
     fever
     post-coagulation syndrome
     pain
   Chronic – fibrotic scarring
     stricture
3. *Coaxial gas jet*
   Abdominal distention with respiratory distress
   Benign pneumoperitoneum
   Hypercarbia (with carbon dioxide gas)

Endoscopic complications

Endoscopic complications occur up to 10 time more frequently with emergency endoscopy for upper gastrointestinal bleeding than with routine endoscopy (1). The bleeding patient is more frightened and less cooperative,

D.M. Jensen and J.M. Brunetaud (eds), Medical Laser Endoscopy. 207-215.

making endoscopic conditions less optimal and perforation risk higher. Less sedation should be employed because of risk of hypotension. Adequate monitoring of blood pressure and cardiac rhythm will aid early detection and treatment of hypotension or significant arrhythmias. Endoscopic trauma may induce active hemorrhage, especially from esophageal varices. A bleeding Mallory-Weiss tear may result from retching during endoscopy. Gastric lavage or endoscopy may induce abrasions or suction artifacts which may be falsely identified as the true bleeding point. Vigorous irrigation and suction of overlying blood clots to allow close inspection of the bleeding point may precipitate active bleeding. Additionally, the prolonged nature of many therapeutic endoscopic procedures increases the risk of complications.

Aspiration during endoscopic laser therapy for upper gastrointestinal hemorrhage has been noted in 1 to 2% of patients by most investigators (2). The potential for aspiration is increased by massive variceal hemorrhage, use of gastric lavage, or when the patient is rolled to various positions during endoscopy. Remember that gastric blood clots pool safely in the fundus in the left lateral decubitus (standard endoscopic) position, whereas aspiration tendency is high in positions that drain the fundus (especially right lateral decubitus position). Aspiration potential is also increased with laser therapy of esophageal cancer, particularly if there is fluid retention above the tumor. Additionally, a partial obstruction may be temporarily converted to a complete obstruction by tissue edema produced by laser treatment. Pietrafitta noted pulmonary aspiration in 17% of laser patients treated by the antegrade method of tumor ablation (3). Laser therapy will increase the likelihood of aspiration unless the obstruction is effectively relieved in a single therapeutic session. Potential for aspiration can be reduced by careful attention to endoscopic suction of fluid, oropharyngeal suction by the assistant, reverse Trendelenburg position (if blood pressure allows), and timely endotracheal intubation when needed to protect the airway. Aspiration is a preventable endoscopic complication if proper precautions are taken.

Thermal complications

Thermal complications may be divided into acute, subacute and chronic categories.

Acutely, the main danger with the laser is vaporization or erosion of tissue. Whereas acute ablation of tissue may be a goal in the treatment of an obstructing malignancy, this tissue cutting effect is distinctly undesirable in the treatment of gastrointestinal hemorrhage. For hemostasis, clinically useful temperature elevations include 60°C for coagulation of tissue protein (producing a visible white spot) and 75 to 90°C for collagen contraction (producing shrinkage of the vessel wall) (4). Water boils at 100°C, and at this temperature, near instantaneous heating of a volume of tissue by the laser causes tissue disruption by rapid expansion of tiny steam pockets in the tissue.

This erosive effect at 100°C is unique to the *rapid* heating produced by the laser or by electrical sparking, whereas simple electrocoagulation (without sparking – as with the BICAP probe or the 'wet' monopolar electrode) or thermal cautery with the heater probe produce *slower* boiling of tissue water at 100°C and do not erode or cut the tissue (5). These non-erosive heater and BICAP probes have been employed effectively for gastrointestinal hemostasis, whereas larger BICAP probes have been developed for tumor therapy (6).

Erosion of tissue by the laser may produce acute perforation of the target wall or induced bleeding by eroding a vessel wall (7). In treatment of peptic ulcers with a sentinel clot which is not actively bleeding, YAG laser may induce active arterial hemorrhage frequently (5). In ablation of neoplastic tissue by YAG laser, there is also the potential for induced bleeding (8).

Acutely during laser treatment, full tensile strength of the target gut wall is maintained unless the tissue is eroded or ablated. Unfortunately, there is considerable difficulty in trying to heat a target blood vessel (with prominent heat sink effect due to rapid blood flow) to 75 to 90°C, yet avoid the dangerous effects of slightly higher tissue temperature elevation to 100°C, especially since there is no tissue 'thermometer' to guide endoscopic laser therapy. Tissue heat production by the laser is primarily a function of power density and time of laser application. Because of the conical shape of the laser beam, power density varies dramatically with treatment distance, which is difficult to assess and control precisely through the endoscope.

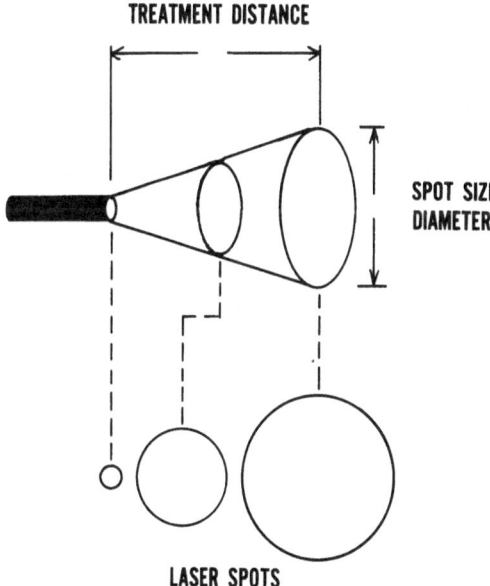

Fig. 17.1. Diagram of a divergent laser light beam, creating laser spots of increasing size with greater distance of the lightguide from the target.

Power density varies tremendously over the treatment range: next to the mucosa, spot size diameter is 0.6 mm; at a distance of 5 cm, spot size is 9.4 mm (15 fold). However, power density is inversely related to the square of the spot radius, so that as spot size diameter varies 15 fold, the power density actually varies *225* fold.

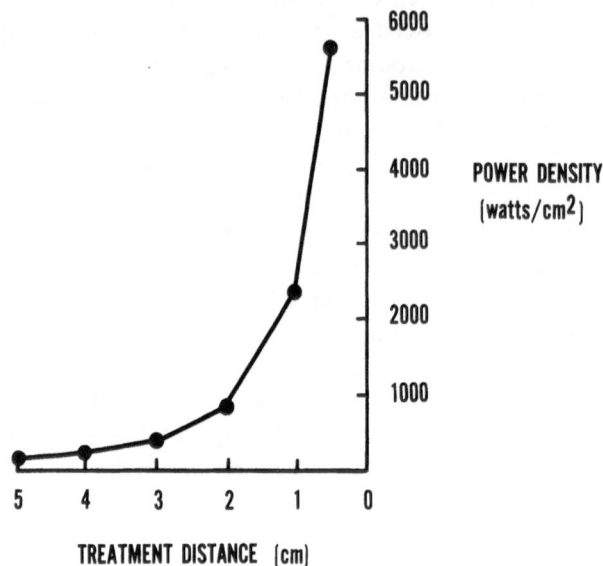

Fig. 17.2. Relationship between laser power density and treatment distance, assuming constant power setting of 75 watts and laser beam divergence of 10°.

Figure 17.2 depicts this relationship between power density and treatment distance. For effective coagulation with the YAG laser, the operator should use 0.5-1.0 second pulses with power density in the 500 to 1000 watt/cm² range, occasionally up to 2000. Above that range, tissue vaporization occurs. As shown in Fig. 17.2, changes in treatment distance between 2 and 5 cm produce relatively small changes in power density. In contrast, for treatment distance less than 1 cm, truly dramatic rises in power density occur with small changes in treatment distance. At a treatment distance of 0.5 cm, power would have to be reduced to 12 watts to maintain a power density of 1000 watts/cm². If the laser fiber tip inadvertently touches the mucosa while firing with 75 watts, the resultant power density would be in excess of 25,000 watts/cm²! For hemostasis, avoidance of excessive power density is critical. For example, if treatment in the duodenum demands a short treatment distance of one centimeter or less, then the power output should be reduced accordingly. The currently available YAG laser lightguide has no safeguard to prevent accidental contact with the mucosa while firing the laser. The operator must pay close attention to endoscopic spot size and treatment distance. When one is uncertain about treatment distance, it can be gauged by lightly touching the adjacent mucosa and then withdrawing the catheter 2 cm before firing.

Subacutely, during the period of 1 to 7 days after thermal treatment, there is cell death and necrosis of tissue heated to 45°C. Necrotic mucosa sloughs, producing ulceration, whereas deeper tissue typically retains some connective tissue matrix. Small ulcerations of normal mucosa in the upper gastrointestinal tract usually heal in a couple of weeks, but may take longer in the colon or with diseased tissue. Prolonged ulceration may occasionally be seen clinically with malnourished patients who have impaired healing. Most of the tensile strength of the gastrointestinal wall is provided by the submucosa. Superficial thermal application does not reduce overall tensile strength subacutely. In contrast, full thickness coagulation of the gut wall produces marked weakness for approximately 7 days (9), directly analogous to the period of poor tensile strength during surgical wound healing. The body typically responds to full thickness gut injury by an effective sealing effort with adherence of fibrinous exudate, omentum and adjacent bowel loops against the damaged area as a bandage. This protective response effectively guards against perforation in most instances, although reduced host defenses can be expected with malnourished, immunosuppressed, or very elderly patients. Additionally, this protective sealing effect can be overwhelmed by increased intraluminal pressure, as by endoscopy repeated during the week following transmural coagulation.

There are two main factors to be considered with perforation risk: target wall thickness and nature of the adjacent structures. Caution is advised with a thin target wall, such as the cecum. Endoscopic overdistention is also an important cause of target wall thinning. An acute stress ulcer, without underlying chronic fibrotic inflammatory changes, may have a particularly thin base, as may an acute Mallory-Weiss tear. In contrast, perforation risk is less with a thicker target such as the stomach, a chronic ulcer with fibrotic base or a bulky tumor.

The consequences of perforation depend upon the nature of the adjacent structures. For example, perforation into the soft tissue surrounding the distal rectum below the peritoneal reflection may have little clinical significance. Caution is advised with target lesions adjacent to the peritoneal cavity (anterior stomach and duodenum, many portions of the colon, etc.). Similarly, the dire clinical consequences of esophageal perforation and mediastinitis demand respect for this organ. Perforation into an adjacent hollow viscus may result in a variety of enteric fistulae.

In YAG laser therapy of gastrointestinal hemorrhage, many investigators have not experienced any perforations, and, in large series, a perforation rate of 1 to 2% has been reported (2). However, in general, the perforation risk is five fold higher in palliative treatment of esophageal tumors. The majority of investigators attending the Washington Laser Symposium reported a perforation rate of 5 to 10% in YAG laser treatment of esophageal cancer (2). This may present after YAG laser treatment as a tracheoesophageal fistula. Caution is advised in treatment of mid-esophageal lesions because of the risk of TE fistula development. The therapeutic endoscopist should be prepared for placement of a prosthetic stent should a tracheoesophageal fistula develop. In addition to free perforation with laser treatment of colonic tumors, rectovaginal, rectovesical and entero-enteric fistulae have occurred (2).

Caution is advised with dilatation procedures following thermal treatment, especially as regards the weakened wall during the week following laser therapy. Problematic areas may be anticipated by careful scrutiny of the CT scan as a guide to wall thickness and tumor asymmetry.

Another subacute thermal complication is delayed hemorrhage. This may follow any thermal treatment, including endoscopic polypectomy or sphincterotomy, as well as laser coagulation (10, 11). If thermal-induced ulceration includes a normal underlying submucosal artery, massive arterial hemorrhage may result 1 to 8 days post-treatment as necrotic tissue sloughs (12). The cause of rebleeding may be difficult to ascertain with a bleeding peptic ulcer, but with a vascular ectasia, delayed hemorrhage due to arterial ulceration may present as truly massive bleeding which is an uncharacteristic bleeding pattern for the particular patient. The incidence of delayed hemorrhage is reported to be higher with YAG laser than with hemostatic devices which produce less tissue injury, such as the heater probe or BICAP (5).

Other subacute thermal effects after laser therapy include the following: fever may be due to thermal necrosis of tissue as well as secondary infection. A 'post-coagulation syndrome', characterized by localized pain and tenderness, fever and leukocytosis in the absence of free perforation or pneumoperitoneum, is due to transmural injury and inflammation or possibly a walled-off perforation. This can usually be managed non- operatively with nasogastric suction and antibiotics, whereas free perforation typically requires surgical intervention. Intractable pain following laser therapy is due to inflammatory changes produced in pain-sensitive tissues, especially at the anus or cricopharyngeus. Odynophagia or heartburn have been noted to occur in up to 20% of patients receiving laser therapy for esophageal cancer (13).

The main problematic *chronic* sequel to endoscopic thermal treatment is stenosis or stricture formation. This may occur following laser treatment of a circumferential tumor, especially if there is mainly submucosal infiltration as opposed to exophytic mucosal tumor. Post-thermal strictures can usually be managed by periodic dilatation, and the new endoscopic balloon dilators are particularly useful in difficult areas such as the colon (4).

Coaxial gas

The last category of complications is related to the coaxial gas jet used with the laser. Although venting and recycling systems are available, there remains a real hazard of bowel overdistention. With the YAG laser, at least 10 cc/sec is recommended to protect the waveguide tip from contamination, and up to 60 cc/sec is often used with endoscopic laser application to clear overlying blood. These figures translate respectively to 36 and 216 liters of gas introduce into the target organ during a one hour treatment session. The potential for inadvertent overdistention is obvious.

If a thermal treatment is applied to an overdistended, thinned out target wall, the incidence of deep tissue damage is greatly increased (7). Although effective recycling of the coaxial gas is helpful, there is no device available to accurately monitor endoscopic distention. Pressure probes are not helpful because a distensible hollow viscus can stretch notably before a significant pressure rise occurs. The most useful way to avoid over distention is to consider this possibility frequently during a treatment, to use manual suction freely, and to avoid visual effacement of mucosal folds.

If the coaxial gas is room air, there is a theoretical concern regarding air embolism, although this has not been reported with endoscopic laser therapy. To avoid this potential hazard and to allow more rapid absorption of the gas, carbon dioxide is often preferred to compressed air. Carbon dioxide absorption and hypercarbia may become significant in patients with chronic obstructive pulmonary disease and impaired carbon dioxide exchange.

Another problem related to the coaxial gas jet is gas dissection through the target wall, producing pneumatosis and/or a benign pneumoperitoneum. In my initial series of 100 YAG laser treatments, there were three instances of pneumoperitoneum found on routine post-treatment x-rays (15). In two of these cases, contrast x-rays revealed no leakage, and there was no abdominal pain, tenderness, ileus, fever, leukocytosis or other untoward effect. In the third case, pneumoperitoneum followed a low energy treatment of cecal angiodysplasia. The surgical specimen revealed prominent retroperitoneal and cecal subserosal pneumatosis and no free perforation, although peritoneal culture grew Escherichia coli in very low titer. Upon filling the resected right colon with water, no leakage of fluid occurred. It was felt that this regional subserosal emphysema represented a dissection of high pressure carbon dioxide gas though a laser induced mucosal erosion, with subsequent rupture of a gas-filled bleb. Dixon, in canine experiments using the argon laser with coaxial carbon dioxide, also observed occasional dissection of gas between layers of the colon, extending into the adjacent mesentery (16). As shown in Fig. 17.3, there is an exponential rise in the force of the carbon dioxide gas jet at close treatment distances and an extremely high pressure results when the gas catheter inadvertently touches the target mucosa. This type of dissecting microperforation and gas leak should be distinguished from a free direct thermal perforation discussed earlier. A similar benign pneumoperitoneum has been described following other endoscopic procedures and can be treated conservatively if appropriately recognized (17).

Concomitant use of high flow coaxial gas jet or water jet irrigation is essential for effectiveness with the argon laser in treating actively bleeding lesions. In contrast, the YAG laser may be used effectively without a coaxial gas jet. With the YAG laser we prefer to use occasional bursts of coaxial gas to clear debris from the fiber tip, rather than employ constant gas flow.

In conclusion, the challenge of the laser endoscopist is to control laser power

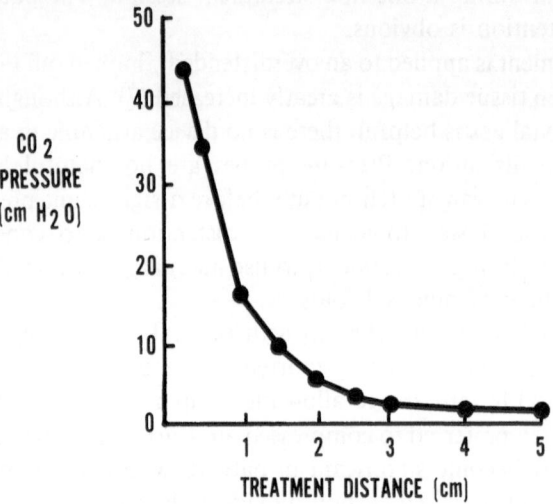

Fig. 17.3. Relationship between coaxial gas pressure and treatment distance. Note the marked increase in CO_2 back pressure with decreasing distance of coaxial gas catheter from the mucosa.

density to avoid unwanted tissue erosion, to limit thermal energy as much as possible to minimize the delayed complications of tissue ulceration, and to control coaxial gas delivery and removal to avoid gaseous complications.

References

1. Gilbert DA, Silverstein FE, Tedesco FJ et al. The national ASGE survey on upper gastrointestinal bleeding. III. Endoscopy in upper gastrointestinal bleeding. Gastrointest Endosc 1981;27:94-103.
2. Survey of investigators attending the Washington Laser Symposium, April, 1985.
3. Pietrafitta J. Complications of endoscopic laser therapy. Endoscopic laser therapy course, Boston University, July, 1985.
4. Gorisch W, Boergen KP. Heat-induced contraction of blood vessels. Lasers in Surg and Med 1982;2:1-13.
5. Johnston J. Endoscopic thermal treatment of upper gastrointestinal bleeding: Overview and guidelines. Endoscopy Review 1985;vol.2, No. 3:12-33.
6. Johnston J, Wuint R, Petruzzi C et al. Development and experimental testing of a large BICAP probe for palliative treatment of obstructing esophageal and rectal malignancy. Gastrointest Endosc 1985;31:127(abstract).
7. Johnston JH, Jensen DM, Mautner W et al. Argon laser treatment of bleeding canine gastric ulcers: Limitations and guidelines for endoscopic use. Gastroenterology 1981;80:708- 16.
8. Groisser V. YAG laser therapy of adenocarcinomas of the rectum and colon. Endoscopic laser therapy course, Boston University, July, 1985.
9. Johnston J, Rawson S. Marked weakness of the intestinal wall following experimental transmural thermal coagulation. Gastroenterology 1985;88:1435.
10. Shinya H, Wolff W. Colonoscopic polypectomy: Technique and safety. Hospital Practice 1975;10:71-78.
11. Friedman C. A new complication of endoscopic papillotomy. Gastrointest Endosc 1983;29:62.

12. Johnston J. Complications of endoscopic laser therapy. In: Fleisher D, Jensen D, Bright-Asare P, eds. Therapeutic laser endoscopy in gastrointestinal disease. Boston: Martinus Nijhoff, 1983;173.

13. Dwyer R. Single session therapy of esophageal cancer. Endoscopic laser therapy course, Boston University, July, 1985.

14. McCray R. Laser therapy of rectosigmoid cancer. Endoscopic laser therapy course, Boston University, July, 1985.

15. Johnston JH. Complications following endoscopic laser therapy. Gastrointest Endosc 1982;28:135.

16. Dixon JA, Burt RW, Rotering RH et al. Endoscopic argon laser photocoagulation of small sessile colonic polyps. Gastrointest Endosc 1982;28:162-65.

17. Katz D, Cano R, Antonelle M. Benign air dissection of the esophagus and stomach at fiberesophagogastroscopy. Gastrointest Endosc 1972;19:71-74.

18. LASER BRONCHOSCOPY: AN AMERICAN EXPERIENCE

KENNETH R. CASEY

Endobronchial surgery for both benign and malignant disease has been performed ever since the development of the open tube bronchoscope by Jackson (1). The application of this technique was limited by its difficulty and problems with hemorrhage. Because of the poor prognosis of bronchogenic carcinoma, endoscopic surgery was largely limited to non-malignant lesions such as granulomas and benign adenomas. Refinements in tools, including electrocautery and cryotherapy increased the utility of endobronchial surgery to some degree but it remained a procedure practised in highly specialized referral centers. The development of laser technology, particularly the Nd:YAG laser, with the capability of fiberoptic delivery systems has greatly increased the interest in endobronchial surgery in both tertiary referral centers and community hospitals.

The first use of laser light for endobronchial treatment involved the carbon dioxide (CO_2) laser (2). This instrument is capable of great precision because of its sharply attenuated tissue penetration. It is not compatible with existing fiberoptic systems, however, which limits its usefulness to the proximal portion of the tracheobronchial anatomy. Because of its tissue penetration characteristics, the CO_2 laser has minimal hemostatic properties. Consequently, the CO_2 laser is very useful for the treatment of small neoplasms, such as carcinoma of the larynx and relatively avascular obstructing lesions of the proximal trachea, such as webs and granuloma (3). This discussion will be concerned primarily with the Nd:YAG laser and its use in the lower respiratory tract.

Early developments in laser bronchoscopy

By far the greatest use of the Nd:YAG laser in bronchology (in part reflecting the early approved protocols) has been the palliative treatment of obstructing bronchogenic carcinoma. This work was pioneered by two groups in France beginning in 1977 (4, 5). Excellent results in large numbers of patients were reported by these groups which stimulated interest in Great Britain, Germany, and Japan. Beginning in 1981 several groups in the United States have been actively involved in Nd:YAG laser bronchoscopy. The early experience in this country produced reports which detailed dramatic complications, including

D.M. Jensen and J.M. Brunetaud (eds), Medical Laser Endoscopy. 217-231.
© 1990 Kluwer Academic Publishers, Dordrecht

fires and exsanguinating hemorrhage. Although much remains to be learned of the indications, safety, and efficacy of this procedure, in a short span of time Nd:YAG laser bronchoscopy has been approved by the FDA and appears to have become an established therapeutic tool for surgery of the airway. Numerous courses are held each year to teach principles of laser physics and biophysics to prospective laser bronchoscopists and to provide 'hands-on' experience with the laser. The University of Utah Laser Institute has trained 125 individuals in the past two years. Well over 1000 otolaryngologists, thoracic surgeons, and pulmonologists have attended such courses to date. It is likely that within two years most medium to large-sized hospitals in the United States will have the capability to perform laser bronchoscopy.

It is therefore timely to consider the indications, complications, and safety problems associated with laser bronchoscopy. Which lesions can be effectively treated with laser bronchoscopy? How large is the population of patients who might benefit from this treatment? Can laser bronchoscopy be performed with an adequate measure of safety? Is a rigid or flexible bronchoscope preferable? The following discussion will attempt to answer these questions based on the experience at the University of Utah Laser and Endoscopic Surgery Laboratory and the published reports form other centers.

Nd:YAG laser-tissue interaction

The greatest number by far of laser treatments in the lower respiratory tract have been done with the Nd:YAG laser. A limited number of treatments with the argon laser for specific indications have been performed (6, 7). There are several unique aspects of the interaction of the Nd:YAG laser with tissue which must be kept in mind to appreciate the potential benefit and hazard of using this laser in the airway. The extinction length, the thickness of material which absorbs 90% of the intensity of the light, in water for the Nd:YAG laser is 60 mm or approximately 2000 times greater than the 0.03 mm extinction length for the CO_2 laser. The Nd:YAG laser is very poorly absorbed in tissue and therefore there is considerable scattering of energy backward and sideward, especially in the particulate and in homogeneous medium of biological tissue. This effect causes the Nd:YAG laser to spread as it passes through tissue. The nature of Nd:YAG laser-tissue interaction has been recently reviewed by Polanyi who pointed out the following features of this phenomenon (8). Virtually all of the observable effects of the Nd:YAG laser on tissue are caused by thermal reactions. The absorption of Nd:YAG laser light is color dependent with darker tissues including blood absorbing light more strongly. A complex group of changes occur in the tissue. Cellular water reaches 100°C and vaporizes. Particulate elements are coagulated. As coagulation and desiccation continue the tissue becomes carbonized. In the early stages of this process the tissue may become lighter in color and therefore reflection may increase and absorption decrease. With carbonization absorption increases dramatically. With sufficiently high power density tissue may reach the point of combustion, producing sparks. Most studies of laser tissue interaction are based on simple models of uniform density. The production of temperatures greater than 100°C and particularly the production of sparks have been poorly studied because of the difficulties inherent in modeling complex systems.

Because of the characteristic scattering of Nd:YAG laser radiation, the point of maximum temperature may be just below the surface. Tissue water located there may rapidly vaporize and expand explosively. The resulting 'pop' can be very dramatic and has been referred to as the 'popcorn effect'. The tissue injury produced by the Nd:YAG laser extends deeply and widely into the surrounding tissue. The involvement of surrounding tissue may not be apparent; consequently the effect of Nd:YAG laser cannot be accurately assessed visually. Since the thermal energy is distributed widely, the rate of temperature rise is relatively slow. Consequently, a large volume of tissue can be devitalized with relatively little tissue being removed by direct vaporization; an ideal characteristic for a tumor debulking tool.

There is a wide area of coagulation surrounding the tissue cylinder of direct impact which creates the well-known hemostasis capability of the Nd:YAG laser. It should be obvious from this discussion that the Nd:YAG laser must be used with great caution in areas requiring precision such as the tracheo-bronchial tree.

University of Utah experience

Since October of 1982, we have performed 42 Nd:YAG laser bronchoscopy treatments for 31 patients. The majority of these patients have had malignant obstruction of the central airways (Table 18.1).

Table 18.1. University of Utah experience.

Bronchogenic carcinoma	
Squamous cell	16
Small cell	1
Adenocarcinoma	1
Total lung CA	**18**
Melanoma	3
Metastatic breast cancer	2
Hypernephroma	2
Embryonal cell cancer	1
Total malignant	**26**
Miscellaneous benign lesions	
Tracheal stenosis	3
Hamartoma	1
Sclerosing hemangioma	1
Total benign	**5**
Total	**31**

Ninety percent of these treatments have been done with the flexible fiberoptic bronchoscope in the Laser and Endoscopic Surgery Unit. The laser used was either the MediLas 2 or the Cooper/Molectron 8000. Because of the nature of the experimental protocol we were using, most of these patients were in the far advanced stages of bronchial carcinoma. Approximately 40% of patients evaluated for treatment were rejected. Patients were not treated if they failed to meet the criteria listed in Table 18.2.

Table 18.2. Laser bronchoscopy for malignant disease selection of patients.

1. All other reasonable therapy has failed, is likely to fail, or is associated with unacceptable complications.
2. There is an identifiable bronchial lumen.
3. The axial length of the endobronchial component is less than 4 cm in length.
4. The obstruction of the airway should be largely the result of endobronchial tumor rather than extrinsic compression.
5. The tumor does not overtly invade other structures in the thorax such as the esophagus, pericardium, and especially vascular structures in close apposition to the involved bronchus.
6. There should be evidence that recoverable functioning lung is present beyond the obstruction.

The approach to laser bronchoscopy that we have developed include fiber optic bronchoscopy through an endotracheal tube specifically developed for bronchoscopy (Xomed, Inc.). Following a routine clinical examination, an attempt is made to evaluate extent of disease. The patient is evaluated by bronchoscopy in the usual manner using topically applied anesthesia. If the endoscopic appearance confirms the clinical indications for treatment, it is carried out subsequently under general anesthesia. Frequently, we perform the laser bronchoscopy on the following day after extensive, detailed discussion of the indications, risks, and potential benefit of therapy with the patient and his family. Intravenous anesthesia is generally induced intravenously with methohexital (Brevital) and maintained with fentanyl (Sublimaze). Non-flammable inhaled agents other than nitrous oxide (which supports combustion) can also be used. Careful radiographic evaluation of the extent and location of obstruction is essential. Ventilation-perfusion scans are of no value in assessment of tumor involvement of the vasculature because the circulation may be greatly decreased in response to airway obstruction and the resulting alveolar hypoxia. One patient in our series had a complete left mainstem obstruction associated with less than 5% of the pulmonary circulation going to the left side. Following successful relief of the bronchial obstruction the perfusion increased to 35%. We have found hypocycloidal bronchial tomography to be helpful.

In our early experience, laser power of 60 to 80 watts given in 1.0 second pulses was employed. Because of the high incidence of severe complications observed at other laboratories, the power has been markedly reduced. It is rarely necessary to use more than 40 watts. The goal of treatment with the fiberoptic technique is coagulation of visible tumor and avoidance of extensive carbonization. The coagulated tumor can them be removed mechanically with minimal bleeding. It is often necessary to do repeated treatments to achieve satisfactory opening of an obstructed bronchus.

We defined a good response as restoration of the bronchial lumen to greater than 80% of normal. A fair response was a bronchial lumen of 40 to 80% of normal, and less than 40% or the residual presence of obviously untouched tumor was a poor response. In 26 patients with malignant disease the immediate results were good in 3; fair in 10; and poor in 13. The results in the 2 patients with benign neoplasms were good. Three patients with tracheal stenosis have had acceptable short term results. However, each of these patients with bottleneck tracheal stenosis resulting from prolonged endotracheal intubation have required additional procedures for more definitive treatment. We have stopped using the Nd:YAG laser for this condition because it is though to be better managed with the CO_2 laser. The assessment of results is subjective and limited to short-term follow-up. It is clear from this group of patients, however, that a good short-term response is not necessarily related to prolonged survival, which probably reflects the advanced nature of the tumors in these patients.

The longest survival of any of the patients in the malignant disease group has been 10 months. This figure is somewhat less than that reported in other series. In general patients treated in the United States have had more advanced disease than those treated in Europe. To date there is no published controlled study of survival following laser bronchoscopy. In fact, there is surprisingly little data available regarding the natural history of endobronchial carcinoma untreated following radiation therapy. Until the development of laser bronchoscopy, there was no practical means of treating post-radiation recurrences of malignant airway obstruction. Therefore, these patients were followed radiographically rather than endoscopically.

Interestingly, although about 50% of our patients with malignant airway obstruction experience symptomatic improvement, it did not appear to be closely correlated to the response to therapy assessed endoscopically or radiographically. These patients are frequently desperate and highly susceptible to a 'placebo' effect. This is a factor which should be kept in mind when evaluating subjective responses to treatment.

It is apparent that our experience using laser bronchoscopy in patients with advanced carcinoma has been less than gratifying. The following case histories suggest applications in which laser bronchoscopy represents a clear advantage over previously available therapeutic techniques.

Plate 42 and 43 in the atlas contains pre- and post-treatment endoscopic photographs of the right mainstem bronchus of a 19 year-old female. A large tumor was completely obstructing the bronchus. Biopsy presented a confusing dilemma to the pathologist. After several weeks it was finally concluded that the pathology was consistent with an endobronchial hamartoma but that it was probably malignant. Because of the location of the tumor surgical treatment was not an option. She was treated with the Nd:YAG laser with remarkable results. Luckily, the stalk of this polypoid tumor was transected by the laser and the entire bulk of the tumor was removed with rapid resolution of obstructive symptoms. After three months the tumor was found to be recurring. At that time she underwent a carinal resection with apparently complete removal of abnormal tissue. This surgery would have been extremely difficult if not impossible at the time of initial presentation.

The second patient, whose endoscopic photographs are shown in Plates 44 and 45 in the atlas is an 82-year-old gentleman who presented to the Salt Lake City Veterans Administration Medical Center with acute respiratory failure associated with consolidation and collapse of the right lung, high fever, and hypoxemia requiring 80% oxygen to maintain adequate arterial saturation. He was started on mechanical ventilation and underwent a diagnostic bronchoscopy which revealed a virtually complete obstruction of the right mainstem bronchus by poorly differentiated squamous cell carcinoma. Because of his dependence on ventilatory support and because of the severity of his obstructive pneumonia we felt acute relief of the obstruction by laser bronchoscopy was indicated. Following treatment he remained on the ventilator four days during which he was bronchoscoped daily and plugs of necrotic tumor were removed from the treatment site. His pneumonia improved and on the fifth day he was weaned from ventilator support and began a course of radiation therapy. The laser probably shortened this patient's hospital stay significantly and allowed him to be quickly weaned from mechanical ventilation. Although his survival was short he was able to leave the hospital and arrange his personal affairs.

There have been two major complications in the series of patients treated at the University of Utah. On patient, who was later found to have superior vena caval obstruction, suffered a cardiorespiratory arrest immediately after completion of the procedure because of laryngeal edema. He was successfully re- intubated and resuscitated with no apparent ill effects. Another patient, a 19 year-old traumatic quadriplegic with tracheal stenosis was exposed to the combustion of the fiberoptic bronchoscope and polyvinyl chloride endotracheal tube intra- tracheally (9). This patient developed extensive tracheal stenosis following prolonged endotracheal intubation. At the time of treatment she was dependent on mechanical ventilation and was not felt to be an acceptable candidate for reconstructive surgery. After treating her stenosis for approximately 2.5 hours a bright flash of yellow light was observed. The bronchoscope and endotracheal tube were removed both of which were in flames. The patients was immediately re-intubated and the airways examined. It was then discovered that an assistant had increased the oxygen concentration in the inspired air to approximately 80% during the course of treatment. It was then routine practice in our institution to increase the oxygen level during bronchoscopy on intubated patients. Remarkably enough, she did not appear to suffer any irreversible injury from the incident. She had a functional tracheal lumen of 8mm following treatment; however the stenosis recurred. Ultimately she was treated with CO_2 laser and a stint was put in place for 3 months. Her

222

trachea has been stable for over 24 months.

We have not yet produced massive bleeding. Patients commonly have 100-400 ml of blood loss during the course of the procedure which is of minimal consequence other than it interferes with visualization of the airway structures. Fatal hemorrhage is an ever-present risk. It is of interest to note that one of the patients we chose not to treat because of the advanced state of his tumor died of overwhelming hemoptysis within a few hours of our consultation. Penetration of vascular structures is an uncommon but well described cause of death in patients with lung cancer.

Review of Nd:YAG laser bronchoscopy in the United States

It is not possible to discuss the current status of laser bronchoscopy without briefly mentioning the pioneering work done by two groups in France. Toty et al. reported a large series of 317 treatment sessions in 164 patients in 1981 (4). Dumon et al. reported the experience of more that 205 treatments in 111 patients in March 1982 (5). This group accumulated a series of more than 1500 treatments from several laboratories (10). One of the earliest reports of Nd:YAG laser bronchoscopy in the United States, described the first 22 patients treated by McDougall and Cortese (11). Two of these patients died because of uncontrollable hemorrhage. Similar results were reported by Arabian and Spagnolo (12). They had two deaths in the first 20 patients treated. Even so, in both of these groups the majority of patients had immediate symptomatic improvement. Unger (13) reported a series of 325 procedures of which the majority were done with the fiberoptic bronchoscope and topical anesthesia. They did not note any occurrence of anesthetic complications. This group claimed that 80% of patients with malignant disease experienced an improvement. They reported 23% of patients with poor results (defined as no restoration of lumen), 30% as fair (partial restoration of lumen), and 47% as excellent (restoration of lumen with improvement in symptoms). These investigators corroborated the observation made in the French series that lesions in the central airways responded better than distal lesions. Eighty-seven percent of the patients with benign lesions had excellent responses and 13% (2 patients) had fair results. Joyner et al. (14) took a somewhat different approach by concentrating on more peripheral lesions using an intrabronchial mapping technique to identify the bronchial lumen distal to the obstruction. Performing 109 treatments in 45 patients using topical anesthesia, they reported 27 patients with obstruction in lobar and segmental bronchi. Of these patients, results were said to be excellent in 19, good in 5, and poor in 3. This series had two patients who expired from intra-airway hemorrhage.

Gelb and Epstein (15) reported a series of 27 lung cancer patients with incomplete bronchial obstruction and 19 patients with complete obstruction. The results were considerably better in the group with incomplete rather than total obstruction. Mean survival for the incomplete obstruction group was 4.9

months ($\pm$ 3.2) compared to a mean survival of only 2.0 ($\pm$ 1.7) for the complete obstruction group. There were two deaths in this series, one of which was related to progressive respiratory failure associated with extensive tumor involvement. The other death was in a patient who experienced an endotracheal fire, although the death seemed to be more closely related to extensive tumor than to the fire.

Kvale et al. (16) reported 99 patients who were considered for laser treatment of whom 55 were treated 89 times. Eight of ten patients with benign disease had satisfactory results. They classified the lung cancer patients into a group treated with the laser at their initial presentation and a group with recurrent tumor. Of the initial treatment group 12 of 13 had satisfactory results. In the recurrent group, satisfactory results were obtained in 22 of 32. They had two deaths, one associated with a fatal arrhythmia and the other with Staphylococcal pneumonia. One patient was reported as a complication because of a near perforation of the esophagus from the trachea. This group had three flash fires but no sustained combustion. Because of concern over vascular penetration this group introduced a method of rapid sequence CAT scans to elucidate the thoracic anatomy.

Much of the early experience in the United States, particularly in centers where pulmonary internists are doing laser bronchoscopy, has involved the use of the fiberoptic bronchoscope. It has been argued by Dumon and his collaborators that there are considerable advantages to the rigid bronchoscope for these operative procedures (10). The arguments in favor of the rigid technique include better control of hemorrhage and more complete debulking of tumor. It is doubtful that any of the massive hemorrhage episodes reported in the above series would have been treatable with the rigid bronchoscope. Nevertheless, it is possible to remove coagulated tumor tissue much easier with the rigid scope. During training courses, it appears that surgeons accustomed to the rigid bronchoscope become comfortable with the laser technique using that instrument much quicker than physicians learning the fiberoptic technique. Common sense suggests that a laser bronchoscopist should have a reasonable level of skill with either procedure. There is now substantial agreement about the importance of decreasing power from the high levels used in the early studies in order to decrease the risk of perforation and combustion (17).

Summary of indications and Complications

Table 18.3 presents the present indications for Nd:YAG laser bronchoscopy. Benign endobronchial lesions are quite rare. There are occasional patients with granuloma, amyloidosis, polyposis, etc. who could be treated endoscopically without the need for thoracotomy. 'Bronchial adenomas', such as carcinoid tumors and cylindromas are not truly benign but have a variable potential for malignant behavior. Consequently, in the absence of contraindications for surgical resection, these tumors should be removed by a conventional operation. For reasons suggested in the discussion of Nd:YAG laser-tissue interaction, the CO_2 laser appears to be the preferable tool for laser treatment of tracheal stenosis and other lesions of the trachea which are not bulky or highly vascular.

Table 18.3. Indications for laser bronchoscopy.

1. Benign endobronchial lesions
2. Tracheal or bronchial adenomas in patients in whom surgery presents a high risk
3. Tracheal stenosis
4. Metastatic cancer to the airway with obstruction of bleeding.
5. Bleeding after biopsy of endobronchial lesions.
6. Bronchogenic carcinoma which is immediately life-threatening because of airway obstruction or bleeding (before radiation of chemotherapy).
7. Bronchogenic carcinoma which is recurrent or unresponsive to 'conventional' therapy.

Patient selection is a critical factor in the management of patients with malignant bronchial obstruction. A variety of approaches to evaluating these patients have been presented including rapid sequence computerized axial tomography with contrast media, hypocycloidal chest tomography, intra-bronchial injection of contrast media, and endoscopic staging. A very strong selection criteria should be the duration of apparent bronchial obstruction. If the airway has been blocked for more than a few weeks, it is unlikely that significant pulmonary function is recoverable. From an ethical standpoint one must consider two poles of a debate concerning the medical management of patients with terminal cancer. On the one hand is the philosophy of doing everything possible. On the other hand, one could argue that the expense, discomfort and considerable risk of laser bronchoscopy are seldom justifiable in light of the limited benefit which has been demonstrated. We have to date generally tried to perform the procedure unless the risk-benefit scale was strongly balanced to the contrary. As data confirming limited benefit are reported it seems clear that the number of patients in whom this aggressive treatment is warranted is small.

Table 18.4 presents the major complications of Nd:YAG laser bronchoscopy. The largest number of adverse outcomes has been associated with anesthesia complications. This reflects the fact that patients considered for laser bronchoscopy are frequently debilitated. Although there are minimal data available comparing the complications of the two techniques, one advantage of the flexible fiberoptic bronchoscope is that the level of anesthesia need not be as deep as with the rigid bronchoscope. Consequently, the risk of anesthetic complications is probably less. It is essential to closely monitor cardiopulmonary function, including continuous monitoring of arterial oxygen saturation, during these treatments as would be done during any major surgical procedure.

Table 18.4. Complications of laser bronchoscopy.

1. Massive hemorrhage
2. Endotracheal combustion
3. Anesthesia complications:
   cardiac arrhythmias
   hypoxemia
   carbon dioxide retention, etc.
4. Retained secretions
5. Infection (local and/or disseminated)
6. Bronchial perforation without hemorrhage:
   pneumothorax
   pneumomediastinum, etc.
7. Diffuse alveolar injury from smoke inhalation

Two unique and dramatic complications deserve to be discussed in detail – specifically endotracheal combustion and massive hemorrhage. The three mechanisms through which and endoscope might be ignited, direct impact, reflected light and sparks, are illustrated in Fig. 18.1.

Our study of the combustion incident at the University of Utah included creating a model system (Fig. 18.2) in which a flow of gas with a known oxygen concentration was passed around a piece of tissue, used as a laser target, toward the bronchoscope. In this model we were able to create fires with O_2 concentrations as low as 30-35%.

The investigation was limited by the number of surplus bronchoscopes available for destruction. Based on this observation it seems most likely that indirect ignition of the bronchoscope by sparks is the most common cause of

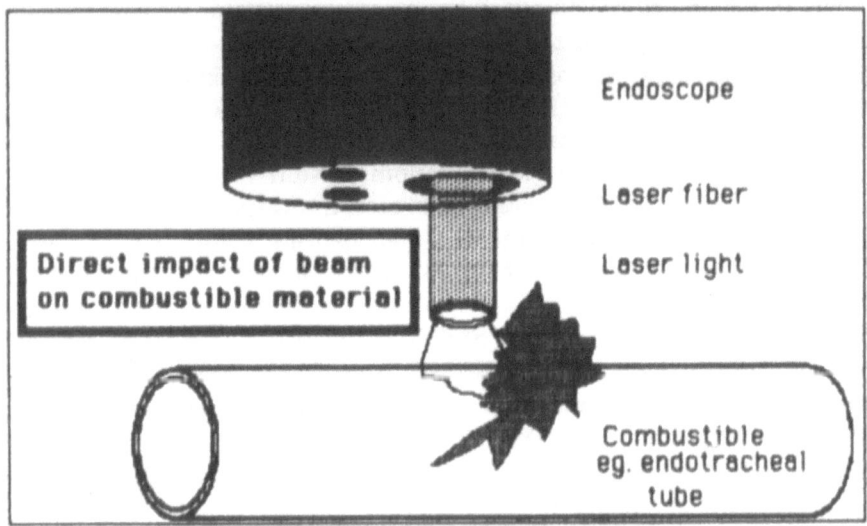

Fig. 18.1A. Direct impact of laser on combustible material.

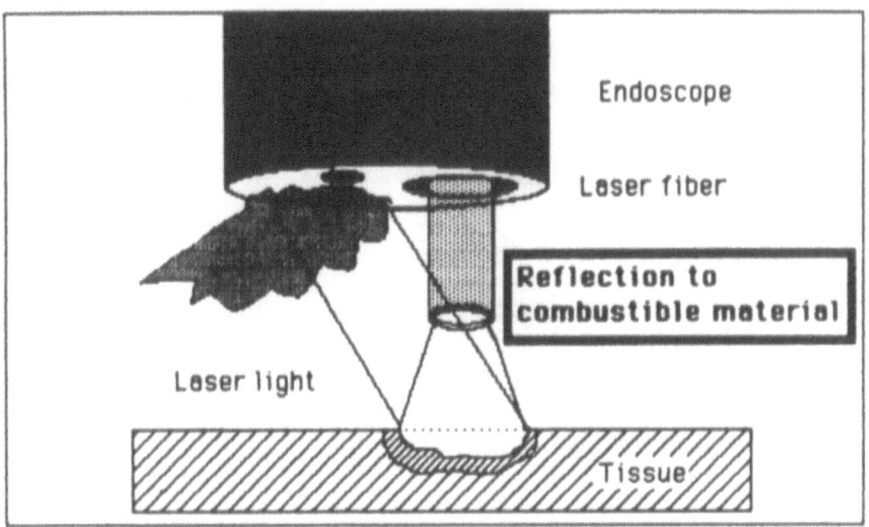

Fig. 18.1B. Reflection to combustible material.

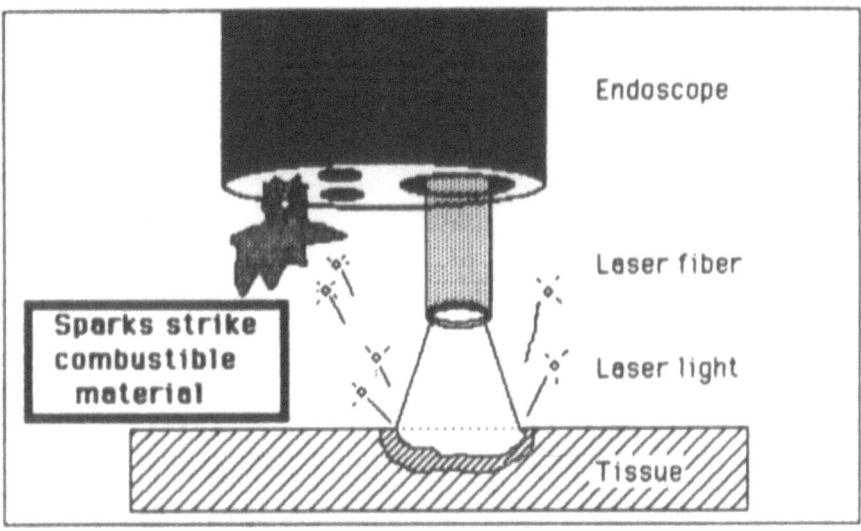

Fig. 18.1C. Sparks strike combustible material.

fires. We have therefore suggested the steps listed in Table 18.5 to avoid this serious complication.

The oxygen concentration is a major risk factor for fires. We minimize the amount of oxygen present in the microenvironment of laser impact by using an inert coaxial gas, helium. Nitrogen could also be used and is considerably less expensive. Helium has the advantage of greater heat dissipating capacity. Carbon dioxide should not be used as the coaxial gas in bronchoscopy because

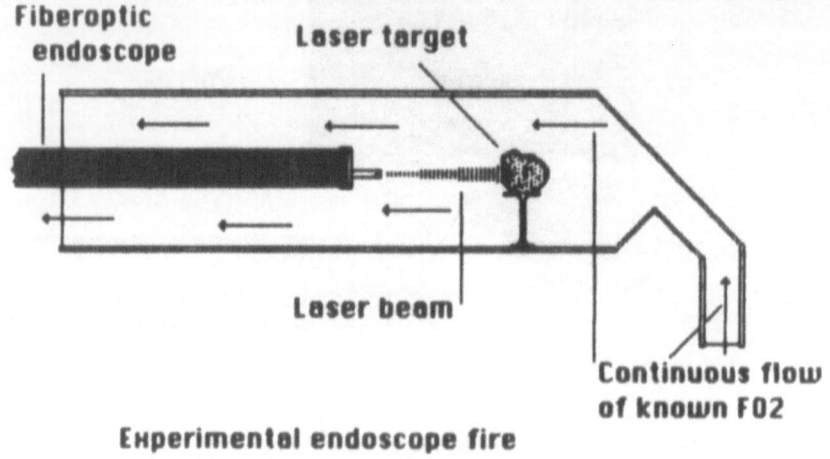

Fiberoptic endoscope

Laser target

Laser beam

Continuous flow of known F02

Experimental endoscope fire

Fig. 18.2. Experimental bronchoscope.

Table 18.5. Endotracheal fires during Nd:YAG laser bronchoscopy.

A. Factors responsible for fires
    1. Enriched oxygen atmosphere
    2. Combustible material
    3. Intense heat
    4. Enclosed space

B. Principles to follow to avoid fires
    1. Lowest possible oxygen concentration
    2. Helium flush of operative field
    3. Meticulous preparation of laser fiber tip
    4. Maintain clear field of vision
    5. General anesthesia
    6. Work at greatest possible distance from the bronchoscope
    7. Avoid extensive carbonization of tissue
    8. Close cooperation of the operating team

it will cause increased PCO_2. This is particularly the case in patients under general anesthesia who are unable to increase their ventilatory rate. We closely monitor arterial saturation with a pulse oximeter (or ear oximeter). The inhaled FiO_2 is under continuous control by an assistant. When the laser is being used, the FiO_2 is 21% until the patient's arterial blood begins to show significant desaturation (SaO_2 of less than 88%). At that point the laser is withdrawn and optimal oxygen loading is resumed.

The incidents of massive hemorrhage that have occurred seem to be related to penetration of the bronchus and creation of a broncho-vascular fistula. It is difficult to predict the precise relationship between vascular structures and the bronchus in cancer patients. The anatomy is often distorted by the tumor, collapse, and radiation. Comprehensive knowledge of thoracic anatomy and

CAT scans may be of some value to avoid dangerous areas. However, the risk of massive bleeding cannot be completely eliminated. As discussed above, with the Nd:YAG laser it is difficult to control the depth of penetration. The most effective way to decrease the incidence of massive bleeding is to keep the power density low and the pulse duration less than 1.0 second. The end-point of treatment should be coagulation rather than carbonization. It must be pointed out that this conservative approach may result in less complete removal of tumor tissue and a more rapid recurrence of obstruction.

Future directions in laser bronchoscopy

There are few current accepted strong indications for laser bronchoscopy and the risk of complications is high. Consequently, it would be appropriate to consider limiting the proliferation of medical centers doing Nd:YAG laser bronchoscopy.

Controversy will persist over the indications for laser bronchoscopy until controlled trials can be designed to objectively evaluate the response to treatment, particularly in malignant airway obstruction (18). From the experience to date, it does appear that laser bronchoscopy offers considerable palliative benefit in carefully selected patients. However, this type of laser surgery will remain a secondary form of treatment because it cannot destroy tumor tissue outside of the airway. As currently practised, laser bronchoscopy involves a marginally acceptable risk of complications and a rate of response which is often disappointing. Combining Nd:YAG laser bronchoscopy with other modalities may enhance its value. There is preliminary experience which suggests that using the laser *before* radiation for obstructing tumors is associated with a better survival (16). As in one patient in our series, laser bronchoscopy may be useful acutely to relieve the immediate threat to life of an obstructed bronchus making more definitive surgery possible. It is possible that the Nd:YAG laser can be used in conjunction with photodynamic therapy with hematoporphyrin-derivative or other exogenous chromophores. For example, there is evidence from some investigators that PDT is hazardous in far advanced bronchogenic carcinoma. It is possible that initial relief of obstruction with the Nd:YAG laser may make subsequent PDT feasible.

At the present time it does not appear the Nd:YAG laser bronchoscopy will have dramatic influence on the care of patients with airway lesions. The value in lung cancer patients is strictly palliative and of limited duration, although in a small number of carefully selected patients the palliative benefit is dramatic. The rare patient with benign neoplasia or inflammatory obstruction of the trachea or bronchus will be well treated with laser bronchoscopy. The availability of a fiberoptic delivery system for the CO_2 laser may be useful for some patients currently being treated with the Nd:YAG laser. There has been minimal data published which address the question of 'should' we use the laser in bronchology. To date there have been no controlled studies demonstrating benefit from laser bronchoscopy in *any* population of patients. The data available are directed at 'how' to do the procedure. Some of these technical concerns with the Nd:YAG laser are summarized below.

1. There is a long learning 'curve' during which the incidence of serious complications is greater than after a given team has learned to work together with precision and caution. The learning curve is probably less dramatic using the rigid bronchoscope. The fiber optic technique is difficult to learn and requires considerable endoscopic experience and skill. The fiberoptic bronchoscope can be used to perform laser bronchoscopy if it is used with great skill and great caution. It is probably inherently more risky in novice hands than the rigid bronchoscope.

2. There is an unavoidable risk of combustion during laser bronchoscopy. For upper airway procedures in which the Nd:YAG laser or CO_2 laser are being used, specially designed endotracheal tubes are essential. The fiberoptic bronchoscope, with or without an endotracheal tube greatly increases the risk of fire. The risk of fire is related to the concentration of oxygen in the airway, the power density of the laser, and the light absorbing characteristics of the tissue (e.g. the degree of carbonization). Avoidance of high FiO_2, extensive carbonization, and high power density are vital. Close cooperation of the operating team, the use of non-flammable anesthetics, and adequate anesthesia also decrease the fire hazard.

3. There is a serious risk of penetration of the bronchus resulting in pneumomediastinum, pneumothorax, and particularly broncho-vascular fistula formation. Several patients have died from massive intra-operative or post-operative hemorrhage.

4. Decreasing the power density used with the aim of coagulation rather than vaporization reduces the risk of penetration and combustion. A setting of 25 to 40 watts with a pulse duration of 0.5-1.5 seconds is adequate for the majority of laser applications.

5. Careful selection of the patients is important since treatment of extensive, complete luminal obstruction is unlikely to produce satisfactory palliation.

6. Some technique to elucidate the juxtaposition of the involved airway and surrounding chest structures should be undertaken such as rapid sequence contrast chest computerized tomography, hypocycloidal tomography of the tracheobronchial tree, or intra- bronchial injection of water-soluble contrast media. In any event, the distal portion of the left mainstem bronchus and both upper lobe bronchi are dangerous locations for treatment because of the proximity of the pulmonary arteries. The posterior wall of the trachea and proximal mainstems should be approached with caution because of risk of esophageal penetration.

7. Because of the high risk (and limited indications), laser bronchoscopy is best restricted to referral medical centers with a team of personnel experienced in laser bronchoscopy. It is unlikely that small hospitals will be able to maintain a sufficient number of patients to maintain the high level of skill necessary.

8. The introduction of new techniques of photodynamically mediated laser effects promises substantial advantage over the current thermal laser-tissue interaction.

References

1. Poyd AD, Spencer FC. Endoscopy: bronchoscopy and esophagoscopy. In: Sabiston DC Jr, Spencer FC, eds. Gibbon's Surgery of the chest, 4th edition. Philadelphia, Saunders. 1983;60-70.
2. Strong MS, Vaughan CW, Polanyi T, Wallace RA. Bronchoscopic carbon dioxide laser surgery. Ann Otol 1974;83:769-776.
3. Mc Elvein RB, Zorn GL Jr. Indications, results, and complications of bronchoscopic carbon dioxide laser therapy.
Ann Surg 1984;199:522-525.
4. Toty L, Personne C, Colchen A, Courc'h G. Bronchoscopic management of tracheal lesions using Nd:YAG laser. Thorax 1981;36:175-178.
5. Dumon JF, Reboud E, Garbe L, Aucomte F, Meric B. Treatment of tracheobronchial lesions by laser photoresection. Chest 1982;81:278-284.
6. Williams I, Radcliffe G, Hetzel M, Millard J. Tracheal rhinoscleroma treated by the argon laser. Thorax 1982;37:638-639.
7. Millard FJC, Hetzel MR, Williams I, Bridges C. Endoscopic argon laser treatment of bronchial carcinoma. Thorax 1981;36:235.
8. Polanyi TG. Physics of surgery with lasers, Clinics in Chest Medicine. June 1985, pp. 179-202.
9. Casey KR, Fairfax W, Smith S, Dixon J. Intratracheal fire ignited by the Nd:YAG laser during treatment of tracheal stenosis. Chest 1983;84:295-296.
10. Dumon JF, Shapshay S, Bourcereau J, Cavaliere S, Meric B, Garbi N, Beamis J. Principles for safety in application of Nd:YAG laser in bronchology. Chest 1984;86:163-168.
11. McDougall JC, Cortese DA. Nd:YAG laser therapy of malignant airway obstruction, a preliminary report. Mayo Clin Proc 1983;58:35-39.
12. Arabian A, Spagnolo SV. Laser therapy in patients with primary lung cancer. Chest 1984;86:519-23.
13. Unger M. Nd:YAG laser therapy for malignant and benign endobronchial obstructions. Clinics in chest Med 1985;6:277- 290.
14. Joyner LR Jr, Maran AG, Samara R, Yakaboski A. Nd:YAG laser treatment of intrabronchial lesions: a new mapping technique via the flexible fiberoptic bronchoscope. Chest 1985;87:418-427.
15. Gelb AF, Epstein JD. Laser in treatment of lung cancer. Chest 1984;86:662-666.
16. Kvale PA, Eichenhorn MS, Radke J, Miks V. YAG laser photoresection of lesions obstructing the central airways. Chest 1985;87:283-288.
17. Brutinel WM, Cortese DA, McDougall JC. Bronchoscopic phototherapy with the Nd:YAG laser. Chest 1984;86:158-159.
18. Beamis JF, Shapshay S. More about the YAG. Chest 1985;87:277- 278.

19. NEODYMIUM-YAG-LASER TREATMENT OF BENIGN AND MALIGNANT TRACHEO-BRONCHIAL LESIONS

C. PERSONNE, A. COLCHEN, G. VOURC'H,
J.F. DUMON AND A. MERIC

Laser, in bronchology, was first tried in 1974 by Strong, who used a carbon dioxide laser coupled to a rigid bronchoscope (1). In 1978 the Paris team first used the Neodymium-Yttrium-Aluminum-Garnet laser (Nd- YAG) which is much better suited to endoscopic requirements than the CO_2 laser because of the flexible fiber (2).

Our two teams, working in Paris and Marseilles, have carried out about 5000 endoscopic resections of tracheo-bronchial lesions and tumors (3, 4, 5). In the past few years, the number of publications on laser in bronchology has greatly increased. But, apart from that of Strong (6), the series reported are small. Major technical problems have impeded a widespread use of the method (7, 8, 9, 10, 11, 12).

In the present chapter, the techniques and indications of our two groups will be analyzed and discussed. Our twin experiences are parallel but similar. The differences will be discussed. They underscore essentially technical details.

Material and methods

Indications for our two series are presented in Table 19.1: 2898 patients had 4928 endoscopic resections, over a 9 year period for our two Nd:YAG laser units (Nov. 1978 to Oct. 1987 for Paris; Apr. 1980 to Oct. 1987 for Marseilles).

Table 19.1. Paris (Personne) and Marseilles (Dumon) indications and total cases.

Indications	Paris	Marseilles
Cancers	967	513
Mod. malignant tumor	64	39
Benign tumor	85	51
Stenoses	525	190
Granulomas	228	74
Miscellaneous	29	133
Patients	1898	1000
Sessions	3204	1724

D.M. Jensen and J.M. Brunetaud (eds), Medical Laser Endoscopy. 233-245.
© 1990 Kluwer Academic Publishers, Dordrecht

Apparatus

Both groups used a French Nd:YAG laser (YM 100 Cilas). It provides an input of 50 watts in continuous burst or 100 watts in pulses of 0.3 seconds. The duration of the pulses is adjustable, but the interval between two pulses is 2 seconds. The fiber is made of flexible quartz (600 microns). It is inserted in a sheath of Teflon of 2 mm diameter, and can be easily mended by any hospital technical department.

Endoscopy and anesthesia in Paris

At the time of the first endoscopic resections in patients in Paris the rigid bronchoscope was selected as Toty has done in the course of his previous animal experiments. Ever since, we have used rigid bronchoscopes in nearly all our patients. Over several years, various improvements have been made in our technique, and a special bronchoscope has been manufactured (Storz). Within the lumen of the bronchoscope, three channels have been welded: one to convey the light fiber, the other for jet ventilation, the third one to fit a constant suction catheter, reaching beyond the distal end of the bronchoscope (Fig. 19.1).

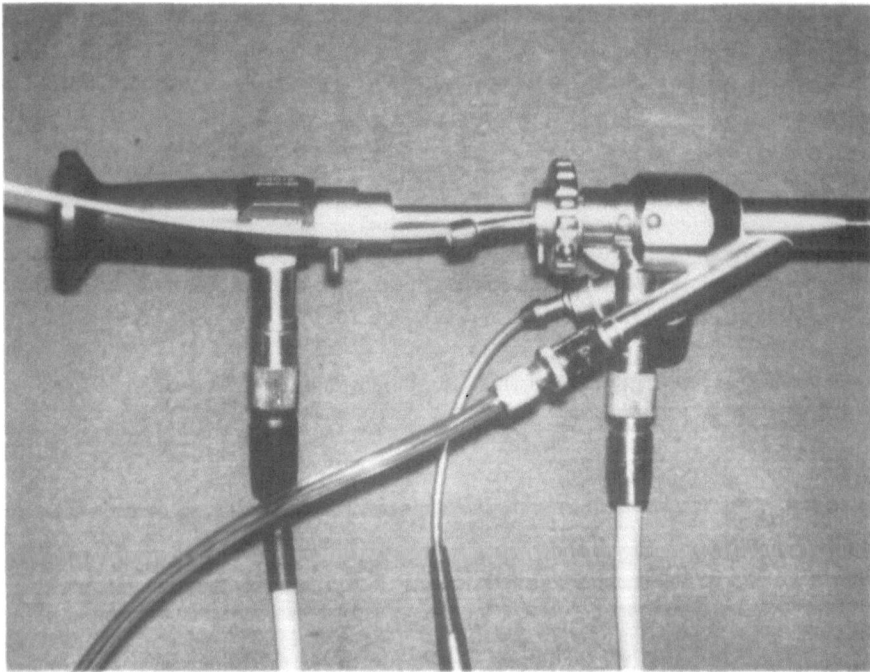

Fig. 19.1. Bronchoscope used by the Paris team. These channels are incorporated inside the tube for light, Sanders ventilation, and permanent suction. The laser fiber coupled with the optics is adjustable.

The fiberscope alone is used only for minor, selected indications such as iatrogenic granulomas sprouting around a chronic tracheostomy ostium. On the other hand, the fiberscope inserted within the rigid bronchoscope is mandatory to deal with distal lesions, or those sited in an upper lobe bronchus.

For anesthesia, intravenous short acting drugs are given (methohexital or propanidid) with occasional narcotics (Alfentanyl). Muscle relaxation is achieved by a suxamethonium infusion in order to achieve a complete immobility of the target. For ventilation we use the Sanders injector, with a 50% mixture of oxygen and nitrogen (13). Although reported by others (14), no case of ignition or explosion has been observed. None of our endoscopic equipment is flammable. This form of jet ventilations safe for the most dangerous cases. As soon as the bronchoscope is inserted and jet ventilation used, the patient's condition always improves even if apparently desperate. High frequency jet-ventilation has been tried since 1983. The main advantage provided is the nearly complete immobility of the chest wall and bronchial tree, but it cannot be used in case of major obstruction since it leads to a dangerous increase in Pa CO_2 (15). Following the resection the patients are monitored in a recovery room. The duration of hospitalization is 2 to 4 days.

Table 19.2. Complications of the Paris series.

Immediate complications	
Deaths	5
Hemorrhage > 250 cc	12
Mediastinal emphysema	5
Delayed complications	
Deaths	20
Pneumothoraces	22

Complications of the Paris Series

The complications of the Paris series are reported in Table 19.2. A total of 25 deaths occurred. The five deaths from massive hemorrhage were due to the laser itself: in four the hemorrhage was due to massive tumor necrosis at the carina and probable involving the pulmonary artery. The fifth patient expired from perforation of the innominate artery during the ninth endoscopic treatment of a patient whose airway had been maintained for 17 months. The twenty delayed deaths were due to obstructions which could not be relieved by laser retreatment. They are both failures and complications of the method but, above all, errors in selection. Those 25 deaths (0.7% of all sessions, 1.3% of all patients) were all in patients with cancer. This reflects the severity of the indications met with and accepted (281 patients were admitted as extreme emergencies, with acute asphyxia and sometimes comatose). Our complication rate of treatment must be considered in light of 58 patients who died on their way to the hospital.

The 22 pneumothoraces were not due to the laser itself but the jet ventilation. All were quickly diagnosed and easily treated. None occurred during the past six years with our increasing use of high- frequency jet ventilation. Some post-operative febrile infections were easily treated. No case of delayed bleeding has been observed. The development of fibrinoid membranes on the resection surfaces can be a complication which one must be aware of. If large and loose, they may induce severe dyspnea the day after resection. They are easily removed with a fiberscope. Endoscopic control must be systematic after all resections.

The techniques used in Marseilles are similar to those used by the Paris group, although there are some differences. General anesthesia and rigid tube are used in high risk cases such as tracheal or main bronchial tumors and tracheal stenoses. However, 20% of the total cases are performed under local anesthesia, by fibroscopy, particularly when the lesion is small (small peripheral tumors, granulomas, stitches) (16). The anesthetic technique does not include curarization or jet ventilation. The patients are left on spontaneous breathing. An EFER bronchoscope was made to provide close circuit ventilation in case of hypoxia or cardiovascular complications (Fig. 19.2).

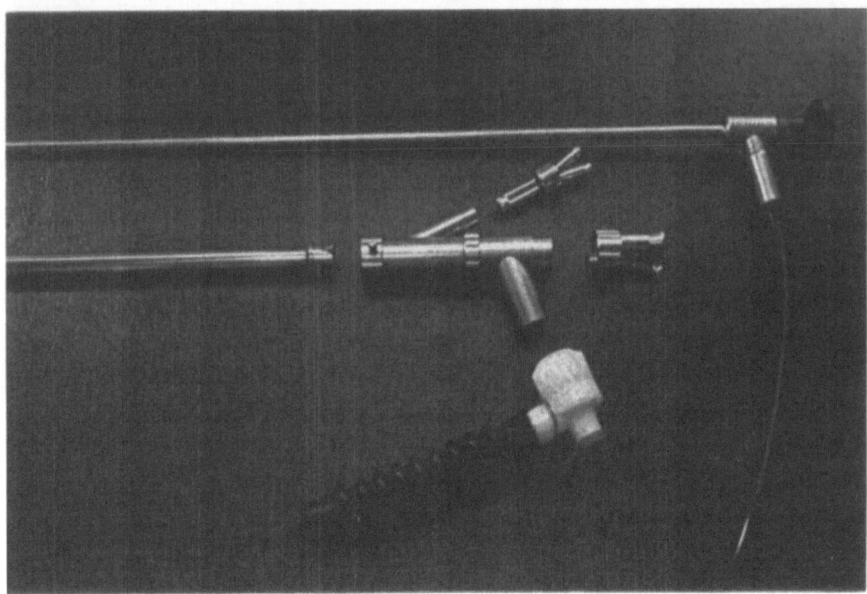

Fig. 19.2. Bronchoscope used by the Marseilles team. On the same head several tubes may be adapted (3 to 9mm). There is an adjustable ventilation connection.

The fiber is left free in the bronchoscope. One or two single use catheters are introduced near the fiber in order to clear blood and smoke during the procedure. The laser is always used at a power lower than 50 watts with pulses that average 0.7 seconds. The number of pulses is kept to a minimum and the tip of the bronchoscope being used to complete the resection.

Table 19.3. Complications of the Marseilles series.

Immediate complications	
Cardiac arrests	2
Severe hypoxemia	4
Hemorrhage > 250 cc	14
Mediastinal emphysema	2
Delayed complications	
Deaths	3
Pneumothoraces	3
Infections	3
Hemorrhage	1

Complications for Marseilles are summarized in Table 19.3. The Marseilles group considers hemorrhage to be the major risk, on account of the hypoxia induced (over 700 ml in 3 cases), and warrants the use of the rigid bronchoscope. Priority must be given by the anesthetist to provide adequate ventilation until the blood gases are back to normal.

As for technical maneuvers, we can only summarize them, and point out some basic notions. 1) The tip of the fiber must never touch the target. It must be kept between 5 to 10 mm from it in order to achieve the best efficiency. 2) To achieve coagulation, the best is to withdraw the tip of the fiber, rather than reducing the power. 3) Continuous burst must be restricted to tumors, especially cancers. This achieves quicker destruction. Pulses are preferable for iatrogenic lesions since they generate less heat and avoid adding thermal injury to a stenotic lesion. 4) Charred surfaces must be removed once established because carbonization impedes further laser photocoagulation. 5) The main difficulty to be met when resecting obstructing cancerous lesions is to assess their exact extension. Very often the endoscopist sees only the tip of the tumor. Unable to pass it, he cannot assess its extension. For example, a tracheal tumor which at first sight seems more or less spherical. However, as the resection proceeds, it may be found to involve the carina and one or both main bronchi (Fig. 19.3A). Another one which starts with a polypoid growth ends up with an unmanageable external compression (Fig. 19.3B). Resection with the laser may take up to an hour. Sometimes it is necessary to pass distal to the tumor and perform the resection while withdrawing the bronchoscope.
6) Whatever the difficulties met with, it is most important that an adequate airway should be restored at the end of the session. An overly timid or impossible resection may worsen the situation. One session should achieve as much as possible, especially if the respiratory situation is serious.

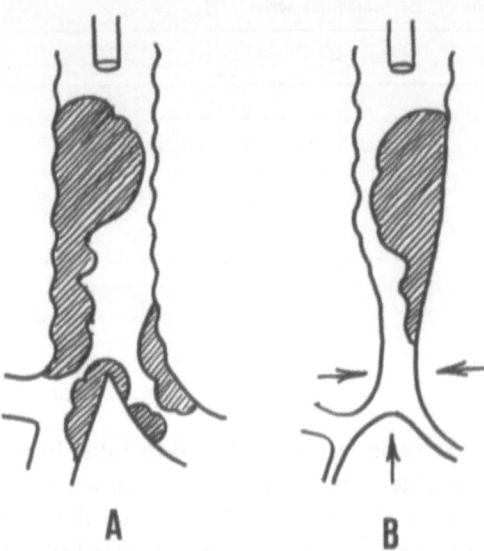

Fig. 19.3. Two cases of cancers which appear similar to the endoscopist: A) extensive spreading: the resection is possible and efficacious; B) an underlying external compression makes the resection useless.

Discussion of indications

There is general agreement upon indications for endoscopic resections in bronchology. Strong had already considered them in his pioneer article (1). As reported in the present paper, indications can be classified below.

1) Benign tracheobronchial tumors

These are exceedingly rare. The least rare of these are lipomas and solitary papillomas. However, most of them have mixed histology, which makes their classification difficult. They are usually round, of beige color, poorly vascularized, with a thin pedicle, and are well suited to endoscopic resections. Unfortunately, their growth is usually distal and the pedicle is not easy to visualize. Therefore, one must often resort to total destruction instead of complete extraction. The stem of implantation must be destroyed carefully to prevent recurrence. In our series, there has been no recurrence during four years mean follow-up. For this particular indication, endoscopic laser resection must achieve a radical cure and takes the place of traditional surgery, which should no longer be resorted to except for the rare benign, iceberg-like tumors and for tumors stemming from a segmental bronchus of an upper lobe which is difficult to reach. Refer to Plates 1-2 in the Atlas as an example of treatment of a leiomyoma. A similar technique would be used for treatment of other benign pedunculated tumors.

Diffuse papillomatosis differs whenever it affects a child or an adult. In the adult form, even when the tuft of papillomas are widely spread, their total number usually does not exceed 20 to 30. Two or three sessions should be enough to treat them, destroying both papillomas and their stalks. The procedure may be curative: 4 cases of the Paris series have no recurrence 2 and 3 years later.

In the childhood form, tracheobronchial localization is always the spread of a laryngeal growth, which made a tracheostomy compulsory in earlier years. The tracheal spread is such that no normal structure can be found throughout the tracheal tree. In such conditions, no radical resection is possible. All one can do is to resect the predominant ones for palliation. Recurrence is common. Radical cure of children papillomatosis can only be medical. Interferon may be a possible solution.

Tracheobronchial amyloidosis is a unique disease never associated with systemic amyloidosis. It induces multiple obstructions of various bronchi. The amyloid deposits, consisting in bloated plaques, spreading more or less towards the two bronchial trees, lead to progressive occlusion of all lobar orifices. So far, no medical treatment has been found for this rare disease. Laser resection can restore the patency of most obstructed ones. Those are unusual and difficult procedures, since one has to perform a careful and tangential planing. Among the 16 cases treated in Paris, 11 had a good result (no recurrence in 4 years), 5 had a poor result (immediate recurrence or little improvement). In one case of extensive amyloidosis, we treated both sides in a same session. This was a mistake because the patient had to be put under artificial ventilation for several weeks.

2) Moderately malignant tumors

The routine management for carcinoids and adenocystic carcinomas is surgical. Their thick stalk and their tendency to spread beyond the bronchial wall warrant an endoscopic resection only in cases where a standard surgical resection is impossible. However, laser resection of pedunculated carcinoids is feasible. Refer to Plates 48 and 49 in the atlas for an example of carcinoid treatment. Also, laser destruction of an obstructing tumor can be effective for relief of atelectasis and drainage of infected secretions prior to a sleeve-resection. Some patients are inoperable owing to advanced or concomitant major medical conditions. Although palliative endoscopic laser resection may only bring them a long respite, for their tumors are slow growing. Iterative endoscopic procedures may extend their life for several years.

Adenocystic carcinomas are often inoperable when diagnosed because of extensive involvement of the trachea and the carina, or spreading tumor islets which preclude surgical resection. Laser abrasion followed by irradiation, is a feasible alternative.

Although recurrences following surgery are rare with carcinoids, they are common with adenocystic carcinomas. Those recurrences are often amenable to endoscopic resection. Those are the cases in which laser is invaluable, since the growth does not recur for some months following each session. In the Paris series 22 cases of carcinoids and 11 of adenocystic carcinomas are followed for 3 years or more with examinations ever 6 months.

The technical difficulties met during photocoagulation vary whether one deals with carcinoids or adenocystic carcinomas. With adenocystic carcinomas, the main problem is the bulk of the tumor, its extension, and sometimes the degree of obstruction. But the reduction in size of the adenocystic carcinomas following the impact of the laser beam is usually rapid and bloodless. On the other hand, the resection of carcinoids is always risky. Severe bleeding may occur at any moment, particularly when one resects the base of the tumor, blood can obscure the target. The risk of severe bleeding mandates the use of strict operative protocol, which shall be discussed with the technique.

3) Cancers

Photocoagulation can only be palliative. Nevertheless, this indication is the most common in laser bronchology. Refer to Plates 50-53 in the Atlas for examples of cancer treatment via bronchoscopy. Such treatment may be the most rewarding, since this method provides a solution to an intractable situation. Endoscopic laser resection may overcome a desperate asphyxic episode, prolong survival, and lay the path to a more radical form of treatment. It is impossible to detail all specific indications, so varied are the histology, topography and evolution of cancers. We can just give hints as a result of our experience: a) Overcome asphyxia in a case of 'not yet diagnosed' cancer. This presentation is common for cancers of the trachea or the carina. The chest X-ray can be normal and progressive dyspnea may be attributed to asthma. Fibroscopy can be performed when tracheal obstruction is nearly total. A single laser session may restore the respiratory condition, permitting more radical treatment to be undertaken immediately. b) Prolong the life of previously treated patients whose cancer has otherwise become intractable. They represent a class of patients, either inoperable, already operated upon, or treated with radio and/or chemotherapy. When the respiratory problem is predominant and due to an obstruction of the trachea or one of the main stem bronchi, an endoscopic resection can provide many months survival. Recurrence of the dyspnea indicates the need for another resection and further palliative. Several of our patients have been kept alive for one to two years following five to ten laser sessions while they would have died prior to the laser era. The evolution of the cancer determines the timing of further laser sessions. Our shortest interval has been one month. c) Relieve total atelectasis in a respiratory cripple who cannot survive on one lung only. d) Relieve an atelectasis of a febrile patient prior to chemotherapy. Relief of bronchial obstruction affords the drainage of infected secretions. e) Treat cancers spreading form the neighboring structures (thyroid, larynx, esophagus) to the trachea or main bronchi. For esophageal cancer, one must ascertain that there is no fistula. A laser session would only result in it. If there is no fistula the Laser abrasion must spare a tumoral depth of two to three mm on the membranous face of the trachea. These laser resections for cancer must be carried out only if the growth bulges in the lumen of the trachea and its resection is likely to restore the airway. They must be undertaken only in an operating room, since they may lead to acute respiratory and hemorrhagic complications.

On the other hand, it is not acceptable to treat by laser photocoagulation cancers amenable to other more efficient forms of therapy, such as surgery or radiotherapy. This would deprive the patient of a chance of long-term survival which endoscopic laser cannot provide. Laser is in no way a cancer treatment but only treatment of cancer's obstructive consequences. Therefore, its results cannot be compared to any classical treatment whose aim is to cure the patient.

4) Iatrogenic lesions

Granulomatous lesions and fibrous stenoses following tracheostomy or tracheal intubation of any duration are a heavy price to pay for otherwise successful intensive care treatment. These are the second most common indication in our series.

Granulomas may lead to major respiratory problems. We do not include the small, beadlike warts, often seen around recent or healed tracheal ostium, but the more bulky ones that induce obstruction. We see several forms: a) Cherry looking granulomas, that are solitary and originate from a pedicle, like a bell clapper to occlude the vocal cords, or the trachea beyond a tracheostomy tube (Fig. 19.4A).

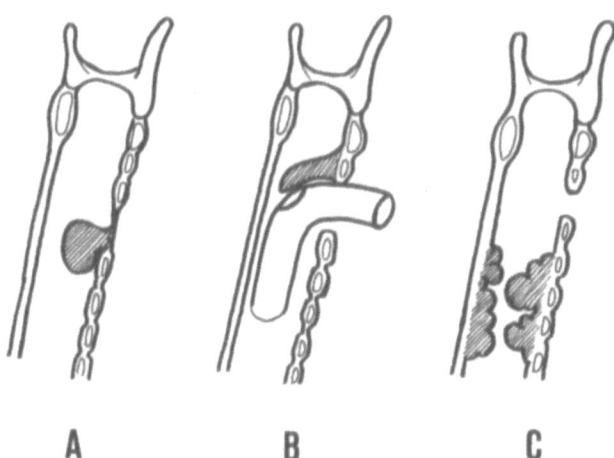

Fig. 19.4. Main types of granulomas: A) cherry like; B) peak like; C) crown of granulomas.

b) Sleeve or crown-like granulomas that induce a true ring-like stenosis at the level of the tube inflation cuff (Fig. 19.4C). c) Peak-like granulomas that sprout from the upper edge of a chronic tracheostomy ostium and progressively occlude the elbow of the tube. Eventually this induces complete obstruction and precludes closure of the tracheostomy (Fig. 19.4B).

Whatever the type of granuloma, resection by laser must be complete. The outcome depends upon whether the tracheostomy tube can be removed. If it must be kept inserted, every effort should be made to find a better tolerated material. Refer to Plates 54 and 55 in the atlas for an example of granuloma treatment.

Iatrogenic stenoses represent the most important not only because of their number but also for the problems they cause. At first sight, they appear to be a particularly good indication. Although the immediate results are usually excellent, recurrences are common.

Laser treatment of a stenosed trachea is usually easy and quick. The extent of the stenosis is of small importance. For the narrowest ones with a lumen of only about 2 mm we achieve the most spectacular results. When the lumen achieved appears to be inadequate (60% of the initial lumen), the rigid bronchoscope may be pulled through like a bougie to restore an adequate lumen.

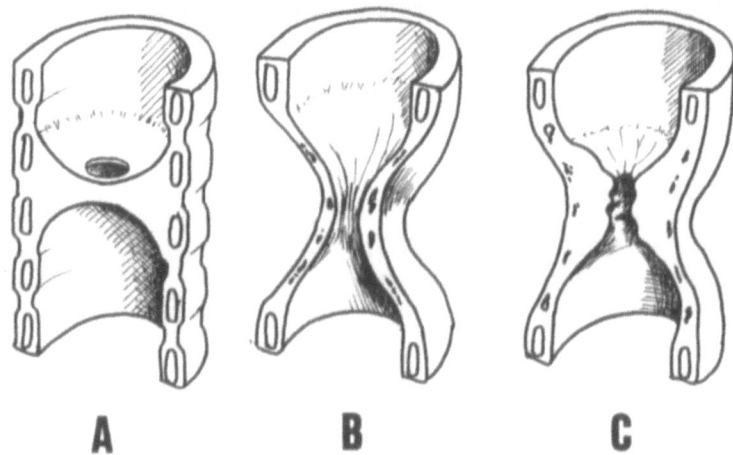

Fig. 19.5. Main types of stenoses: A) true diaphragm; B) parietal collapse; C) most usual association of collapse and fibrous ring.

Unfortunately, recurrence of stenosis within 6 to 8 weeks is common. Corticosteroids administered either parenterally or as a spray may prevent recurrence in some cases. Failures are common, since the crux of the matter is anatomy itself. Sleeve resections have shown that in the vast majority of cases the stenoses are not endoluminal bur parietal (Fig. 19.5). Although the endoscopist thinks he is dealing just with a diaphragm, true diaphragms are very rare which spring from mucosa or submucosa (Fig. 19.5A). When they are seen, they are obviously the best indications for laser resections. Much more often, the stenosis involves the tracheal wall itself and its cartilage rings. Excessive pressure of the cuff leads to an ischemic necrosis of the rings, sometimes extending several centimeters. In the most severe cases there is complete malacia of a circumferential portion of the trachea (Fig. 19.5B). This obviously is beyond the scope of any endoscopic resection. But in the great majority of cases, those different types of lesions are complex, a narrowing of the tracheal wall being accompanied by a fibrous flange (Fig. 19.5C). Those are the cases in which the immediate result is excellent, but which always recur 2 to 3 months later. Refer to plates 56 and 57 in the atlas for an example of tracheal stenosis treatment.

It is not easy for the endoscopist to assess and treat most stenotic lesions of the trachea. Tomographies and even better xerographies, provide useful data, particularly on the possible incarcerated cartilage rings, but they are far from being always reliable. In fact, the most useful element is the length of the tracheal segment which had to be photocoagulated. The length corresponds rather well to the extent of damage inflected upon the cartilage rings. When the endoscopic laser resection involves less than 15 mm, 50% are successfully treated. For lesions over 30 mm, recurrence is the rule (Fig. 19.5).

When the stenosis recurs, a new endoscopic resection is quite possible and there may be good immediate results. But, long-term success is negligible. However, in some selected cases it is warranted to keep the trachea patent by laser resections. Such is the case of patients undergoing prolonged intensive care, when a major surgical procedure is planned. The sleeve resection of the trachea is undertaken last. As a rule, it is better to consider a standard surgical resection following the first relapse. A new laser session performed 4 to 5 days before, provides both surgeon and anesthetist with remarkable comfort and safety. Instead of operating on a patient in respiratory distress, with bronchial tree flooded with secretions, one can deal with a patient with a clear trachea, under normal intubation.

Special mention must be made of stenoses or a ring of granulomas that develop on the surgical suture following a sleeve resection. This is an excellent indication for laser, since the stenosis is a short one, sprouting from a strong, firm, cartilage structure. In one single session, the granulomatous flange or the stenosis can be cleared and any suture material can be removed.

Discussion of methods

Various types of lasers are still used for endotracheal and bronchial resections. The choice of the apparatus is not always intentional, but based upon the availability of one laser machine. The same laser may be in use by other subspecialists. For some time, the CO_2 laser was the only laser available. In spite of the qualities of the beam, its use in bronchology is obviously limited. Since it follows a straight pathway, one must use a coupler with the rigid bronchoscope and aim with a biomicroscope over a distance of 30 cm or even more (18). In spite of some interesting trials, the use of the CO_2 laser is limited to some subglottic or tracheal lesions.

Endoscopic argon laser has seldom been used for bronchology. Most authors feel that the power delivered is inadequate for laser bronchology (10).

The Nd-YAG laser is the only one currently suited because of its power and transmissibility through a flexible fiber which are essential for bronchologic surgery.

The choice of the endoscope is, by far the most important technical problem. The more widespread use of laser in our speciality has been considerable hampered by the deliberate use of the fiberscope. But year by year, paper after paper, the rigid tube gains ground (19).

We choose the rigid bronchoscope because of its safety and ease of use for most laser cases. Its only real drawback is that it looks obsolete. But its advantages for an endoscopic resection make its use compulsory in the vast majority of cases. There is far better vision through a rigid telescope. One can quickly clean the telescope and immediate return on the target. There is absolute steadiness of the tube and of the fiber when aiming at a lesion. There are excellent facilities for ventilation, which can be adjusted to meet any requirements. There is the possibility of removing tumor fragments with large biopsy forceps. Also, there are several possibilities of controlling a hemorrhage and this is the crucial point. A suction catheter is always present near the lesion to clear the blood. But should bleeding be profuse, the rigid tube allows a set of maneuvers which would be impossible with a fiberscope. Insertion of adrenalin-soaked cottonoids and suction through a large bore catheter (5 to 6 mm) are easy. As a last resort, one can block a main bronchus (or bypass a tracheal tumor) to achieve ventilation of the healthy lung. One must always bear in mind that an endobronchial hemorrhage may lead to death by anoxia in a few minutes from as little as ten millimeters of blood (13). Any lesion (tumoral or not) which appears to be amenable to easy, quick resection, may induce unexpected bleeding, compelling one to achieve rapid and efficient maneuvers.

Many teams have used or still use the fiberscope in two ways. 1) Under local analgesia, the fiberscope may enable the resection of minor lesions (16). Our two teams use it in such cases. 2) Other teams use the fiberscope through a tracheal tube under general anesthesia. Although this technique makes the cleaning and reinsertion of the fiberscope easier, it jeopardizes the ventilation, owing to the bulk of a fairly large fiberscope. It provides no safety. In case of trouble, it is recommended to remove both tube an fiberscope, and replace them by a rigid bronchoscope, which means a loss of time at the worst possible moment. Why not use a rigid tube straight away?

It is unlikely that indications for thermal lasers in bronchology should increase. Laser treatment will remain more palliative than curative. New technical advances will undoubtedly be made such as new laser sources, tunable lasers, and also more flexible fibers. For our two teams these new developments may not change the overall results because these depend upon the frequency of emergency procedures, the bad condition of our patients, and the high risk of laser resection. The main contribution of the Nd-YAG laser is that we have been able to treat these specific bronchologic cases. At the present time Nd-YAG laser is the only non- surgical treatment available for many patients with stenotic or obstructing malignant tracheobronchial lesions.

References

1. Strong S, Vaughan CW, Polanyi T. et al. Bronchoscopic carbon dioxide Laser Surgery. Ann Otol 1974;83:769-776.
2. Toty L, Personne C, and Colchen A. Utilsation d'un faisceau Laser YAG à conducteur souple pour le traitement endoscopique de certaines lésions trachéo-bronchiques. Rev Fr Mal Resp 1979;7:57- 60 et 475-482.
3. Personne C, Colchen A, Toty L and Vourc'h G. Endoscopic laser resections in bronchology. New frontiers in laser medicine – Ecerpta Medica edit., Amsterdam, 1983 Intern Congr 609, 280-287.
4. Dumon JF, Reboud E, Garbe L et al. Treatment of tracheo- bronchial lesions by laser photoresection. Chest 1982;81:278-284.
5. Personne C, Colchen A, Leroy M et al. Indications and technique for endoscopic laser resections in bronchology. J Thorac Cardio- vasc. Surg 1986;91:710-715.
6. Shapshay S and Strong S. Tracheobronchial obstruction from metastatic distant malignancies. Ann Otol Rhinol Laryngol 1982;91:648-651.
7. Laforet E, Berger R, and Vaughan C. Carcinoma obstructing trachea. Treatment by laser resection. N Engl J Med 1976;5:294-341.
8. McDougall JC and Cortese DA. Nd-YAG laser therapy of malignant airway obstruction. Mayo Clin Proc 1983;58:35-39.
9. Brutinel WM, Mc Dougall JC, and Cortese DA. Bronchoscopic therapy with Nd-YAG laser during intravenous anesthesia. Chest 1983;84:519-521.
10. Hetzel M., Millard F, Ayesh R et al. Laser treatment for carcinoma of the bronchus. Br Med J 1983;286:12-16.
11. Elvein R and Zorn G. Treatment of malignant disease in trachea and main-stem bronchi by carbon dioxide Laser. J Thorac Cardiovasc Surg 1983;86:858-863.
12. Warner ME, Warner MA, and Leonard FF. Anesthesia for Nd-YAG laser resection of major airway obstructing tumors. Anesthesiology 1984;60:232-235.
13. Toty L, Personne C, Colchen A, and Vourc'h G. Bronchoscopic management of tracheal lesions using the Nd-YAG laser. Thorax 1981;36:175-178.
14. Casey KR, Fairfax WR, Smith SJ et al. Intratracheal fire ignited by Nd-YAG laser during treatment of tracheal stenosis. Chest 1983;84:295-296.
15. Vourc'h G, Fischler M, Michon F et al. Manual jet- ventilation versus high frequency jet ventilation during laser resection of tracheo-bronchial stenosis. Br J Anaesth 1983;55:973-975.
16. Dumon JF, Reboud E, Meric B et al. Bronchofibroscopie et laser YAG-Nd. Rev Fr Resp 1981;9:76.
17. Personne C, Colchen A, Toty L et al. Indications et limites de la résection endoscopique en laser dans les sténoses trachéales (et leur récidive après chirurgie). Ann Chir Thor 1981;8:613-620.
18. Ossoff R and Karlan M. Universal endoscopic coupler for carbon dioxide laser surgery. Ann Otol 1982;91:608-609.
19. George PJM, Garrett CPO, Nixon C et al. Laser treatment for tracheo bronchial tumours: local or general anaesthesia. Thorax 1987;42:656-660.

20. THE NEODYMIUM-YAG LASER IN UROLOGY

A. HOFSTETTER AND E. KEIDITSCH

Biophysical basis

Conversion of light energy into heat is the basis for the use of lasers as cutting or coagulation instruments. The degree and extent of the thermal effects depend upon the laser beam geometry, the energy and the wavelength of the incident light as well as the optical and thermal properties of the tissue (1, 2, 3).

The three laser systems which are most frequently used in surgery at present – the CO_2 the argon and the neodymium-YAG (Nd-YAG) – show clear differences in their thermal behavior due to the different absorption and scatter. Both the absorption and scatter of the light in the tissue are strictly dependent on the wavelength. Since the CO_2 laser beam is strongly absorbed by water, and the water content of the tissue is known to be very high, this light (with a wavelength in the middle infrared region) is almost exclusively absorbed. The scatter is so slight that it can be neglected. The light energy is completely converted into heat at the surface of the tissue. The CO_2 laser is thus very suitable for tissue resection, i.e. it constitutes a cutting tool with limited depth of laser penetration. Plate 58 in the Atlas shows the typical histological changes after an incision with a CO_2 laser in the bladder wall of a rabbit. In a widely gaping tissue defect with deposits of carbonized material at the margins, a coagulation necrosis of slight extent with evaporation cavities is found between the fibers, which appear to be distorted. The radiation is completely absorbed in a very thin layer of about 0.1 mm (4). The argon laser, whose wavelength is between 458 and 515 nm, is hardly absorbed by water, but is very strongly absorbed by the red pigment of blood hemoglobin. Argon laser is absorbed by the tissue to a smaller extent than the CO_2 laser. With argon laser irradiation there is a shallow coagulation effect in the tissue associated with relatively slight tissue resection. Plate 59 in the atlas shows the histologic effects after irradiation of the bladder wall with argon laser in the rabbit (4, 5). Only minor zones of coagulation necrosis with destruction of the superficial epithelium, a thickening of the connective tissue (in which the collagen fibers are partly destroyed), and moderately pronounced interstitial edema were found under the light microscope. Only the muscle strands which are very near the mucosa are included in the necrosis (4). The tissue- resection effect becomes larger when the dose of radiation is raised, whereas the zone

D.M. Jensen and J.M. Brunetaud (eds), Medical Laser Endoscopy. 247-256.

of necrosis continues to appear to be only very slight.

The wavelength of the Nd-YAG laser (1064 nm) is in the near infrared range. In this region, the absorption of the tissue is very slight, since the transmission in water is very high. Scatter is of considerable importance with Nd-YAG and leads to a homogeneous distribution of the irradiation in the tissue. There is a profound heating effect with only slight destruction of the tissue surface. With Nd-YAG laser both the forward and the backward scatter are very pronounced. Depending upon the qualities of the bladder tissue, 30-40% are measured as back-scatter *in vivo* and 20-30% as forward scatter with a tissue thickness of 2 mm (3). The irradiation with 40 watts causes a relatively large area of the bladder wall tissue to be homogenously destroyed with only slow warming of the tissue surrounding the immediate area. Depending on the exposure time, a depth of coagulation necrosis of 4-5 mm can be attained, without a temperature of more than 100° C arising at the tissue surface.

Plate 60 in the atlas shows the effect of Nd-YAG laser radiation on the rabbit bladder. Under the light microscope, a sharply delimited coagulation necrosis is found comprising all wall layers. In the irradiated region, there is significant edema, especially in the region near to the surface. Punctiform or clumped protein precipitates can also be discerned between the deeper layers and the smooth musculature. The tissue resection effect is minimal (4). These histological investigations show the typical effect of Nd-YAG laser on the bladder, manifested by deep penetration and homogenous coagulation of the entire bladder wall tissue. Such effects are desirable for endoscopic treatment of bladder tumors.

Radiation dose

We have employed the Nd-YAG laser for destruction of bladder tumors since June 1, 1976. Contact-free destruction of carcinoma tissue is an important feature distinguishing this technique from conventional methods. Using water as a flushing fluid for the bladder and with a laser power of 40 watts, the depth of tissue coagulation is about 4 mm.

Losses during irradiation arise from heat conduction and absorption of the scattered light in the adjacent tissue. The intestine bordering on the posterior wall of the bladder is especially endangered. We performed animal experiments to study this problem, using spatial and chronological temperature profiles at the bladder wall serosa. The purpose was to determine optimal irradiation doses which on the one hand could radically destroy bladder tumors and on the other hand cause as little damage as possible to the surrounding tissue. We found that the directly irradiated area of the bladder wall did not correspond to the areas of necrosis obtained. In bladders of different thickness, we varied laser parameters such as power, irradiation time, and irradiation distance and found that the zone of bladder necrosis could be twice as large as the directly irradiated area of the bladder wall. This was attributable to the scatter of the

Nd-YAG laser in the bladder tissue as well as heat conduction (6).

Our experimental investigation and clinical controls on intraoperatively exposed bladders have given us some therapeutic guidelines. For complete homogenous coagulation of a 4-6 mm thick bladder wall using water as a flushing fluid and an irradiation distance of 1 mm, a Nd-YAG power of 45 watts is required with an irradiation time of about 4-5 sec. For determination of the tumor or bladder wall thickness, we have applied endovesically ultrasound probes with A or B modes (7).

Laser instruments

For endoscopic application of the Nd-YAG laser, special laser urethrocystoscopes were developed in collaboration with the companies Wolff and Storz. At the beginning of our work, a biconical quartz glass fiber developed by Nath was available as transmission system for the Nd-YAG laser. This system was very sensitive to mechanical strain (8), and required rigid endoscopes with lens systems, prisms and protective windows. These systems naturally had numerous refractive surfaces which has a negative effect on the transmission of the laser beam. Moreover, they had to be constantly kept clean during the operation by means of a gas stream or water flushing .

Since 1978, a highly flexible, teflon-coated quartz glass fiber of high mechanical stability has been available to us. We were consequently able to dispense with the original rigid endoscopes since it was now possible to direct the flexible quartz glass fibers to almost any point of the bladder with an Albaran system (9).

In external application of the laser, a hand-focusing portion with a light conductor was used. This is protected over its entire length by a metal-plastic tube. It is also possible to connect the Nd-YAG laser via a light conductor and a controllable adapter to a conventional surgical microscope for microsurgery.

As a consequence of the biophysical properties of the Nd:YAG laser and the surgical instruments available today, the Nd:YAG laser has found a firm place not only in urology (10, 11), but also in many other surgical disciplines.

Surgical procedure

a) Endoscopic Laser Application

For the endoscopic laser application, the patient is brought into the lithotomy position similar to any other transurethral operation. General anesthesia is not necessary. We usually carry out the endoscopic operations using diazepam or methohexital. To distend the urinary bladder during the endoscopic operation, we use sterile 0.9% saline solution, but is also possible to use sterile water. Figure 20.1 shows a schematic representation of endoscopic laser irradiation in the water-filled bladder. Water filling has the great advantage of keeping the target lesion clean during treatment. Flushing away blood or loose tissue during the operation permits efficient coagulation of the bladder lesion. The effectiveness of the irradiation can be discerned as a white coagulum of the irradiated tumor tissue.

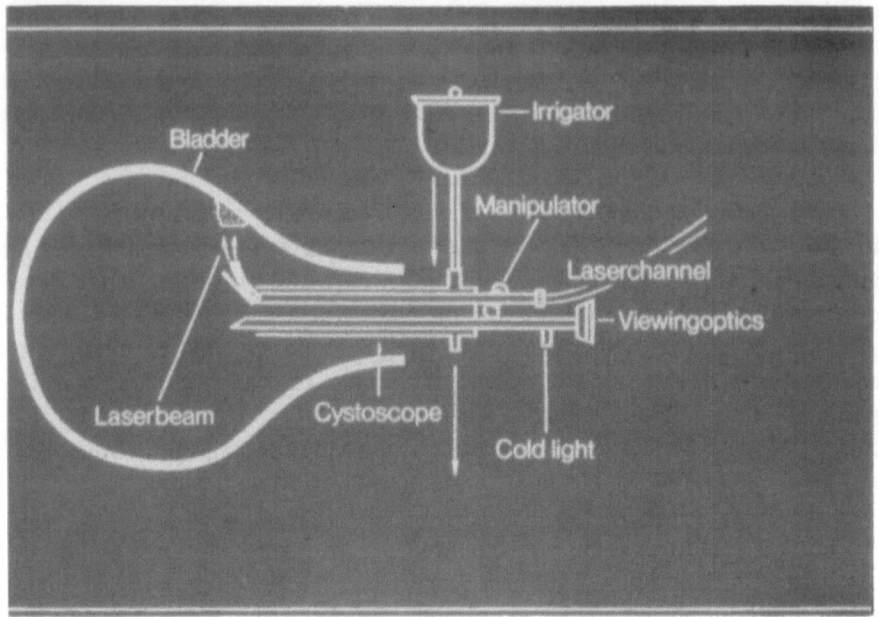

Fig. 20.1. Schematic representation of urologic laser endoscopy.

The endoscopic destruction of larger bladder tumors takes place in three steps. When the tumor is larger than a fingertip, the exophytic portion is first resected with the electric loop deep into the bladder wall after coagulation of edges of the tumor. Then the base and edges of the tumor are postcoagulated with the Nd-YAG laser. Smaller tumors are primarily destroyed with the Nd-YAG laser. In these cases, we first irradiate to a white coloration the tissue surrounding the tumor for about 0.5-1 cm in order to close off the afferent blood vessels and lymphatics. Afterwards, the tumor is coagulated directly. Before laser treatment, biopsies are taken from the tumor bed or from the edge of the tumor and the tissue immediately surrounding the tumor. This procedure is supplemented by 'quadrant biopsy'.

In very small tumors in which a biopsy would be tantamount to a primary tumor extirpation, the Nd-YAG laser irradiation is done first. Immediately after the laser irradiation, the tumor is pulled up with a biopsy forceps. This tissue removed immediately after the Nd-YAG irradiation can be unequivocally verified and classified histologically.

Plate 61 in the atlas shows a typical papillary tumor of the bladder near to left ostium. The histology of the tumor (grade I-II) is shown in Plate 62 in the atlas. Nd-YAG laser treatment was administered and follow-up appearance at 3 months is shown in Plate 63.

Since no or only very insignificant hemorrhage occurs with Nd-YAG laser irradiation, we have dispensed with routine transurethral catheter after the operation. This is important in avoiding nosocomial infections.

The patients should be observed for one to two days after the operation to detect possible intestinal perforation. This is particularly important when large areas are irradiated at the posterior wall of the bladder. With a radiation dose up to 45 watts using water as a flushing fluid, we have not observed a single intestinal perforation after irradiation of several thousand bladder tumors. In seven years only two cases of small intestinal perforations occurred after irradiation using too high a power (about 80 watts). Clinically, these perforations were manifested with signs of acute abdomen within 12 hours after the laser irradiation.

b) Open Laser Application

Laser application during surgery can be carried out whenever the tumor tissue can be reached directly by the laser beam. Hand pieces are useful for these treatments. The use of a gas stream on the side facilitates hemostasis in severe hemorrhage. This is of special significance in operations on the corpora cavernosa or the glans penis. In open work with the Nd-YAG laser protective goggles must be worn. According to the investigations of Frank (10), it is not necessary in endoscopic laser application.

Clinical results

Bladder tumors. Since 1976, we have treated more than 500 patients with urinary bladder tumors of the stages pT_A, pT_1 and pT_2 with the Nd-YAG laser. The advantages of this technique are in the contact free tumor destruction under excellent visual conditions. No or only insignificant hemorrhages result during the operation. The operation does not require general anesthesia, as mentioned above. In most cases, light sedation is sufficient, so that the operation can also be carried out in ambulatory patients. Postoperative catheter treatment is usually not necessary, so that nosocomial infections can be largely avoided. Electrolyte-free flushing solutions which may be very expensive can be replaced by sterile water, thus reducing costs.

Apart from these advantages, the question as to the degree of efficacy of the Nd-YAG laser compared to conventional transurethral resection techniques was studied. In a prospective, randomized study, we compared the efficacy and recurrence rates of the Nd-YAG laser with transurethral resection. Patients with urothelial carcinomas (n = 65, 38 men: 27 women, average age: 68 years) of the stages pT_A-pT_2, N_O, M_O, were included in the study. Patients were randomized to laser or transurethral resection treatment. In addition, adjuvant chemotherapy with mitomycin C (20 mg/14 days for six months or two years) was administered 8 days after the operation. Control groups (laser or TUR alone) did not receive chemotherapy. The study was commenced on September 1, 1981.

Table 20.1. Primary tumors.*

Number:	40 (m = 23, f = 17)	
Age:	Males	45 – 81 years, $\bar{x}_m$ = 66.5 years
	Females	54 – 84 years, $\bar{x}_f$ = 69.1 years

*(pT_A – pT_2, N_O, M_O)

Table 20.2. Transitional cell carcinomas.

	Laser group				TUR group			
pT/G	1	2	3	n	1	2	3	n
A	7	3	0	10	7	5	0	12
1	4	3	1	8	1	0	3	4
2	0	0	2	2	1	2	1	4

Classification and incidence distribution of transitional cell carcinomas in 20 (m = 12,f = 8) patients of laser group and 20 (m = 11,f = 9) patients of TUR group of a randomized trial.

Table 20.3. Results of randomized trial.

	Laser chemotherapy (n = 15)	Laser (n = 5)	TUR + chemotherapy (n = 12)	TUR (n = 8)
Recurrence of a tumor	1	1	3	2
Recurrences/100 pt mos	0,35	0,95	1,8	3,5
Mean follow-up months	19,33	21,0	13,7	7,13
Deaths	1(14mo,CV)	–	–	–
Recurrence of a tumor after 12mos f/u	0,0	0,0	6,7	54,5
Recurrence of a tumor after 12mos f/u (E.O.R.T.C.)	–	–	17	58,3

Therapeutic results after Nd:YAG laser coagulation versus TUR in Table 20.2.

The patients were divided into groups with primary tumors (Table 20.1) and relapse tumors (Table 20.5). The classification of primary tumors is shown in Table 20.2 and the classification of relapse tumors in Table 20.6. The therapeutic results in primary tumors is shown in Table 20.3. You can see that the laser application with and without chemotherapy is superior to TUR with and without chemotherapy according to relapse rate (P<0.0001). These results have been confirmed by others.

Table 20.4. Growth of primary tumors.

	TUMOR GROWTH		
	before therapy		after therapy
Laser + TUR	multiple	7	1 (h,Ch +)
(n = 13)	localized	6	0
Laser	multiple	1	0
(n = 7)	localized	6	1 (h,Ch – –)
TUR + TUR	multiple	10	2 (Ch +, Ch –)
(n = 16)	localized	6	1 (Ch +),
			1(o,Ch –)
TUR	multiple	1	0
(n = 4)	localized	3	1 (Ch +), 0

Legend: Ch + = with chemotherapy; h = heterotopic;
Ch – = without chemotherapy; o = orthotopic

Table 20.5. Relapse tumors.*

Number:	25 (m = 15, f = 10)	
Age:	Males	40 – 79 years, $\bar{x}_m$ = 62.1 years
	Females	53 – 83 years, $\bar{x}_f$ = 72.1 years

* (pT_A -pT_2,N_0,M_0)

Table 20.6. Transitional cell carcinoma distribution.

	Laser group				TUR group			
pT/G	1	2	3	n	1	2	3	n
A	3	3	0	6	1	3	0	4
1	5	6	3	14	1	0	0	1
2	0	0	0	0	0	0	0	0

Classification and distribution of transitional cell carcinomas in 20 (m = 12,f = 8) patients of laser group and 5 (m = 3,f = 2) patients of tur group.

Table 20.7. Therapeutic results after Nd:YAG laser coagulation versus TUR in Table 20.6.

	Laser + chemotherapy (n = 15)	Laser (n = 5)	TUR + chemotherapy (n = 1)	TUR (n = 4)
Recurrence of a tumor	5	5	1	3
Recurrences/100 pt mos	2.7	8.6	7.1	7.6
Mean follow-up months	12.3	11.6	14.0	9.83
Deaths	1 (12mo,Ap)	–	–	–

Table 20.4 shows the growth of primary tumors before and after treatment. It is interesting that there was never a change from a localized tumor to multiple tumors after laser application in contrast to TUR.

The therapeutic results in relapse tumors are shown in Table 20.7. Although laser application together with chemotherapy was quite different than the other groups, too few patients are included for a statistical significance.

Table 20.8. Growth of relapse tumors.

	TUMOR GROWTH		
	before therapy		after therapy
Laser + TUR	multiple	10	2 (h,Ch+,Ch−)
			3 (h,Ch+,Ch+,Ch+)
	localized	22	2 (o,Ch+,Ch+)
Laser	multiple	1	1 (o,h,Ch−)
	localized	2	0
TUR + TUR	multiple	1	1 (o,h,Ch−)
	localized	1	1 (h,Ch−)
TUR	multiple	1	1 (o,h,Ch+)
	localized	2	1 (o,Ch−)

Ch+ = with chemotherapy;   h = heterotopic;
Ch− = without chemotherapy;   o = orthotopic.

Table 20.7 shows the growth of relapse tumors before and after treatment. A change from multiple to localized tumors was seen in three cases in the laser group.

Other Tumors

Besides the destruction of urothelial carcinomas of the urinary bladder, we were also able to destroy corresponding tumors in the ureter () successfully in (Plates 64-65 in Atlas) patients in whom a more radical surgical procedure was not indicated. Tumors of the urethra, particularly condylomata acuminata, can be treated excellently with the Nd-YAG laser (Plates 64-65 in Atlas). The results in penis carcinomas we treated indicate the importance of open Nd-YAG laser (Table 20.9).

Critical evaluation of ND-YAG laser application

With endoscopic Nd-YAG laser application, tumors up to the size of fingertips can be destroyed with simultaneous interruption of the lymphatics and blood vessels supplying the tumor.

When the exophytic portion of the tumor is larger, a conventional transurethral resection should be carried out. The 'second session' in conventional transurethral resection can be replaced by Nd-YAG laser application. It is a

Table 20.9 Clinical results obtained from neodymium-YAG-laser treatment of malignant penile tumors

Tumor classification	# pts	Age yrs	F/U to 12-83 monts	Local recurrences	Palpable lymph nodes
Laser irradiation					
T_1, N_0, M_0	8	40-82	31-54	3 ($2T_{1s}$, $1T_1$)	1
T_2, N_0, M_0	5	53-81	28-51	0	0
Laser + lymphadenectomy					
T_1, N_2, M_0	1	48	56 + *	0	0
T_2, N_2, M_0	1	59	27	1 (T_1)	0
Laser + lymphadenectomy + chemotherapy					
T_2, N_3, M_1	1	59	30 +	1 (T_1)	fixed lymph nodes-pockets
T_2, N_2, M_0 (melanoma)	1	61	23 +	0	0

*bladder cancer

much less radical procedure than TUR. Other advantages of laser application compared with standard therapy are no hemorrhage with treatment, local anesthesia, and shorter operation times.

The main indications for Nd-YAG laser application are tumors of the glans penis, the penis shaft, and bladder, especially multiple small tumors of early stage.

The reason why the Nd-YAG laser is being accepted slowly in our specialty despite these advantages is probably due to the high purchase cost as well as some distrust of new technologies by urologists. Also, additional training and experience with lasers is required prior to initiating this work in urology. Although our non-randomized clinical experience is large and now routine, comparison of laser treatment with standard treatments is only now being evaluated. The number of cases is small and the duration of following in our randomized prospective study is still too short to make a final appraisal. Several such studies should be carried out.

References

1. Blazek V. Reflektions-, Transmissions- und Absorptionsverhalten von biologischem Gewebe für elektromagnetische Strahlung im sichtbaren und nahen IR-Bereich. Biomed Techn 1975;20, Erg.-Bd.
2. Fine S, Klein E. Biological effects of laser radiation. In: JH Laurence and JW Gofman Eds: Advances in Biological and Medical Physics, New York, Academic Press 1965:10.
3. Halldorsson Th, Lengerhoic J. Thermodynamic analysis of laser irradiation of biological tissue. App Optlcs 1978;17,3948
4. Keiditsch E, Langer R, Staehler G, Hofstetter A. Morphologischer Veränderungen an der Kaninchenharnblase nach Laserbestrahlung. Verh Dtsch Ges Path 1977;61,367

5. Staehler G, Hofstetter A, Gorisch W, Keiditsch E, Mussiggang M. Endoscopy in experimental urology using an argon-laser beam. Endoscopy 1976;8,1

6. Pensel J, Hofstetter A, Keiditsch E, Staehler G. Wärmeleitung auf der Blasenrückwand während der endoskopischen Laserbestrahlung. 3rd Intern Congr Laser Surgery, Graz 1979

7. Pensel J, Rothenberger K, Hofstetter A, Frank F. A-Bild- Sonographie zur Messung der Harnblasenwandstärke. Fortschr Med 1980;98,1066

8. Nath G, Gorisch W, Kiefhaber P. First laser endoscopy via a fiber optic transmission system. Endoscopy 1973;5,208

9. Hofstetter A, Frank F. Ein neues Laser-Endoskop zur Bestrahlung von Blasentumoren. Fortschr Med 1979;97,232

10. Hofstetter A, Frank F. Der Neodym-YAG laser in der Urologie. Editiones Roche, Basel 1979

11. Schulmann CC. Early adjuvant adriamycin in superficial bladder cancer. 33rd Kongress d. Deutschen Gesellschaft fur Urologie, Cologne 1981.

21. ENDOSCOPIC LASER SURGERY IN UROLOGY: THE AMERICAN EXPERIENCE

JOSEPH A. SMITH, JR.

Endoscopy has been a fundamental part of urology since its inception as a surgical specialty and helped lead to the development of urology as a separate discipline. The sophisticated instruments and endoscopic expertise of urologists have led to many innovative therapeutic and diagnostic advances in urologic surgery. Presently, there is virtually no portion of the urinary tract from the urethral meatus to the renal papilla which is not accessible for endoscopic examination and treatment.

Because of these factors, adaptation of laser energy to urology has been a natural evolution. Only minor modifications in standard urologic endoscopic equipment are necessary in order to apply laser energy within the urinary tract. In addition, once the basic physics and tissue interaction are understood, the technical factors necessary for urologists to become proficient laser surgeons are not difficult. Nevertheless, despite a recent rapid increase in the number of urologists performing laser surgery, interest in lasers has evolved relatively slowly among urologists in the United States compared to some centers in Europe. Thus, American urologists have sometimes been criticized as being 'behind' their European colleagues.

For the most part, this criticism is unjustified. Laser surgery has been met with healthy scepticism among urologists in the United States. Electrical diathermy has been a successful means of treatment for a number of lesions within the urinary tract for over forty years. Thus, in order for lasers to develop a position of permanence in urology, they must not only be safe and effective but better than existing techniques. Interest in laser surgery has increased at a phenomenal rate among urologists in the United States and clinical experience is being gained in a number of different areas. It seems a relative certainty that, because of their unique physical properties and tissue effects, lasers will become an integral part of clinical practice for most urologists.

Urethra

Although intraurethral extension of condyloma acuminata is relatively uncommon, treatment by standard methods has been disappointing. Intraurethral 5-Fluorouracil cream is effective in removing some of these lesions. Electrocautery resection generally is unsatisfactory because the irregular

D.M. Jensen and J.M. Brunetaud (eds), Medical Laser Endoscopy. 257-268.
© 1990 Kluwer Academic Publishers, Dordrecht

thermal injury which results from treatment is prone to cause stricture formation. A number of investigators have reported excellent results using neodymium:YAG laser treatment of condylomata extending along the entirety of the urethra (1,2). Even for lesions at the urethral meatus, stenosis or stricture has not been observed. Accordingly, laser treatment is already accepted in most centers as the preferred form of therapy for intra-urethral condyloma acuminata.

A more common and more perplexing problem in urology is benign stricture of the urethra. Strictures tend to occur posteriorly near the bulbous or membranous urethra and may be either post- inflammatory, post-traumatic, iatrogenic (usually due to prolonged Foley catheter drainage) or of unknown etiology. After standard treatment either by dilatation or urethrotomy, the recurrence rate is disturbingly high.

Because of evidence that the thermal injury which results from neodymium:YAG laser irradiation may heal with less collagen deposition and more elastic fibers than a comparable electrical injury (3), we initiated a clinical trial at the University of Utah using neodymium:YAG lasers as treatment for benign urethral strictures (4). All patients had failed standard therapy including urethral dilation and internal urethrotomy. The laser fiber was inserted through a standard cystoscope and energy applied to the entire circumference of the stricture. Generally, a power output of 45 watts was used and each area treated for approximately three seconds. A small metal guide was inserted through the lumen of the urethra prior to treatment but a Foley catheter was not used postoperatively. Because the neodymium:YAG laser has a few properties of immediate tissue vaporization, urethral dilation was performed after the laser treatment. The thermally coagulated areas underwent a secondary slough approximately one week later (Fig. 21.1).

Although immediate results were good, nine patients (55%) developed stricture recurrence within six months of treatment. These results are probably not unlike those which could be expected from internal urethrotomy without a laser. No treatment complications were observed except for one patient who required temporary catheterization because of urethral occlusion from some of the sloughed tissue six days after treatment.

Shanberg and Tansey have reported their experience with 24 patients (5). Initially, their treatment regimen was similar to the one which we described. However, recently, they have not attempted complete removal of all of the strictured area but have performed radial incisions using the neodymium:YAG laser. In their experience with 24 patients, 50% have developed recurrence of their stricture. However, all of their patients had failed multiple previous treatments using conventional therapy.

Presently, it seems fair to state that treatment with a neodymium:YAG laser has not demonstrated any definitive advantages over standard therapy for benign urethral strictures.

On the other hand, although it is difficult to draw conclusions from non-randomized series, almost half of the patients treated remain free of recurrence

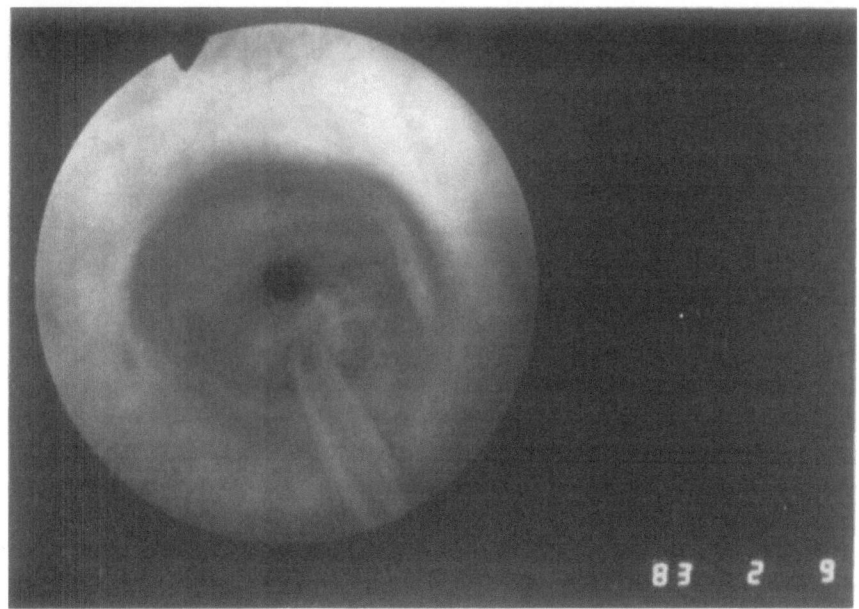

Fig. 21.1A. Fibrous stricture of posterior urethra. A Nd:YAG laser fiber is positioned for treatment.

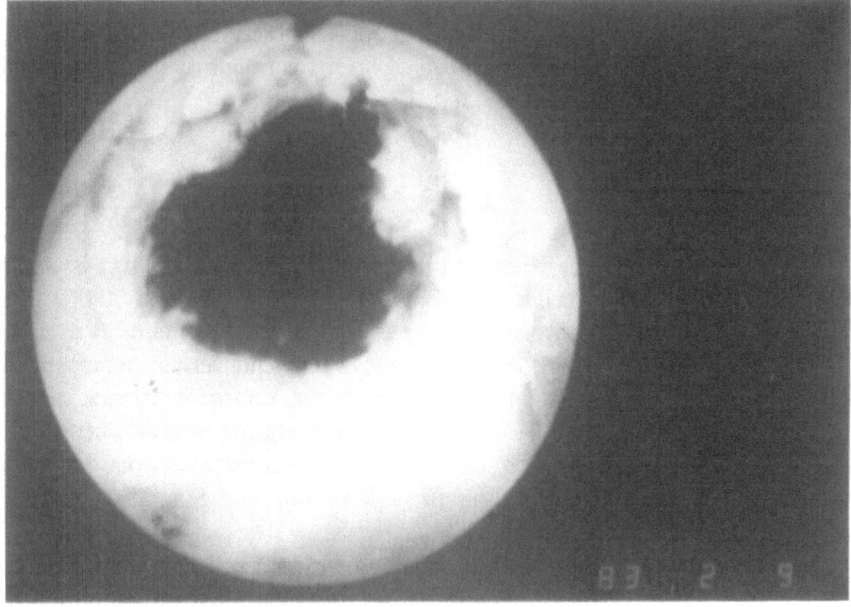

Fig. 21.1B. Immediately after treatment, the thermally coagulated, irregular tissue around the circumference of the stricture is evident.

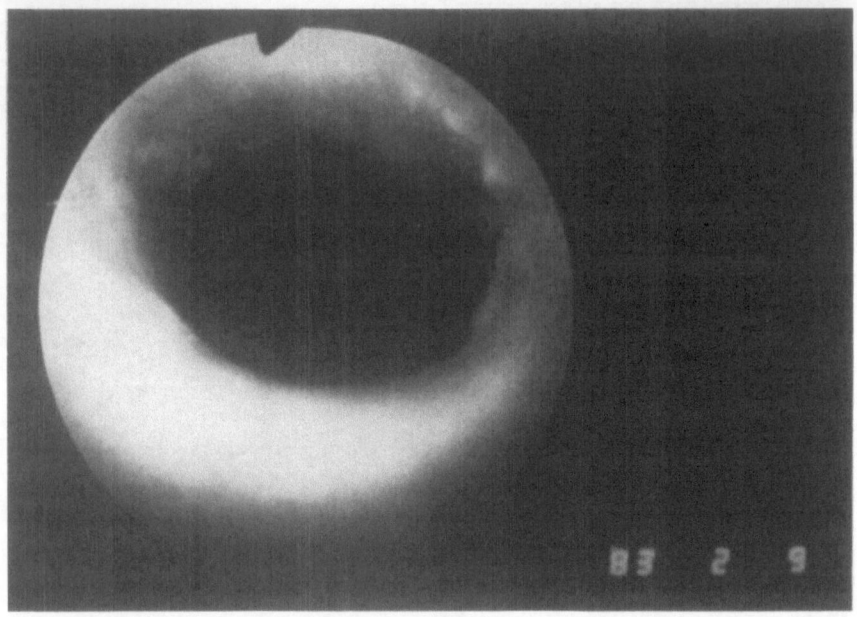

Fig. 21.1C. Six weeks later, the necrotic tissue has sloughed and a normal caliber lumen is present. (Reprinted with permission of J. Urol.)

and all had failed previous conventional therapy. Further clinical studies of neodymium: YAG laser treatment of benign urethral strictures seem warranted but adaptation of carbon dioxide laser energy to cystoscopes via a fiber conduction system or a CO_2 laser cystoscope as described by Willscher (6) may prove to be a more promising form of laser treatment of benign urethral strictures.

Bladder

The greatest clinical experience and potential for lasers in urology is in the treatment of transitional cell carcinoma of the bladder. Almost 30,000 new cases of bladder cancer occur yearly in the United States. The majority of these are of a relatively low grade and low stage where endoscopic management becomes the primary form of treatment. However, tumor recurrence can be expected in some 50 to 70% of patients necessitating repeat operations. Treatment by standard techniques with electrocautery resection generally requires two or three days of hospitalization as well as a general or regional anesthetics.

The high recurrence rate of superficial transitional cell carcinoma of the bladder after electrocautery resection is, for the most part, probably due to dysplastic changes throughout the bladder epithelium and carcinoma in situ. However, experimental evidence and clinical observation suggest that at least some of the recurrences are due to implantation of viable tumor cells which may become dislodged at the time of electrocautery resection (7). Since lasers are capable of thermally coagulation bladder tumors without direct tissue contact, it has been suggested that the recurrence rate after laser treatment may be less than with standard therapy (8). Because of differences in patient population and selection criteria, this is a difficult issue to resolve without randomized trials. However, there is an increasingly large clinical experience with laser treatment of superficial bladder tumors in the United States. We have treated 64 patients at the University of Utah using either neodymium:YAG laser or argon laser irradiation. Twenty-four patients (35%) have developed a recurrence with a period of follow- up ranging from 3 to 42 months (9,10). Shanberg, Malloy and Tansey have found tumor recurrence in only 7 (13%) of the 52 patients whom they have treated (11). Partial explanation for this difference may lie in the fact that some of the patients in the latter series were being treated for their initial tumor rather than for recurrent lesions. In North America, Stein (12), Aledia (13), and McPhee (14) have also reported experience with laser treatment of bladder cancer. Nevertheless, due to variation in patients selection, definitive conclusions regarding the impact of laser treatment on recurrence rate in superficial bladder tumors cannot be made at this time.

Although no decided treatment advantages are evident, there does appear to be several practical advantages for laser treatment compared to standard

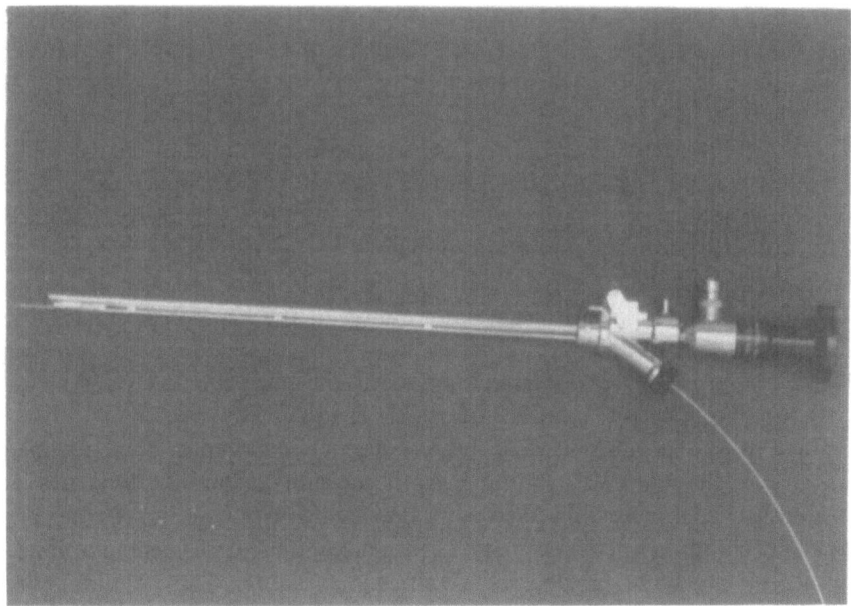

Fig. 21.2. Cystoscope with laser bridge. The laser fiber is inserted through the working channel and the fiber tip deflected with modified Albarran apparatus. (Courtesy American Cystoscope Makers Incorporated.)

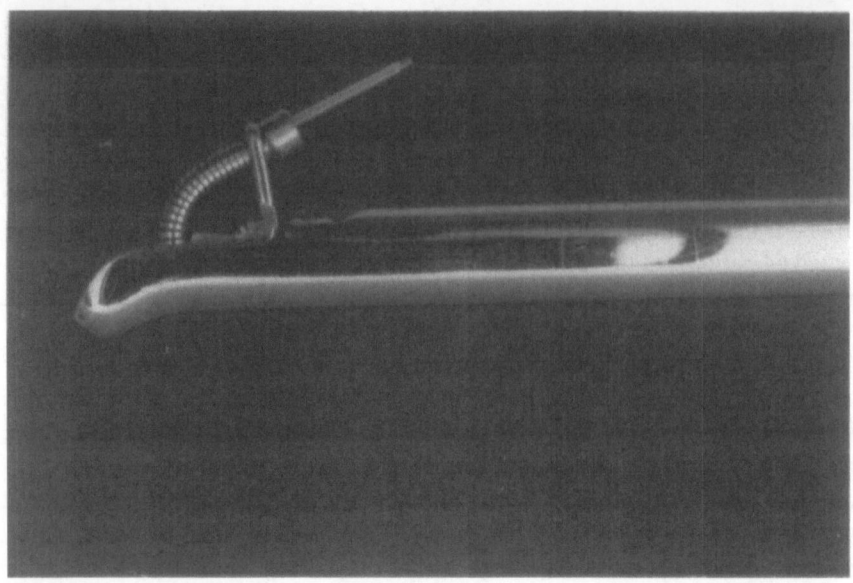

Fig. 21.3. Exaggerated Albarran deflection device. When used with a 120° viewing telescope, lesions at the bladder neck can be treated directly. (Courtesy Storz Instrument Company).

electrocautery. In general, laser fibers can be inserted through standard cystoscopic equipment (Fig. 21.2). A modified Albarran tip is used to direct the laser energy (Fig. 21.3). If desired, a sedative can be administered but a general or regional anesthetic is unnecessary. Usually, patients are able to perceive some slight discomfort when the laser energy is applied but tolerate the procedure well without anesthesia. Superficial tumors can be identified by a typical papillary appearance (Fig. 21.4). In addition, voided urinary cytology is useful in excluding high grade tumors (Fig. 21.5). For superficial bladder tumors, we have used a power output of 35 to 40 watts and treated each area for two to three seconds. A white discoloration of the tumor indicative of adequate thermal coagulation is visibly evident.

Using these laser specifications, perforation of the bladder or small bowel is extremely unlikely and Foley catheter drainage of the bladder is not necessary (15). Bleeding is usually negligible or nonexistent and patients are discharged from the outpatient area immediately after treatment.

There have been no reports of major complications due to laser treatment of superficial bladder tumors among American investigators. In our series, no complications have been observed other than some irritative voiding symptoms which are common after cystoscopy. In particular, there have been no instances of either immediate or delayed significant bleeding. Thus, although no definitive treatment advantages have been established for laser therapy of superficial bladder tumors, there are decided practical advantages which appear to make the procedure less morbid than alternative therapy and, perhaps, more cost effective (16).

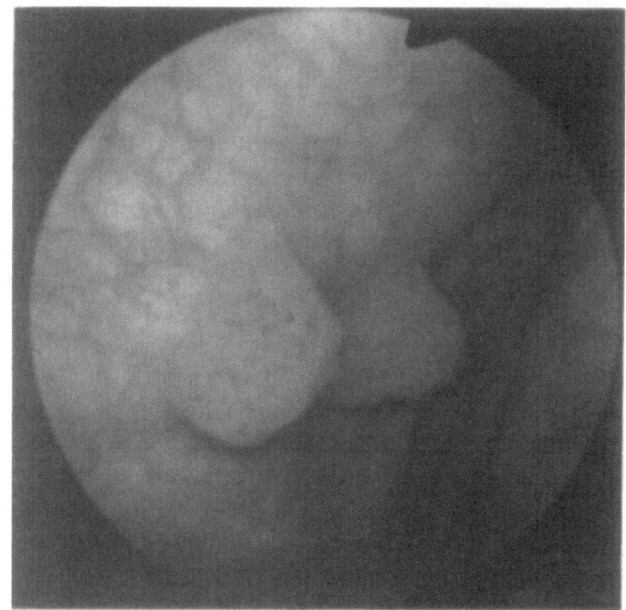

Fig. 21.4. Typical, papillary appearance of low grade, low stage transitional cell carcinoma of the bladder.

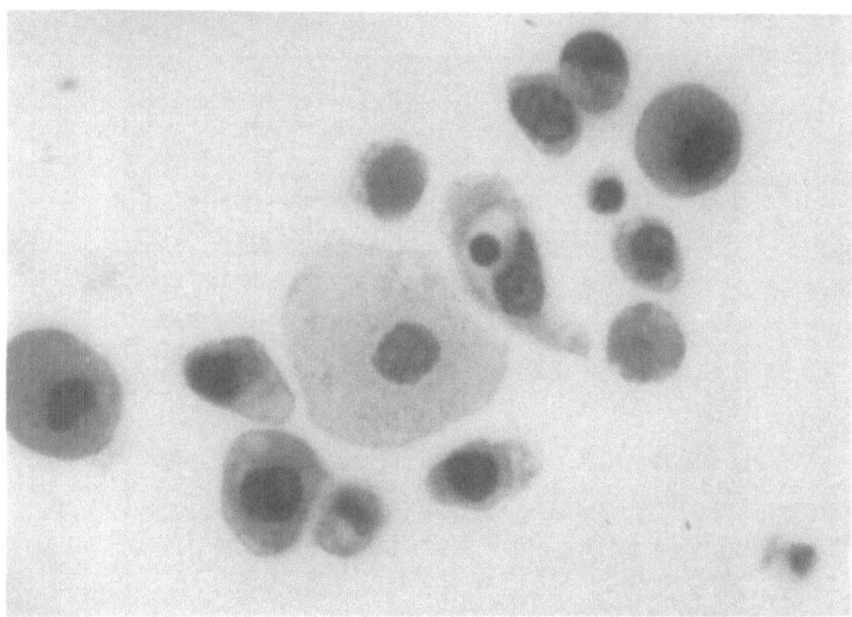

Fig. 21.5. High grade, malignant transitional cells in voided urine. Detailed histologic examination, sometimes not possible after laser treatment, should be performed on high grade tumors.

Invasive bladder cancer

Issues of treatment cost and patient convenience become less important when discussing invasive bladder cancer. Even after conventional therapy consisting of radical cystectomy with or without irradiation, five year survival rates of only 50% can be anticipated when transitional cell carcinoma invades the muscle of the bladder wall (17). Additionally, endoscopic management of these tumors has been unsatisfactory since removal of large portions of the bladder wall using electrocautery results in gross urinary extravasation. Under controlled conditions, a neodymium:YAG laser is capable of inducing a transmural coagulation of the bladder wall without damage to adjacent organs, in particular the small bowel (18). Therefore, theoretically, muscle invading bladder tumors could be treated endoscopically with the neodymium:YAG laser. Appropriately, treatment to date has been limited to patients who are not candidates for cystectomy because of age, health or metastatic disease or to those who refuse standard treatment. Using a power output of 45 to 50 watts with a treatment duration of around 3 seconds for each area, we have treated 15 such patients (Fig. 21.6). The total amount of energy has varied depending upon the size of the tumor but has been as high as 27,000 joules. Despite these higher power densities and total amounts of energy delivered, no instances of bladder or bowel perforation have occurred. Unlike superficial bladder tumors, treatment has been performed under regional or general anesthesia and a Foley catheter has been left indwelling overnight. No problems with immediate or delayed bleeding have been encountered.

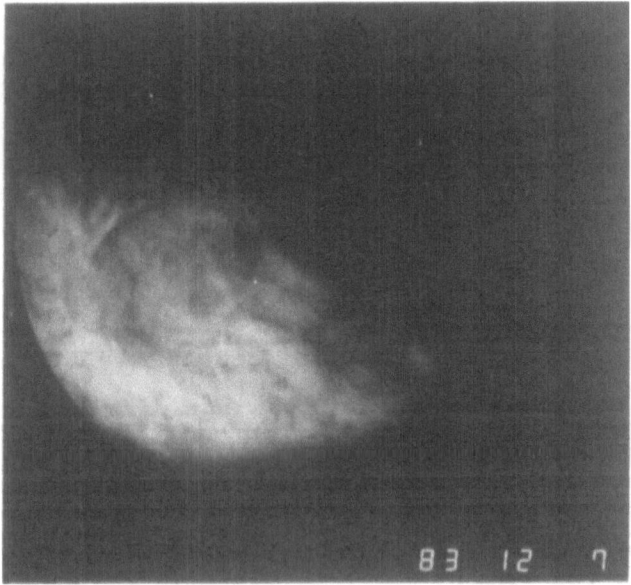

Fig. 21.6A. Flat, irregular appearance of high grade, invasive transitional cell carcinoma of the bladder.

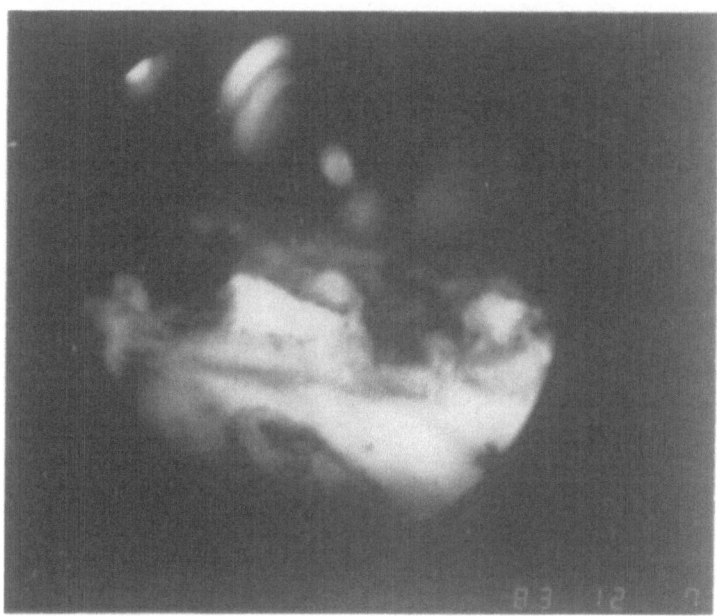

Fig. 21.6B. After Nd:YAG laser treatment, irregular thermal necrosis of the tumor surface is evident. Visible control of tissue effects is not as precise as with treatment of superficial, papillary tumors.

Cystoscopy has been repeated at three month intervals and appropriate biopsies and voided cytology obtained. Tumor persistence and, therefore, treatment failure was detected at three months in four patients and in another patient at the six month evaluation. The other patients remain apparently free of tumor for periods of follow-up of 3 to 22 months.

Based upon tissue properties, neodymium:YAG laser irradiation is theoretically an attractive way to treat muscle invading bladder tumors. Although our early results are somewhat encouraging, no conclusions can be drawn without longer follow-up and larger patient populations. Thus, until further information is available, laser treatment should not be recommended to patients with muscle invading bladder tumors in lieu of potentially curative alternative therapy.

Ureter and upper collecting system

Over the past several years, rigid instruments have become available for transurethral endoscopic visualization of the entire ureter and upper collecting system. In addition, these instruments have a working channel which will accept up to a 5 French laser fiber. Potentially, therefore, the entire upper urinary collecting system is accessible for delivery of laser energy.

A number of lesions which occur in the ureter, renal pelvis, or intrarenal

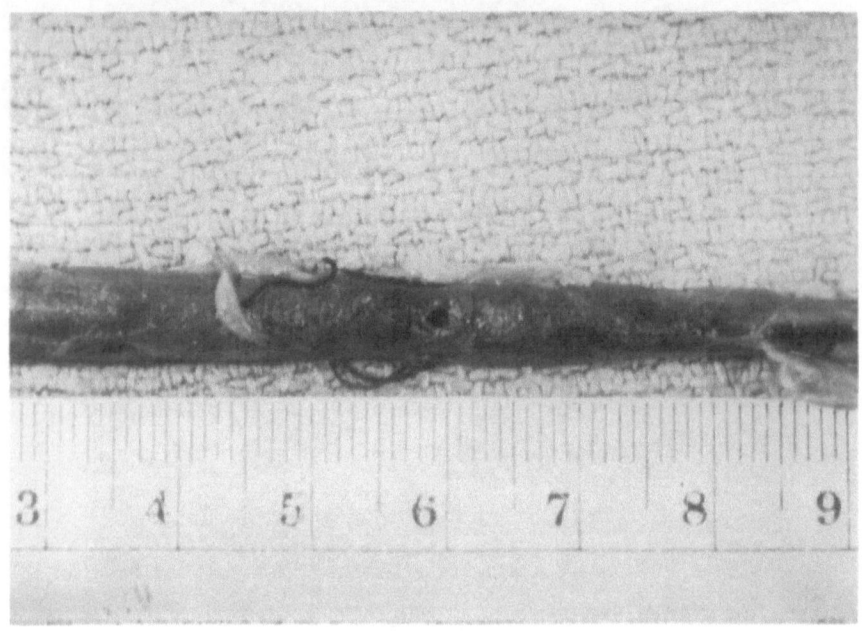

Fig. 21.7A. Gross perforation of canine ureter after Nd:YAG laser energy, 35 watts, 2 seconds.

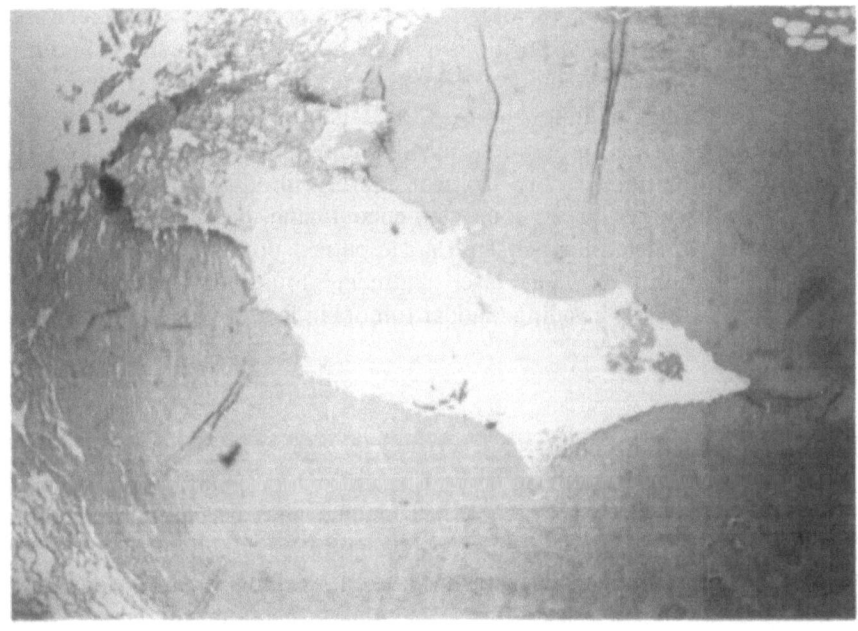

Fig. 21.7B. Histologic examination shows thermal injury extending through entire ureteral wall and into peri-ureteral tissues. (Reprinted with permission, J. Surg. Onc.).

collecting system potentially are amenable to treatment with a laser, including transitional cell tumors. However, the thin wall of the ureter makes it more liable to perforating injury that the bladder. In order to evaluate dosimetry specifications for treatment of ureteral lesions, we applied laser energy to canine ureters through an open ureterotomy. At a dose of 35 watts for 2 seconds, ureteral perforation was encountered invariably when the laser energy was delivered with the fiber at a perpendicular angle to the ureteral wall (Fig. 21.7). Higher power settings (60 watts) of short duration (0.5 seconds) created an injury which extended into the muscle of the ureter without perforation (19).

Several observations seem pertinent. First of all, laser doses which are safe in the bladder may be excessive when applied to the ureter. However, tangential application of the laser energy with a resultant larger spot size and decreased power density as would be expected when working through a ureteroscope would greatly decrease the chances of perforation. In addition, some degree of ureteral distention and surface cooling would be expected from the irrigating fluid used during ureteroscopy (20).

Clinical experience with laser treatment of upper urinary tract lesions is quite limited. Malloy has reported two patients with transitional cell tumors of a solitary kidney who underwent laser treatment immediately prior to partial nephrectomy (21).

We have treated three patients with tumors of the intra-mural ureter without complications. In addition, we have treated two patients with tumors of the renal pelvis although in neither case was the treatment sufficient for complete tumor destruction or able to obviate the need for additional surgery.

Endoscopic laser treatment of upper urinary tract lesions through either a ureteroscope or a percutaneously placed nephroscope is an exciting and potentially promising possibility. However, much greater clinical experience is needed as well as investigational studies to establish proper dosimetry specifications.

References

1. Smith JA Jr and Dixon JA. Laser photoradiation in urologic surgery. J Urol 1984;131:631.
2. Stein BS and Kendall AR. Lasers in urology: Laser therapy. Urology 1984;23:411.
3. Hofstetter A and Frank F. The neodymium:YAG laser in urology. Edition's Roche, F., Hoffmann-LaRoche and Co., Basel, Switzerland, 1980.
4. Smith JA Jr and Dixon JA. Neodymium:YAG laser treatment of benign urethral strictures. J Urol 1984;131:1080.
5. Shanberg AM, Chalfin SA, and Tansey LA. Neodymium:YAG laser: New treatment for urethral stricture disease. Urology 1984;24:15.
6. Willscher MK, Filoso AM, Jako GJ, Olsson CA. Development of a carbon dioxide laser cystoscope. J Urol 1978;119:202.
7. Soloway MS and Masters S. Implantation of transitional tumor cells on the cauterized murine urothelial surface. Proc Am Asso Cancer Res 1979;20:256.
8. Hofstetter A, Frank F, Keiditsch E and Bowering R. Endoscopic Neodymium:YAG laser application for destroying bladder tumors. Eur Urol 1981;7:278.

9. Smith JA Jr. and Dixon JA. Argon laser phototherapy of superficial transitional cell carcinoma of the bladder. J Urol 1984;131:655.

10. Smith JA Jr and Middleton RG. Bladder Cancer In: Lasers in Urologic Surgery, Edited by JA Smith Jr, Year book Med. Publishers, Chicago, 1986.

11. Malloy TR, Wein AJ and Stranberg A. Superficial transitional cell carcinoma of the bladder treated with the neodymium:YAG laser: A study of recurrence rate within the first year. Abstr Am urol Assoc 79th meeting, 1984:251.

12. Stein BS and Kendall AR. Use of Nd:YAG laser in urology. Ibid. 1984;142.

13. Aledia FT. Treatment of bladder tumor with Nd:YAG laser. Lasers in Med and Surg 1984;3:307.

14. McPhee MS, Mador DR, Tulip J, Ritchie B, Moore R and Lakey WN. Segmental irradiation of the bladder using a Nd:YAG laser. J Urol 1982;128:1101.

15. Smith JA Jr and Dixon JA. Tissue effects of lasers in the genitourinary system. In: Lasers in Urologic Surgery. Edited by JA Smith Jr, Year Book Med Pub, Chicago, 1986.

16. Smith JA Jr. Is a $90,000 laser cost-effective? Abstracts Western Section, Am Urol Assoc 118, Vancouver, 1983.

17. Smith JA Jr, Batata M, Gravstald H, Sogoni P, Herr H, and Whitmore WF Jr. Preoperative irradiation and cystectomy for bladder cancer. Cancer 1982;49:869.

18. Pensel J, Hofstetter A, Frank F, Keiditsch E and Rothenberger K. Temporal and spatial temperature profile of the bladder serosa in intravesical neodymium:YAG laser irradiation. Eur Urol 1981;7:298.

19. Smith JA Jr. Neodymium:YAG laser photoradiation of canine ureters: An analysis of penetration depth and subsequent healing. Surg Forum 1983;34:696.

20. Smith JA Jr and Dixon JA. Laser treatment of the ureter. J Surg Onc 1984;27:168-171.

21. Malloy TR. Treatment of lesions of the upper urinary tract. In: Lasers in Urologic Surgery, Edited by JA Smith Jr, Year Book Med Publishers, Chicago, 1985.

22. ARGON LASER IN UROLOGY

J. BISERTE AND J.M. BRUNETAUD

Introduction

Argon laser is presently used in endoscopic urology for two main indications: endoscopic treatment of bladder tumors and urethral stenosis (Table 22.1). Argon laser is also applied for other secondary indications: microsurgery for correction of male sterility, surgery of the meatus in females, treatment of tumors of penis, and vaporization of venereal condylomas (1-8). The purpose of this paper is to describe the indications, contraindications, techniques and results of endoscopic argon laser treatment in Urology.

Table 22.1. Indications for argon laser in urology.

Endoscopic	Non-endoscopic
Urinary bladder tumors	Micro surgery in male infertility
Urethral stenosis	Female meatus surgery
	Penis tumors
	Condylomata

Current endoscopic and non-endoscopic indications for argon laser in urology.

Endoscopic treatment of bladder tumors

Some urologists use Nd:YAG laser because of its deep coagulation and effective hemostasis. We choose argon laser because of the visibility of vaporization, its superficial coagulation effect, and its safety concerning perforation of the bladder and injury to surrounding organs. Our choice was made after an experimental study that compared argon and Nd:YAG lasers.

Experimental Study in Dogs

An experimental study was performed on the normal bladder of 15 dogs. The bladder was surgically opened. Argon laser (5 Watts with 1 to 5 seconds of exposure) was used on the right side of bladder and Nd:YAG (40 Watts with

D.M. Jensen and J.M. Brunetaud (eds), Medical Laser Endoscopy. 269-277.
© 1990 Kluwer Academic Publishers, Dordrecht

0.2 to 1 second) on the left side. The bladder was initially filled with nitrogen gas, but, in the last 3 dogs, it was filled with water. The probe was placed 2 to 3 millimeters from the wall before treatment. Several shots were delivered with each laser. The laser treatment varied from a single superficial effect to a deliberate perforation, that was then sutured. Autopsy and examination of bladders grossly and histologically were done immediately (4 dogs), on day 7 (6 dogs), and on day 15 (5 dogs). The results are summarized in Table 22.2.

Table 22.2. Experimental study in dogs of argon vs. Nd:YAG lasers.

	Observation	Argon	Nd:YAG
Day 0 (15 dogs)	Superficial coagulation	YES	YES
		5 W, 1 s	40 W, 0.7 s
	Acute perforation	YES	NO
		5 W, 3 s	40 W, 2 s
Day 7 (6 dogs)	Edema (chorion)	NO	YES
	Delayed perforation	NO	NO
	Histology – Inflammation	YES	YES
Day 15 (5 dogs)	Edema (chorion)	NO	YES
	Delayed perforation	NO	NO
	Histology – Inflammation	NO	YES

An acute and chronic gross and histologic study was done comparing argon with Nd:YAG laser photocoagulation of normal canine urinary bladder (non-endoscopic treatment).

The canine bladder wall was thin, about two millimeters. It was not possible to perform acute perforation with Nd:YAG laser, using 40 Watts and 0.7 sec pulses. Superficial photo-coagulation was easy with each laser. Secondary inflammatory reaction was greater with the Nd:YAG laser. On day 15, the right bladder (argon laser) was grossly quite normal. However, the left bladder wall (Nd:YAG laser) was still thickened. There was neither delayed perforation nor perivesical abscess of either the argon or the Nd:YAG treated areas. In conclusion, argon laser photocoagulation was more superficial and easier to control. The inflammatory reaction was less with argon laser and the margin of safety greater.

Endoscopic Laser Technique

Some surgeons use modified cystoscopes for laser endoscopy. We use a standard 21 French cystoscope and a special fiber. The fiber is fixed in a catheter, similar to GI endoscopy. We use a liquid flow instead of gas (Fig. 22.1). The liquid flow protects the fiber tip against contamination from ablated tissue which could damage the fiber. We use a 1.5% glycocol solution, similar to that for prostatic resection. The bladder is filled with the same solution. The procedure is performed under local anesthesia on an outpatient basis (Fig. 22.2).

270

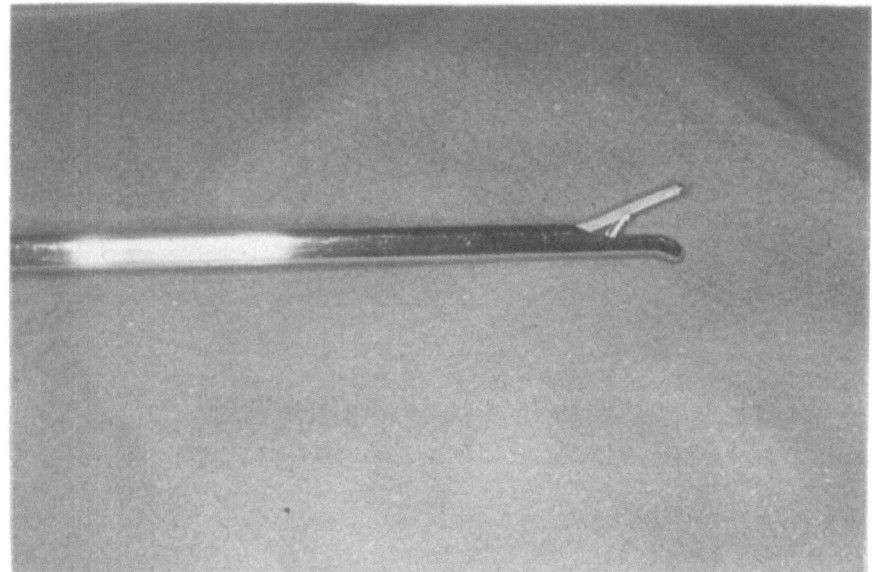

Fig. 22.1. Cystoscope and optic fiber.

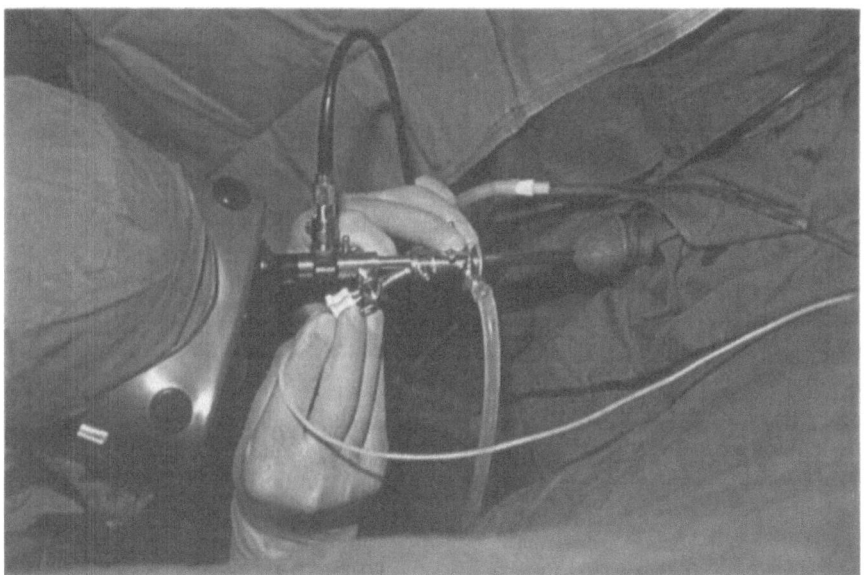

Fig. 22.2. Overall view of cystoscopy.

Our argon laser is a 770 Cooper Lasersonics model (Santa Clara, California). The output laser power is 8 to 10 Watts. The exposure time is controlled by the operator with a foot pedal. The probe is placed in front of the lesion at 2 millimeters treatment distance. The first visible effect is a whitening of the tumor. We vaporize larger portions of the lesion. The tumor base is then widely treated but we always move the laser catheter. We never needed more than two sessions to treat one tumor. Plate 66 in the Atlas shows a typical example of a small bladder tumor before, during and after argon laser treatment. Plate 67 (Atlas) shows a papilloma of the bladder before and after treatment with argon laser. The treatment was accomplished in one session without difficulty.

Indications – Bladder Tumors

Our indications were:
    1) patients with history of low grade, low stage (T0–T1) transitional cell tumor previously treated by multiple electro- resections, and
    2) small tumors (< 1 cm in diameter)

Patients Characteristics

Since 1980, we have treated 88 patients whose mean age was 52 (81 males and 7 females) with endoscopic argon laser. In all 293 tumors were destroyed in 175 sessions. The follow up time is 6 months to seven years (mean follow up: 46 months). The only previous therapy was electrocoagulation. No patient had pelvic irradiation or intra- vesical chemotherapy.

Results

The local relapse rate was about 9% (26/293 papillomas). These local recurrences were probably due to insufficient treatment and happened more frequently in our early experience. The recurrence rate in other areas of the bladder was 67% (59/88 patients). That rate was not improved by laser technique compared to other endoscopic treatment. Some of these remote recurrences were treated by electrocoagulation because of the size or the localization. There were no immediate or long term complications. In particular, we never observed post treatment bleeding or cystitis (See Table 22.3).

Discussion

In Giessen, Germany, Rothauge (9, 10) has been using high power (up to 30 Watts) argon laser photocoagulation since 1976. He treated 101 patients in 185 sessions: 70 sessions with argon laser alone and 115 with electro resection followed by argon laser photocoagulation. There were no complications and he reported 4 local relapses after the 70 laser sessions. His recurrence rate was nearly 40%. In Salt Lake City, Utah, Smith (11) treated 11 patients (9

Table 22.3. Bladder tumors treated by endoscopic argon laser.

Authors	Pts.	Therapy	Tumors	Local relapses	Complications
Biserte J., Lille (France), 1987	88	Laser 10 W	293	26	0
Rothauge C.F. Giessen (FRG), 1978	38	Laser 30 W	41	?	0
Rothauge C.F., 1981	101	Laser	70	4	0
		Laser + TUR	115	0	0
Smith J.A., Salt Lake City (Utah), 1984	11	Laser 5W	9 2 CIS	0 1 cytology +	0 0

Tabulation of clinical results with endoscopic argon laser for bladder tumor treatment. Results are illustrated. TUR is transurethral resection. CIS is Carcinoma *in situ*.

papillomas and 2 carcinomas *in situ*) with a 5 Watt argon laser. He reported no local relapses, 3 recurrences in other areas, and only one complete destruction of the 2 carcinomas *in situ*.

According to the above experiences, there are both advantages and disadvantages of argon laser photocoagulation versus electro- coagulation in the treatment of bladder tumors. The advantages of argon laser are: 1) Treatment is performed under local intra-uretral anesthesia on an outpatient basis. For electro-resection, patients require general anesthesia and hospitalization. In our series, it was necessary to interrupt the argon treatment only once because of patient discomfort. However, the patient who experienced the discomfort had 8 tumors and treatment was interrupted after treatment of the fourth tumor. We related the discomfort mainly to the long duration of the endoscopy rather than the laser treatment itself. In our other cases, only half the patients felt a sensation of warmth during argon laser treatment but were not uncomfortable. Post operative catheter drainage was unnecessary. Patient acceptance was very good. In fact, they were disappointed when a second electro-resection was necessary. 2) Laser coagulation or vaporization is a non-touch treatment. All tumor cells are vaporized. In theory, this should reduce the risk of tumor dissemination to other parts of the bladder, which may occur with a touch method like electrocautery or electro-resection. 3) The inflammatory reaction to argon laser is much lower than electro-resection. Epithelialization is quicker and of better quality. In most of the cases it is impossible to see any scarring after treatment with argon laser. We noted this in patients and previously in canine bladders. This can be an advantage in the treatment of multiple tumors with argon laser. With argon laser treatment, we hope to avoid or to delay sclerosis of the bladder as might occur after multiple electrocautery or electro-resection treatments. 4) Laser treatment is not hemorrhagic. If bleeding occurs, it can be controlled by increasing the laser spot size and treating further. 5) Neither obturator nerve stimulation nor cardiac pacemaker interference occur with argon laser treatment. Both may be problems with electro-resection. 6) No bubbles occur. Bubbles following electro-resection make treatment of the upper part of the bladder difficult.

There are also theoretical advantages of argon laser compared to Nd:YAG laser. 1) Argon laser light is more preferentially absorbed by hemoglobin than Nd:YAG laser. This allows selective treatment of vascular or erythematous lesions such as bladder tumors. 2) With argon laser, we have visible and immediate vaporization without delayed effects as with Nd:YAG laser. With Nd:YAG laser, there is photocoagulation of the tumor but delayed sloughing of tissue. The advantage of argon laser is immediate appreciation of the result of the treatment. 3) The risk of perforation of bladder or adjacent tissue is lower with argon laser than with Nd:YAG, which penetrates deeper. However, even with argon laser some precautions must be taken. These are not to over fill the bladder which results in decreasing of the thickness of the wall; to treat the patient with a dome lesion in the Tredelenburg position; and not to treat lesions in a fixed position but rather use circular motion.

Compared to electro-resection, both lasers have certain disadvantages. After laser coagulation or vaporization, no tissue is available for histologic assessment. Multiple biopsies prior to laser treatment do not necessarily represent the whole tumor and therefore the lesion may be misdiagnosed from the available biopsies. Areas of the bladder such as the neck and the dome may be difficult to get the laser beam perpendicular to the lesion. Laser treatment may not be efficient or complete in these areas.

In conclusion, argon laser photocoagulation and vaporization are safe and efficient for the treatment of superficial bladder tumors. It has theoretical advantages over electro-resection because of lower local recurrence rates, lower risk of tumor spread, and lower risk of bladder scarring or stenosis after multiple treatments. However, this is unproven with any prospective comparisons. At the present time, no controlled trials of argon vs. electro-resection or argon vs. Nd:YAG have been reported for these urologic treatments. The limited penetration of argon laser provides a wider margin of safety than the possible transmural effect of Nd:YAG laser. Finally, the main advantages of argon laser are practical. Treatment is done on an out-patient basis, without general anesthesia and healing is better and quicker than with electro-resection. The best indications for argon laser treatment are: 1) a small, superficial tumor of the posterior wall, even if multiple, 2) large, thin papillary lesion, and 3) tumor near or in the ureteral meatus. Because of the lack of tissue for histologic examination after argon laser treatment and its limited penetration, argon laser should not be used for the treatment of infiltrative lesions even if combined with electro-resection.

Treatment of urethral stenosis

Endoscopic lasers can vaporize circumferential stenoses. This is not possible by any other method, whether surgical or endoscopic. For this purpose, argon laser should be superior to Nd:YAG laser because it vaporizes without delayed effects. However, clinical experience for argon laser treatment of urethral stenoses is less than with bladder tumors.

The first results were reported by Bulow in 1979 with a Nd:YAG laser (12) and Rothauge in 1980 with an argon laser (13-15). They were very encouraging. There were only 6 recurrences after treatment of 40 stenoses by Rothauge with an argon laser. However, Rothauge's results were less encouraging one year later with 36 recurrences after 90 treatments and 126 sessions. Rothauge used a very powerful argon laser (30 Watts) to ablate urethral and periurethral stenoses. His method was to circularly remove the entire stricture area, down to the corpus urethrae spongiosum, so that a smooth transition was created proximal and distal to the stricture. An indwelling catheter was left in for 6 to 8 days.

Our Results

We used a 10 Watt argon laser to treat 4 urethral strictures and 1 bladder neck stenosis. The same instrumentation was employed as for bladder tumors. The procedure required general or regional anesthesia. It was not possible under local anesthesia. The urethral strictures were first dilated with a bougie or balloon dilatation catheter in order to allow cystoscope introduction. Then we attempted to vaporize the whole circumferential fibrotic stricture. But this was never possible and then we realized a laser urethrotomy.

Our results are summarized in Table 22.4.

Table 22.4. Urethral strictures treated by endoscopic argon laser.

Age	Etiology	Localization	Result	Follow-up
40	Post infection	Perineal	Good	6 years
56	Post infection	Perineal	Recurrence	Cold knife urethrotomy
26	Post traumatic	Posterior	Failure	Surgical urethroplasty
50	Post traumatic	Perineal	Failure	Balloon dilatation
54	Post surgical	Bladder neck	Good	6 years

List of patients with urethral strictures treated with 10 Watts argon laser via endoscopy. Etiology, localization, results and follow up are shown.

Our overall impression was that a 10 Watts power output was not sufficient. It was very difficult to realize a single incision. Laser could be superior to other treatments if the whole urethral stenosis was vaporized, what Rothauge names 'recanalization'. Further trials with higher power argon laser need to be performed, in our opinion.

Conclusion

At the present time, it is not proven that argon laser treatment of superficial bladder tumors or urethral stenosis improves the therapeutic results compared to conventional techniques. Prospective, randomized trials are needed to answer these questions. For bladder tumor treatment, argon laser has some practical advantages over electro-resection. Mainly, outpatient treatment is possible and it may also be more cost effective. For urethral stenosis, argon laser is attractive, but results are not yet good. Higher power and better techniques may improve results. Argon laser may be used for other non-endoscopic indications. Microsurgery for male sterility is one. Incision of the epididymis is non-hemorrhagic and the inflammatory reaction is negligible after anastomosis of the epididymis and vas deferens. Surgery of the urethral meatus in the female is another. Treatment of venereal condyloma is also very feasible with argon laser. With new endoscopes such as fibercystoscopes, ureteroscopes, and nephroscopes, other applications of argon laser treatment may be possible. For all these indications, the aim is less inflammatory reaction and quicker healing than with electrocautery, surgery, or Nd:YAG laser.

References

1. Biserte J, Brunetaud JM. Lasers en Urologie. 4th Congress of International Society for Laser Surgery. Tokyo 1981, Proceedings 10-49.
2. Brunetaud JM, Decomps B. Utilisation thérapeutique des lasers. Gaz Méd 1981;88:no.26,3677-3682.
3. Camey M, LeDuc A, Barbegelatta M. La laser et ses applications en Urologie. Concours Méd 1981;103:no.3,181- 186.
4. Bulow H. Present status of endoscopic laser techniques in Urology. Endoscopy 1979;11:no.4,240-243.
5. Bulow H. Present and future plans for laser urological surgery. Lasers surg Med 1981:1(4), 385-390.
6. Hall RR. Report to the standing committee on urological instruments: lasers in Urology. Br J Urol 1982;54(4):421- 426.
7. Hoske HD. Use of lasers in urology with special reference to the therapy of bladder cancer. Z Urol Néphrol 1978;71(5),351- 356.
8. Rothauge CF. Expériences de l'application du laser à l'Argon dans les maladies urologiques. Urologe 1981;20,suppl:333- 339.
9. Rothauge CF, Kraushaar J, Noeske HD. Expériences d'une année de traitement transuréthral par laser de tumeurs vésicales, communication préliminaire. Muench Med Wschr 1977;119(17):593-594.
10. Rothauge CF. La place de l'irradiation laser thrasuréthrale dans le traitement des cancers de vessie. Onkologie 1978;1(5):212- 215.

11. Smith Jr JA, Dixon JA. Argon laser phototherapy of superficial transitional cell carcinoma of the bladder. J Urol April 1984;131:655-656.
12. Bulow H, Bulow U, Levine S, Wurster H, Frohmueller H. L'état actuel de la technique au laser transuréthral pour le traitement de la sténose uréthrale. Urology 1981;20 suppl:328-332.
13. Rothauge CF. Transurethral laser treatment in bladder neoplasm. Helv Chir Acta 1978;45(3):233-236.
14. Rothauge CF. Traitement des sténoses uréthrales par le laser à l'Argon. Helv Chir Acta 1980;47(3-4):401-404.
15. Rothauge CF. Urethroscopic recanalization of urethral stenosis using Argon Laser. Urology (Ridgewood) 1980;16(2):158-161.

23. GYNECOLOGICAL APPLICATION OF LASER ENDOSCOPY

JEAN LUC POULY, GERARD MAGE AND MAURICE A. BRUHAT

Over the past decade two of the most important advances in gynecological surgery were the development of laparoscopic surgical procedures and the use of laser in intra-abdominal gynecological surgery. Laparoscopic surgery still has some limitations, mainly due to the difficulties in achieving complete hemostasis and the risks of extensive tissue damage from electrocautery. So the idea arose to use a laser during laparoscopy to increase the efficiency of surgical laparoscopic procedures. The use of a laser during a laparoscopy was first reported by Bruhat et al. in 1979 (1). But, there are only a few clinical reports because current laser technology does not permit routine or easy use. Laser hysteroscopy has also been reported by Goldrath (2) and Tadir (3).

Problems in development of laser laparoscopy

The first dilemma was the type of laser to use. The CO_2 laser induces destruction of tissue by vaporization. The intracellular and extracellular water boils to form steam, the expansion of which disrupts tissue. A cutting effect occurs only at the impact point as the beam is rapidly and completely absorbed by tissue water. The CO_2 laser induces minimal tissue damage around the impact point. The depth of thermal necrosis is dependent upon the energy density and the exposure time but is usually less than 200 um. Moreover, vessels up to 0.5 mm in diameter may be sealed by this laser to obtain a bloodless section. The CO_2 laser can also induce a very weak tissue coagulation by using low power density that induces absorption of water from the tissue and tissue retraction.

The argon laser beam is mainly absorbed by hemoglobin or pigmented tissue. However, the argon laser can be used with different power densities. Low power density induces photocoagulation and destruction of hemoglobin in tissues. Thermal damage in the surrounding tissue is slightly greater than that induced by CO_2 laser. High power densities are able to cut but the lateral thermal tissue damage is greater than that of the CO_2 laser (4). In our opinion, this limits the use of argon laser to gynecological procedures such as photocoagulation of endometriosis implants.

Nd:YAG laser induces considerable tissue destruction. This laser cannot be used for precise gynecologic surgical procedures via endoscopy and its use near

D.M. Jensen and J.M. Brunetaud (eds), Medical Laser Endoscopy. 279-294.
© 1990 Kluwer Academic Publishers, Dordrecht

vital structures may be hazardous, in our opinion.

For these reasons CO_2 laser is generally considered as the best laser for intra-abdominal gynecological surgery. Unfortunately, no flexible optical fibers are available yet for the CO_2 laser. Argon or Nd:YAG laser have an advantage of easy transmission via optical quartz fibers. The CO_2 laser was the first laser to be used during laparoscopy. Refer to Fig. 23.1 for the CO_2 laser laparoscope connected to the articulated arm.

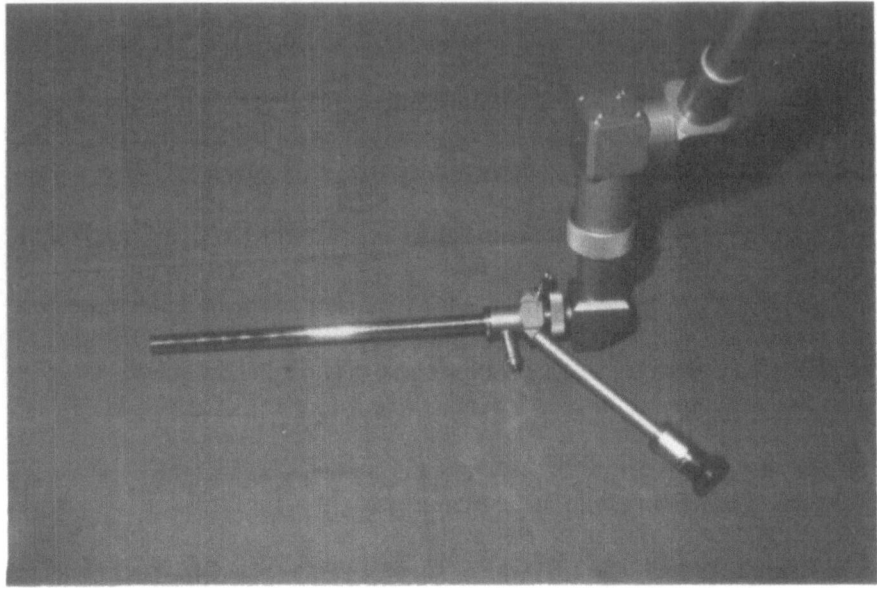

Fig. 23.1. A CO_2 laser laparoscope connected to the articulated arm.

CO_2 laser for laparoscopy

A problem was how to introduce the CO_2 laser beam into the abdomen. It can be introduced through an operative laparoscope or a second puncture. Generally the super-pubic route is more efficient to perform surgical laparoscopic procedures. When we tested the two methods, our conclusion was that the second puncture route was preferable (5). The only advantage of the laparoscopic route was safety: the path of the laser beam must be constantly in view. But this laparoscopic approach permitted only limited laser treatment angles and the range and visibility of the helium-neon red aiming beam was often unclear. To facilitate treatment with the laparoscope CO_2 laser route, a cross hair must be built into the optical channel or an index added at the extremity of the laparoscope. The main advantages of the second puncture route were simplicity in manipulating the laser laparoscopic handpiece and the possibility of many different treatment angles because grasping and moving organs was feasible, sometimes, through a third puncture. Safety was good. The visibility of the helium-neon red aiming beam is generally clear and a guard at the lower end of the probe could be added to avoid tissue damage after the cut is complete. Currently, we recommended the second puncture route for laparoscopic laser. See Fig. 23.2 for an example.

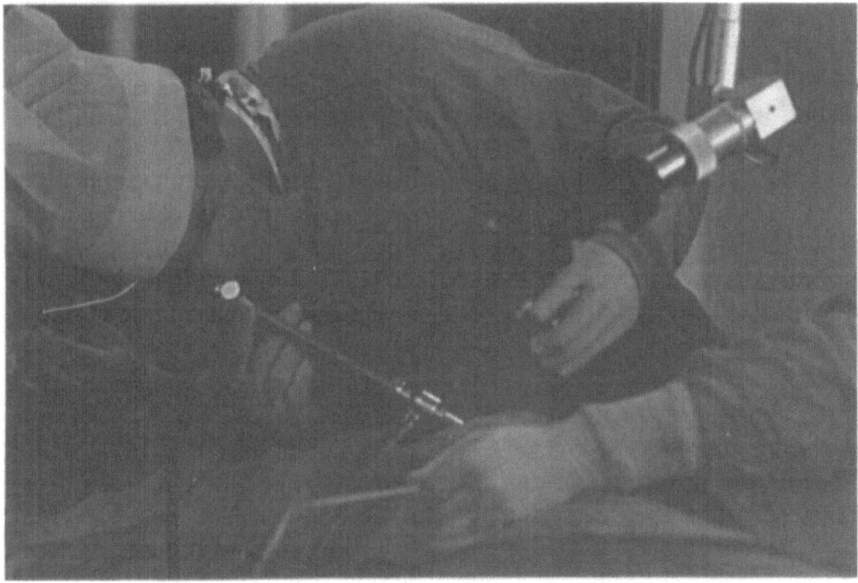

Fig. 23.2. Utilization of a second puncture CO_2 laser.

Another problem is related to the focal length of the CO_2 laser. All the current CO_2 laser probes have a long focal length ranging from 300 to 400 mm. Consequently the diameter of the impact is enlarged to more than 1 mm and the power density is dramatically decreased. One solution to reduce the impact would be to put the lens into the probe and not at the end of the articulated arm. But the difficulties arise from the theoretical diameter of the laser beam before it is focused and from the distortion caused by the articulated arm. Several different solutions include: increasing the diameter of the probe or correcting the beam distortion with a joy stick manipulator or a laser beam translator. However, even if these systems work, they are not suitable for a routine use. Installation can need as long as 30 minutes and can be unsuccessful if the articulated arm causes too much distortion. Another solution is to try a different focal length. For four months, we tested a new CO_2 laser probe with a focal length of 15 cm. This laser does not require a corrective system. This system appears more efficient than the previous ones since the cutting effect is more rapid and assembly of the probe requires only 2 to 3 minutes.

With the long focal length of the CO_2 laser, energy is decreased because of absorption by CO_2 gas used for insufflation. Tadir found on histological examination that the extent of tissue vaporization with CO_2 laser at laparoscopy was one to four times less than at the open laparotomy (6). Daniell reported that with the same probe, tissue effects were greater during laparotomy with 5 watts power than during a laparoscopy with 15 watts power (7). Decreased power density reduces the cutting effect, induces greater tissue thermal damage and moreover eliminates some of the advantages of the CO_2 laser surgery.

CO_2 laser vaporization produces a large amount of smoke that reduced the visibility and must be removed from the abdomen during laparoscopy. Smoke can absorb CO_2 laser energy and also induce moisture on the lens and the mirror. Most of the probes are connected to the insufflation system to avoid this. CO_2 gas blowing down the probe must be associated with aspiration of the smoke. A suction channel can be coupled to the probe, annular (6) or along the laser channel (7). Suction can also be achieved through a special needle that can be put close to the laser impact (J. Daniell, personal communication). The last method efficiently evacuates the smoke. The suction device must be synchronized with the laser to maintain the pneumoperitoneum free of smoke.

Argon laser for laparoscopy

The use of an argon laser during a laparoscopy was first reported by Keye and Dixon (4). They passed a 600 um flexible quartz fiber through the operating channel of a cystourethroscope. This was introduced into the peritoneal cavity through a suprapubic incision. The main advantages of this method is the large range of treatment angles. The intra-abdominal end of the operative channel has a flexible tip that can be directed through a 90°arc by turning a small knob located on the external portion of the probe. It is possible to direct the argon laser beam on the back of the uterus or on the posterior wall of the large ligament with a perpendicular incidence. That is not possible with a CO_2 laser at laparoscopy. Moreover, argon laser energy is not absorbed by the intraperitoneal carbon dioxide and laparoscopic effects are similar to use at laparotomy. Argon laser at lower power coagulates tissue and does not vaporize nor produce smoke.

Argon laser for laparoscopy has some disadvantages. The blue-green aiming beam of the argon laser is difficult to see when the external laparoscopic light is turned on. This is less of a problem when the tip of the laser fiber can be directed to within 1 mm of the lesions to be coagulated. This makes the argon laparoscopic laser a poor tool for precision work in our opinion. Moreover, no laser beam focusing lens can be applied at the end of the quartz fiber. Such focusing is feasible for the CO_2 laser.

During argon laser photocoagulation orange-colored protective goggles must be worn to protect the operator's eyes. That somewhat reduces visualization of the pelvis because there is some color interference. Also, wearing glasses is uncomfortable for a lot of laparoscopists. Protective goggles often must be removed to insure that coagulation is complete. Argon laser mainly coagulates. It does not cut well especially at lower power densities. This is a major disadvantage. The major indication of argon laparoscopic laser is photocoagulation of endometrial implants. It is poorly suited for procedures requiring cutting such as treatment of fimbrial occlusion, uterosacral ligament section or lysis of tubo-ovarian adhesions. One other disadvantage of argon laser is its expense.

Nd:YAG laser for laparoscopy

The use of Nd:YAG laser during laparoscopy was first reported by Lamano (8). The delivery system is similar to that of the argon laser. Most of the problems for laparoscopic use of Nd:YAG laser are similar to argon. But the action on tissues of the Nd:YAG laser may be more problematic for laparoscopic treatment. The depth of tissue coagulation is 4 to 5 mm beneath the surface and the lateral coagulation scattering may be significant. This laser does not cut well even at high power densities. In our opinion, the Nd:YAG laser for laparoscopic treatment can be regarded as a poor precision tool for cutting. Theoretically Nd:YAG laser for laparoscopic coagulation may be dangerous even though Lamano reported no complications for laparoscopic coagulation of endometriosis (8).

Clinical Applications

Laparoscopic laser has been used to perform various procedures listed in Table 23.1.

Table 23.1. Clinical applications of laser for gynecological laparoscopy.

- destruction of endometriosis lesions
- uterosacral ligament section
- neosalpingostomy
- lysis of tubo-ovarian adhesions
- vaporization of uterine or ovarian fibromas
- ablation of ovarian or hydatid cysts
- tubal section

This list may be expanded with more widespread uses of lasers and improvement of equipment.

Uterosacral ligament section

Pelvic pain is a common complaint in gynecological practice. Laparoscopy is generally considered as a diagnostic procedure in these cases but some surgical laparoscopic procedures have been proposed such as anterior uterine ligamentopexy. Uterosacral section has also been advocated in cases of dysmenorrhea and unexplained chronic pelvic pain to interrupt the uterine innervation. It could be performed with CO_2 (9) or argon lasers. This procedure is easily carried out with a second puncture CO_2 laser introduction. By means of a cannula, the uterus is strongly anteverted to obtain a good exposure and tension on the uterosacral ligaments. Then a rectangular portion of each ligament is removed down to a depth of 1 cm and a length of 2 to 3 centimeters with the CO_2 or argon laser. The laser beam must be directed toward the uterus to avoid accidental laser firing of the nearby rectum. Most of the series have never been published but only reported in medical meetings. Pain relief ranges from 70 to 80% for 6 months post-operatively. Feste (9) reported 50 cases among dysmenorrheic patients. The clinical follow-up in 42 patients at 12 months included: 30 (73%) with marked decreased or no pain, 10 (23%) with moderate to some improvement and 2 (4%) with no improvement. We have only performed this procedure in 5 cases with 3 reporting pain relief for 9 months.

In our opinion, there are 3 problems with laser uterosacral ligament section.

First, not all the nerves are cut because the uterosacral ligaments are only partially sectioned and furthermore the uterine innervation has other routes. The etiology of chronic pelvic pain is controversial. Laparoscopic or clinical findings permit specific treatment in some cases. But when no organic lesion is found, it is well established that any surgical procedure or a diagnostic laparoscopy induces pain relief in a large percentage of these cases. This observation leads one to think that this type of chronic pelvic pain has a large functional element. A pain relief rate of 70 to 80% post-operatively is common after any procedure but pain recurrence is frequent after 2 to 3 years of follow-up. No long term data after this laser procedure are yet available. Moreover, no controlled studies have been reported for this method.

Secondly, this procedure could be performed with cheaper techniques such as bipolar coagulation and scissor section or monopolar electrosection.

Thirdly, the uterosacral ligaments are one of the main factors of uterine and pelvic suspension. One can imagine that this procedure might subsequently induce uterine prolapse. We believe that this procedure is often used in America because it is easily performed and because 'Laser procedure' is a magic word. There may be significant placebo effect of laser for relief of chronic pelvic pain.

Endometriosis destruction

Endometriosis is a mysterious disease that induces pelvic pain and/or infertility. The etiology and the pathogenesis remain unclear. The treatment is still not well standardized but mainly depends upon the extent and the type of the lesions, on whether there is associated infertility, and on the physician's experience. Conservative surgery, microsurgery, laparoscopic surgery, danazol, progestins, and estroprogestins are the various treatments and they are often combined. The purpose of treatment is to destroy the ectopic endometrium.

Destruction can be achieved using a laser. Endometriosis treatment is generally considered as the best application of CO_2 or argon laser during intra-abdominal surgery (10). Animal experiments have been reported about the efficacy of destruction of experimental endometriosis with the argon (11) or CO_2 laser (12). Argon laser induced photocoagulation and the CO_2 laser vaporization. Surgical intra-abdominal laser procedures include destruction of peritoneal implants, adhesiolysis and destruction of the internal mucosa of endometrial ovarian cysts.

The purpose of laser laparoscopy is to achieve these procedures without laparotomy. Destruction of endometrial implants is generally easily achieved using a laser laparoscopically. During treatment the CO_2 laser beam must be directed as near to perpendicular as possible on the lesions. Shots with large spot sizes are often better because they cause large areas of destruction. If the lesions have a large surface area, the CO_2 laser beam must be moved continuously to avoid destruction of the underlying tissues. In these conditions, the vaporization of the lesion is more easily controlled than by carefully placed shots. Refer to Plate 69 in the atlas for an example of endometriosis vaporization with a second puncture CO_2 laser probe. Nevertheless all lesions cannot be destroyed for several reasons: sometimes it is impossible to reach the lesions with a direct shot and the mirror-reflected shots are very imprecise and moreover the vaporization of lesions located on the intestinal tract may cause a perforation. Destruction of lesions located on the bladder or along the ureter is possible with the CO_2 laser.

For the argon laser, the flexible fiber enables any lesions to be reached on a perpendicular incidence. The tip of the fiber is directed to within 1 mm of the implants to destroy. Because the tissue effect is coagulation, control of the lesions destruction is difficult. The treatment of endometrial implants on the intestinal tract must be avoided. Destruction of lesions along the ureter and on the bladder is possible, even if the theoretical risk of underlying damage is more elevated than when using the CO_2 laser.

Lamano treated endometriosis via laparoscopy with Nd:YAG laser (8). The technique of treatment was similar to that with the argon laser.

Endometriosis adhesions are thick and vascular. Moreover there is generally no cleavage plane. Lysis of endometriosis adhesions requires a high precision and a good cutting effect. When the intestinal tract is not involved the CO_2 laser is a safe and effective tool. Argon laser for lysis of endometriosis adhesions must be avoided because the cutting effect occurs only at high power densities and can induce thermal damage to the surrounding tissue such as the tube. When adhesions involve the intestinal tract, only the CO_2 laser should be considered, but this still remains a dangerous laparoscopic procedure with a high risk of intestinal perforation.

The adhesions must be put under tension. This is done by moving the uterus with a cannula or by grasping and drawing the pelvic organs with a laparoscopic forceps. The plane of the adhesions must be exposed in the same direction as the laser beam. This is often impossible so that CO_2 laser cannot be applied. On the other hand, argon laser has a poor cutting effect and is more imprecise. For these reasons laparoscopic lysis of endometriosis adhesions is a difficult procedure with the current laser technology. The only adhesions easily removed are those from tubes and uterus or from uterus and ovaries.

Laser laparoscopic treatment of ovarian endometriomas is quite impossible. During a laparotomy this procedure includes cyst opening by laser excision of an elliptical portion of the cyst wall. The chocolate fluid contents are drained. The internal mucosa of the cyst is exposed by eversion. The interior lining is completely destroyed by superficial vaporization with the CO_2 laser treatment. The cyst cavity is finally closed with two suture layers on the cyst wall and the ovarian cortex. This procedure cannot be completely performed during a laser laparoscopy. Opening and draining the endometrioma is easily achieved with any laser. But the destruction of the internal lining is impossible. Eversion of the cyst wall is impossible to maintain, the cyst cavity is often collapsed and cannot be exposed. Moreover, the laparoscopic CO_2 laser does not permit complete destruction because of the limited access of a cyst with the CO_2 laser probe. Laparoscopic argon laser can theoretically carry out this treatment, but complete exposure can be only obtained by introducing at least 2 or 3 suprapubic forceps and that is a very difficult procedure. Finally ovary reconstruction is impossible via laparoscopy and, without it, adhesions can develop.

Consequently the utility of the laparoscopic laser is limited to the destruction of endometriosis implants and to the lysis of adhesions not involving the gastrointestinal tract. These cases generally represent mild or moderate endometriosis in American Fertility Society classification.

The fertility rate is considered as the best data for evaluating the efficiency of a treatment of endometriosis. Initial results are promising (13, 14, 15). Keye (16) reported 47 cases of argon laser laparoscopic treatment and 13 patients had subsequent pregnancies (27.7%). Feste (17) reported 58 cases of CO_2 laser treatment via laparoscopy, 9 patients had an intrauterine pregnancies (45%), 7 delivered or are still pregnant and 2 had abortions. In the orally reported series this rate ranges from 30% to 54%.

The treatment of ovarian or peritoneal endometriosis implants during laparoscopy has been previously reported with monopolar electrocoagulation, bipolar electrocoagulation, thermocoagulation or excision by biopsy. Lysis of adhesions can be achieved with scissors and forceps or by electrocautery. Endometriotic ovarian cysts can be drained and washed, their internal lining can be partially destroyed by electrocoagulation (18, 19).

The results of series with these methods are controversial and this technique that is generally used only in the cases of mild or moderate endometriosis. We obtained an intrauterine pregnancy rate of 33% among 30 patients with severe endometriosis (19). Daniell (20) reported a rate of 57% among 60 patients with mild or moderate endometriosis. Semm reported a rate of 49% among 491 patients for all stages of endometriosis. In these 3 series danazol was associated with the laparoscopic treatment. Without danazol, Sulewski (21) achieved a fertility rate of 47.6% among 42 patients with mild stage and 34.6% among 58 patients with moderate stage. Under similar conditions, Hasson (22) reported a fertility rate of 75% among 8 patients with mild stage. Interpretation of these data is difficult for several reasons. Treatment of stage I or II endometriosis remains controversial. Laparoscopic electrocautery (20), surgery, danazol therapy (23), no therapy (24, 25) seem to result in equivalent fertility rates. Moreover, danazol treatments can achieve different pregnancy rates (23, 26). The fertility rates reported using these other treatment vary greatly. After surgical treatment they range from 62.2% (27) to 73.2% (28), after danazol therapy from 83.3% (29) to 28% (26) and without treatment from 75% (25) to 30.6% (26.). A long follow-up is necessary for controlled studies as a pregnancy can occur as long as 3 to 5 years after treatment. In most series of laparoscopic laser, there was also treatment with danazol. Controlled trials including different treatments will be necessary to determine the best treatment.

Such data for laparoscopic laser may be available in a few years time. Nevertheless treatment of endometriosis by laser laparoscopy must be regarded as a promising procedure. Chong reported a retrospective comparative study: Danazol versus laparoscopic CO_2 laser plus post-operative Danazol in treatment of mild endometriosis. In the first group the intra-uterine pregnancies rate is 45% among 49 patients, after laser application and danazol treatment this rate is increased to 65% among 32 patients (30).

There are three theoretical advantages of laparoscopic laser to treat endometriosis. First, experimental animal studies with the argon (11) and the CO_2 laser (12) have shown that the laser permits precise destruction of endometriosis with minimal subsequent adhesions sequellae. Moreover, the first reported results of intra-abdominal utilization of the CO_2 laser for the severe or extensive stage lead us to think that laser surgery is a real improvement over conventional surgery or microsurgery (10). It is doubtful whether these cases will ever be treated during laparoscopy. Second, the laparoscopic treatment has an advantage because it can be performed during the diagnostic laparoscopy. The cost of this treatment is low apart from the price of the laser generator. Nevertheless lasers are currently available in many large hospitals. Third, laser laparoscopy is an advance over other laparoscopic procedures. The laser is more precise and more effective than electrocoagulation. Adhesions occur less frequently after laser therapy than electrocoagulation. Moreover, risks due to laser application are lower than those of electrocoagulation. For instance destruction of endometrial implants with electrocoagulation is impossible or dangerous when they are located on the bladder, along the ureter or on the intestinal tract. Furthermore laser application for vaporization or cutting provides simultaneous hemostasis that is not achieved during lysis of adhesions with scissors or with electrocautery.

No one can foretell the future role of intra-abdominal or laparoscopic laser in the treatment of endometriosis. Specialists consider laser to be the most suitable surgical treatment and surgery the most effective treatment for severe or extensive endometriosis. There is a debate about treatment of mild or moderate endometriosis. Laser laparoscopy might replace intra-abdominal surgery. Danazol is effective but expensive and chronic treatment is required. No treatment has been advocated in mild cases because fertility rates are similar to Danazol therapy. Prospective controlled trials for different treatment stratified for endometriosis severity are necessary to put laparoscopic laser treatment into perspective.

Laser laparoscopic salpingostomy

Distal obstruction is the most common tubal lesion in mechanical infertility. Salpingostomy can be performed using macrosurgical procedures, microsurgical procedure with microelectrode, laser microsurgery or laser laparoscopic method (31). The purpose is to remove the obstruction by incision of the hydrosalpinges and to maintain the eversion of the fimbria. In the conventional procedure, this last point is generally achieved with microsutures.

The laparoscopic laser salpingostomy was first reported by Daniell (32). It was a logical extension of the intra-abdominal procedure reported by Bruhat and Mage (33). The tube is first distended with dye by transcervical injection and held by a forceps to get a 90° laser exposure angle on the end of the obstructed tube. An incision is made with the focused CO_2 laser beam set on continuous mode with a power of 35 watts. Continuous dye injection is necessary to keep the distal portion of the tube distended as long as possible after the lumen is entered. Nevertheless, when the incision is enlarged, the tube collapses completely. At this time 2 or 3 forceps are used to grasp the edges of the incision. The initial incision is extended always using high power focused shots. One or two additional incisions are made radially in the fimbria to get a large opening of the hydrosalpinx. To improve the safety of this procedure heparinized lactated Ringer's solution is placed in the peritoneal cavity and the uterus is moved and used as a backstop for the laser beam. The eversion of the fimbria must be maintained. This can be accomplished by firing at the hydrosalpinx serosa with very low power density laser shots. The laser probe is withdrawn to provide an unfocused beam, the laser power is decreased to 5 watts and the tube held on a 90° angle from the laser beam. This low power density firing must be applied at the serosal surface from 5 to 15 mm from the cut edges of the hydrosalpinx. The laser must be continuously moved to avoid deep coagulation. This slight superficial coagulation induces a contraction of the serosa and furthermore the cut ends of the tube become everted and rolled back, avoiding an early reobstruction. Refer to Plates 70-72 in the atlas for an example of a laparoscopic salpingostomy with CO_2 laser.

Daniell (32) reported laser laparoscopic salpingostomies among 22 patients that had been previously subjected to terminal tubal surgery. The hysterosalpingogram-documented tubal patency rate was 75% 2 months postoperatively. Within the 12 months postoperatively, 4 women (18.2%) had an intra-uterine pregnancy (3 deliveries and 1 abortion) and 1 patient an ectopic pregnancy. We have little experience of this procedure. Two years ago we performed laparoscopic salpingotomy with CO_2 laser on 4 patients resulting in one ectopic pregnancy and no intra-uterine pregnancies. We stopped this procedure because we felt that the instrumentation was not efficient enough and that an intra-abdominal procedure was more precise. Currently with a new and more efficient probe, a new series of laser laparoscopic salpingostomy has been performed for 4 months. Seven patients were subjected to this procedure and have neither intra-uterine pregnancy nor ectopic pregnancy.

The comparison of the results reported by Daniell (32) with those obtained after an intra-abdominal procedure (33) confirms the efficiency of the laparoscopic procedure. The median intra-uterine pregnancy rate is about 25 to 36% during two years postoperatively for patients who have not had previous tubal surgery, but lower for patients with previous tuboplasties. Lauritsen (34) reported an intra-uterine pregnancy rate of 35.9% among 39 patients subjected to a single salpingostomy versus 13.4 % among 23 patients subjected to a repeated salpingostomy.

Laparoscopic salpingostomy has been reported using electrosurgical procedures (35-37). These small series report different success rates. Fayez (36) obtained two intra-uterine pregnancies (IUP)(10%) and two ectopic pregnancies (EP) (10%) among 20 patients. Mettler and Semm reported 10 IUP (26%) among 38 patients. These results cannot be compared with the series of Daniell (32) because they do not include repeated procedures. Moreover, eversion of the fimbria is difficult to achieve even using bipolar electrocoagulation.

Further clinical studies are required to evaluate the laparoscopic procedure versus the intra-abdominal ones for laser salpingostomy. These comparative studies must stratify patients according to the tubal stage. Intra-abdominal salpingostomies can result in an intrauterine pregnancy rate of 66.6% in the best stage group to 0% in the worst one (38). Series mixing all cases are difficult to interpret. In the most severe stages, the fertility rates after treatment are low because the mucosal tubal lesions are too extensive. Only in the best stages can the operative technique influence the fertility results. In these cases the current results are generally above 45%. This is the success rate which must be achieved to confirm the efficiency of laser laparoscopic procedure.

Laser laparoscopic procedure has three advantages over conventional surgery. The hospitalization time is less: 24 hours versus 5 days after an intra-abdominal procedure. This treatment is performed during the diagnostic laparoscopy, which reduces still further the hospitalization time and avoids a laparotomy. The failures of intra-abdominal neosalpingostomy are due to mucosal tubal lesions or to the occurrence or recurrence of tubo-ovarian adhesions. Any laparoscopic procedure has less risk of adhesions than surgery. Nevertheless, a laparoscopic procedure will never be as precise as an intra-abdominal one. Certainly, the rapid development of *in vitro* fertilization and embryo transfer methods and laser laparoscopic methods will reduce the number of infertile women being subjected to multiple surgical procedures.

Tubo-ovarian adhesiolysis

Pelvic adhesions are frequent among infertile women. They are often associated with tubal blockage, but can exist with normal patent tubes. In these cases, they are sequellae of peritoneal inflammations, such as appendicitis, peritonitis or post-operative infections. Tubo-ovarian adhesions can induce infertility because they disturb the tubal or the ovarian functions. They can be removed using macro or microsurgical procedures, conventional laparoscopic methods or laparoscopic laser.

The laparoscopic CO_2 or argon laser can be used for lysis of pelvic adhesions. No precise technique can be described as it depends on the localization, the extent, the type of adhesions and the skill of the surgeon. Before cutting, adhesions must be set in tension, by grasping and pulling or pushing the pelvic organs with laparoscopic forceps. To avoid uncontrolled shots at the end of the section, one must add a guard at the end of the laser probe. This guard also makes it possible to maintain the adhesions to be fired at a direct angle. Not all adhesions can be removed. Those including the intestinal tract must be sectioned only if they are thin and long to avoid any risk of gastrointestinal perforation. Also, thick adhesions between the tubes and ovaries cannot be sectioned without a risk of tubal injury. Refer to Plates 73 and 74 in the atlas for an example of lysis of adhesions with the CO_2.

No large series have been reported of this procedure. Only Feste (14) reported 7 treatments and obtained 6 intrauterine pregnancies (85%). Comparison with series using other procedures is difficult because large numbers of unselected cases are included (36, 37, 39, 40). The intrauterine pregnancy rates ranged from 30% to 60%. In our experience the laparoscopic CO_2 laser is only one of the instruments suitable for adhesiolysis and pure laser adhesiolysis will be an uncommon procedure. But it is certain that the laser represents a real advance as it permits simultaneous cutting and hemostasis. So it can replace partially conventional laparoscopic procedures using scissors and/or electrocoagulation for intra-abdominal adhesiolysis. The theoretical advantage of the laser procedure is the decreased recurrence rate that has been reported for intra-abdominal laser adhesiolysis (41) and for laparoscopic procedures and simultaneous section and hemostasis. But other methods can achieve the same result such as thermocoagulation or adnexal infiltration with Ornipressin (synthetic vasopressin from Sandoz laboratories, Basel, Switzerland)(42). Larger clinical studies and prospective comparison with other techniques are necessary to evaluate the efficiency of laser laparoscopic adhesiolysis. Major progress in the future would certainly be the pharmacological prevention of the occurrence or the recurrence of adhesions.

Other procedures

Some other procedures have been occasionally reported but still remain to be evaluated in large series: vaporization or resection of uterine or ovarian fibromas, resection of ovarian cysts and section of hydatid cysts. Tubal section has been reported by Tadir (6) but is not valuable as the spontaneous repermeabilization rate was high.

The future of laser laparoscopy

The future of laser laparoscopy may be envisaged as different technological developments: to get better tissue-laser interaction, to enhance the manipulation, and consequently to increase the operative indications of this new surgical endoscopic tool.

Other laser generators

Two different evolutions can be imagined. First would be the utilization of a superpulsed CO_2 laser whose cutting effect appears to be more efficient than continuous wave CO_2 laser even if the current technology is still imperfect and induces non-uniform thermal damage (43). Secondly, use of a laser with variable wavelength may make it possible to obtain variable biological effects harnessed through the same system by changing the wavelength of the laser generator.

The waveguided CO_2 laser

Currently the use of the laparoscopic CO_2 laser is greatly limited as the probe must be connected to the articulated arm. A waveguided CO_2 laser will make it possible to connect the laser generator directly to the probe. Very small waveguided lasers will be available soon. Some prototypes are 27 mm in diameter, 250 mm in length and weigh no more than 190 grams (44). This system is more easily manipulated than standard CO_2 lasers. Moreover, this system results in a thinner diameter laser beam that permits the intra-abdominal introduction through thinner probes without corrective systems. The laser beam can be focused by a lens set into the probe. The beam will be much smaller than in the current technology and will provide very high power densities even if a large part of the laser energy is absorbed by the CO_2 gas of the pneumoperitoneum.
The pneumoperitoneum may be established with a different gas that avoids this absorption of the CO_2 laser wavelength. An inert gas such as azote (nitrogen) may be used without reducing the safety.

The development of optical fiber for the CO_2 laser wavelength would also permit improved manipulation of the laparoscopic CO_2 laser. This could be introduced into the abdomen in the same way as the argon laser.

Future prospects in clinical application of laser laparoscopy

We are unable to imagine all the future procedures but want to speculate about two points. The development of the laser technology and *in vitro* fertilization methods should lead to a simplified management of distal tubal blockages. The laparoscopy for tubal evaluation would be performed to recover preovulatory oocytes and to perform a laser laparoscopic salpingostomy in good prognosis stage (38). No more salpingostomy requiring a laparotomy would be performed. Failures of the laser laparoscopic procedure will be included in an *in vitro* fertilization program with ultrasonically guided percutaneous aspiration of follicles. Peritoneal phototherapy using hematoporphyrin derivatives and laser exposure could have a future for management of advanced ovarian carcinoma. By the means of repeated laser laparoscopy, it may be possible to decrease the tumor volume and furthermore to enhance the efficiency of adjuvant anticarcinomatous chemotherapy.

Laser hysteroscopy

Laser hysteroscopy was first reported with Nd:YAG laser by Goldrath (2) and CO_2 laser by Tadir (3).

Goldrath introduced the Nd:YAG laser into the uterus through an optical fiber via the operative channel of an hysteroscope (2). He used it to destroy all the endometrium in women complaining of drug-resistant menorrhagia. The fiber end has to be almost in contact with the endometrium. The procedure was performed by distending the uterine cavity with a 5% dextrose in physiological saline. Experimental and clinical studies reported the safety of this method. Clinical results among 22 patients appeared promising as the women become hypomenorrheic or amenorrheic. Hysterectomies were avoided. Endometrial biopsies demonstrated that only small amounts of endometrium survive cytogenic stroma was sparse and only rare endometrial glands are present. The epithelium rested directly on the myometrium. To our knowledge, no further studies on this procedure have been reported since the initial publication in 1981.

Tadir developed a hysteroscope for CO_2 laser application (3). This hysteroscope includes four channels, a 4 x 5 mm one or laser beam delivery, a 1 mm one for smoke evacuation, a 2 mm viewing lens and fiberoptics for illumination. The hysteroscope is connected to the articulated arm through a coupler containing a 300 mm focusing lens. Corrective systems are adapted as for the CO_2 laser laparoscope. Smoke evacuation is obtained by opening a valve on the hysteroscope. Tadir tested the equipment on uteruses that had been removed by hysterectomy. Currently preliminary clinical experiences are under way. CO_2 laser hysteroscope may be useful for excision or vaporization of intrauterine adhesions, uterine septum, submucous fibroid and endometrial polyps. The future of laser hysteroscopy application may be for evaluation and the destruction of dysplasic endometrium as it is currently performed for cervical intraepithelial neoplasia.

References

1. Bruhat MA, Mage G, Manhes H. Use of CO_2 laser via laparoscopy. In: Laser Surgery III, Proceedings of the III International Society for Laser Surgery, edited by I Kaplan. Tel Aviv, 1979;p274-276.
2. Goldrath MH, Fuller TA, Segal S. Laser photovaporization of endometrium for the treatment of menorraghia. Am J Obstet Gynecol 1981;140:14-19.
3. Tadir Y, Raif J, Dagan J, Zuckerman Z, Ovadia J. Hysteroscope for CO_2 laser application. Lasers Surg Med 1984;4:153-156.
4. Keye WR, Dixon J. Photocoagulation of endometriosis with argon laser through the laparoscope. Obstet Gynecol 1983;62:383-386.
5. Pouly JL, Mage G, Manhes H, Bruhat MA. Utilisation du laser CO_2 par coelioscopie. Laser Medical 1981-82, ed. Masson, Paris, p 17-21.
6. Tadir Y, Kaplan I, Zuckerman Z, Edelstein T, Ovadia J. New instrumentation and technique for laparoscopic CO_2 laser operations: A preliminary report. Obstet Gynecol 1984;63:582-585.
7. Daniell J, Brown D. CO_2 laser laparoscopy: Initial experience in experimental animals and humans. Obstet Gynecol 1982;59:761-764.
8. Lamano JM. Photocoagulation of early pelvic endometriosis with Nd:YAG laser through the laparoscope. Lasers Surg Med 1984;3:328.
9. Feste JR. CO_2 laser neurectomy for dysmenorrhea. Lasers Surg Med 1984;3:327.
10. Chong AP, Baggish MS. Management of pelvic endometriosis by means of intra-abdominal CO_2 laser. Fertil Steril 1984;41:14-19.
11. Keye WR, Maston GA, Dixon J. The use of argon laser in the treatment of experimental endometriosis. Fertil Steril 1983;39:26-29.
12. Chaubard T, Mage G, Richard E, Pouly JL, Bruhat MA. Utilisation du laser CO_2 dans le traitement de l'endometriose: Experimentation chez la lapine. J Gyn Obst Biol Reprod 1984;13:861-866.
13. Kelly RW, Robert DK. CO_2 laser laparoscopy: A potential alternative to danazol therapy in the treatment of stage I or II endometriosis. J Reprod Med 1983;28:638-643.
14. Feste JR. Laser laparoscopy: A new modality. Fertil Steril 1984;41:74S.
15. Martin DC. Interval use of the laser laparoscope for endometriosis following danazol therapy. Fertil Steril 1984,41:74S.
16. Keye WR. The use of argon laser laparoscopy in the treatment of infertility. Lasers Surg Med 1984;3:327.
17. Feste JR. Laser laparoscopy: A new modality. Lasers Surg Med 1984;3:327-328.
18. Pouly JL, Mage G, Manhes H, Bruhat MA. La coelioscopie opératoire. Encyclop Méd Chirur 1985 Ed. Editions Techniques Paris, In Press.
19. Manhes H, Mage G, Pouly JL, Bruhat MA. Techniques et résultats du traitement coelioscopique de l'endométriome ovarien: à propos de 30 cas. Gynécologie 1980;31:149-52.
20. Daniell J, Christianson C. Combined laparoscopic surgery and danazol therapy for pelvic endometriosis. Fertil Steril 1981;35:31-35.
21. Sulewski SM, Curcio FD, Bronisky C, Stenger VG. The treatment of endometriosis at laparoscopy for infertility. Am J Obstet Gynecol 1980;138:128-132.
22. Hasson HM. Electrocoagulation of pelvic endometriotic lesion with laparoscopic control. Am J Obstet Gynecol 1979;135:115-121.
23. Dmowski WP, Cohen MR. Antigonadotropin (Danazol) in the treatment of endometriosis: evaluation of post-treatment fertility and 3 years follow-up data. Am J Obstet Gyncol 1978;130:41-49.

24. Portuondo JA, Echanojauregui AD, Herran C, Alisarte I. Early conception in patients with untreated mild endometriosis. Fertil Steril 1983;39:22-25.
25. Schenken RS, Malinak LR. Conservative surgery versus expectant management for the infertile patients with mild endometriosis. Fertil Steril 1983;37:183-192.
26. Buttler L, Wilson E, Belisle S et al. Collaborative study of pregnancy rates following Danazol therapy of stage I endometriosis. Fertil Steril 1984;41:373-376.
27. Guzick DS, Rock JA. A comparison of danazol and conservative surgery for the treatment of infertility due to mild or moderate endometriosis. Fertil Steril 1983;40:580-586.
28. Buttram VA. Conservative surgery for endometriosis in the infertile female: a study of 206 patients with implications for both medical and surgical therapy. Fertil Steril 1979;31:117-122.
29. Cohen MR. Laparoscopic diagnosis and pseudomenopausal treatment of endometriosis with danazol. Clin Obstet Gynecol 1980;23:901-917.
30. Chong AP. Danazol versus carbon dioxide laser plus post-operative Danazol: Treatment of infertility due to mild endometriosis. Laser Medicine & Surgery News 1985;3:22.
31. Daniell JF. The role of laser in infertility surgery. Fertil Steril 1984;42:815-822.
32. Daniell J, Herbert CM. Laparoscopic salpingostomy using CO_2 laser. Fertil Steril 1984;41:558-563.
33. Mage G, Bruhat MA. Pregnancies following salpingostomy: comparison between CO_2 laser and electrosurgical procedures. Fertil Steril 1983;41:472-475.
34. Lauritsen JG, Pagel JD, Vangsted P, Starup J. Results of repeated tuboplasties. Fertil Steril 1982;37:68-72.
35. Gomel V. Salpingostomy by laparoscopy. J Reprod Med 1977;18:265-269.
36. Fayez JA. An assessment of the role of operative laparoscopy in tuboplasty. Fertil Steril 1983;39:476-479.
37. Mettler L, Giesel H, Semm K. Treatment of female infertility due to tubal obstruction by operative laparoscopy. Fertil Steril 1979;32:384-388.
38. Mage G, Pouly JL, Bouquet de JJ, Chabrand S, Bruhat MA. Obstructions tubaires distales: microchirugie ou fécondation in vitro. J Gyn Obst Biol Repr 1984;13:933-937.
39. Gomel V. Salpingo-ovariolysis by laparoscopy in infertility. Fertil Steril 1983;40:607-611.
40. Bruhat MA, Mage G, Manhes H, Soualhat C, Ropert JF, Pouly JL. Laparoscopic procedures to promote fertility: Ovariolysis and salpingolysis; results of 93 selected cases. Acta Europ Fertil 1983;14:113-116.
41. Scheidel P, Wallurener G, Hepp H. CO_2 laser in treatment of pelvic adhesions: experimental results; in Laser Surgery vol. 3 part 1, ed: Kaplan I, Jerusalem, Academic Press 1979, p. 269-270.
42. Manhes H, Mage G, Pouly JL, Ropert JF, Bruhat MA. Améliorations techniques du traitment coelioscopique de la grossesse extra-utérine. Nouvelle Presse Médicale 1983;12,22:1431-1432.
43. Bellina JH. Application of the CO_2 laser to the infertility surgery. Surgical Clinics of North America. 1984;64:899-904.
44. Bourez J, Triboulet JP, Balester L, Lemaire J, Herlemont F. Fundic vagotomy by waveguided CO_2 laser: experimental study of a new technique in dogs. Lasers Surg Med 1984;4:345-352.

24. PHOTODYNAMIC THERAPY:
BASIC ASPECTS AND TISSUE INTERACTION

JEFFREY J. GILBERTSON AND JOHN A. DIXON

Photodynamic therapy (PDT) describes the use of photochemically active compounds (photosensitizers) in conjunction with applied electromagnetic radiation to treat cancer. Photosensitizers used in this form of treatment have been selected from a large family of photochemically active compounds for their ability to generate chemical species capable of influencing biological systems. In both man and animals a number of endogenous and exogenous compounds, notably many porphyrins, have been found to possess two attractive properties: 1) the ability to concentrate or be retained in malignant tissue to a greater extent than most normal tissue; and 2) the ability to generate cytotoxic species *in vivo* in response to application of appropriate wavelength visible light.

The development of PDT as a clinical tool is a result of the synthesis of separate lines of research into each of these two properties. In 1924, the Frenchman Policard (1) noted that certain human and animal tumors would spontaneously fluoresce under ultraviolet illumination, a finding he attributed to high endogenous porphyrin levels in the tumors. German workers (2) in 1942 noted similar red fluorescence in rat tumors after systemic injection of hematoporphyrin, a compound derived from hemoglobin.

This affinity of hematoporphyrin for tumor tissue was generalized to a number of induced and transplanted mouse tumors by Figge in 1948 (3). He also noted accumulation of porphyrin in inflammatory, reticuloendothelial, and rapidly growing tissue and recognized the potential for tumor detection by detection of fluorescence.

Hematoporphyrin derivative (HPD) appeared in the literature in 1960 (4), the result of acid treatment of hematoporphyrin by Lipson. This substance, actually a mixture of compounds, was shown to have better tumor localizing ability than hematoporphyrin. Because HPD also emitted a red fluorescence under UV light, researchers pursued its use as a diagnostic tumor localizing compound. In 1964, Lipson (5) reported an 80% correlation of tumor fluorescence with biopsy-proven cancer in patients with suspected bronchogenic carcinoma. This experience was supported by other workers in a variety of tumors (5, 6, 15).

In 1962, Winkelman (7) introduced tetraphenylporphine sulfonate (TPPS), the first of several synthetic porphyrins used for tumor localization. In 1983, Dougherty (8) identified dihematoporphyrin ether (DHE), the so-called 'active

D.M. Jensen and J.M. Brunetaud (eds), Medical Laser Endoscopy. 295-311.
© 1990 Kluwer Academic Publishers, Dordrecht

ingredient' in the mixture of compounds referred to as HPD.

The second property noted in the porphyrins is their ability to generate cytotoxic species after activation by visible light. In 1900, Raab (9) noticed that acridine dye and visible light would kill paramecia when neither would alone. The first attempt to treat cancer by this means was in 1902 when Von Tappeiner and Jesionek (10) used topical eosin and sunlight to effect regression of skin tumors. Although they were apparently successful they published no further results. In 1908, Hausmann (11) reported murine skin photosensitivity after subcutaneous hematoporphyrin administration and in 1913 Meyer-Betz (12) reported cutaneous photosensitivity in himself after auto-inoculation with hematoporphyrin. These findings lay dormant until 1966 when Lipson (13) reported the first treatment of cancer with this technique. In 1972 Diamond (14) brought the two lines of research together again with the observation that systemically administered hematoporphyrin could result in necrosis of a subcutaneously implanted glioma after exposure to white light. Over the next few years pioneering work by Dougherty, Kelly, Snell and Tomson, (16-18) revealed that numerous compounds, including several dyes, appeared capable of photodynamically inducing tumor regression.

The first documented eradication of experimental tumor was reported by Dougherty (19) and associates in 1975 after the treatment of mammary tumor-bearing mice with hematoporphyrin derivative and red light. The first human bladder tumor treated was reported in 1976 by Kelly and Snell (20). They noted destruction of tumor histologically after HPD followed by white light. Significantly, normal portions of bladder epithelium were unaffected. Continued research into improved photosensitizers, light sources and light delivery systems will be discussed below.

Sensitizers

The ideal photosensitizing compound for PDT would be a nontoxic, pure, inexpensive, highly tumor-selective material. In addition, its absorption spectrum should be maximum at the wavelength of maximum tissue penetration (650-1000 nm) (21). Unfortunately, none of the sensitizers currently in use fit this demanding profile. HPD, until recently the most popular photosensitizer, is a mixture of a number (at least eight) of porphyrins and porphyrin aggregates (22). The major components of HPD, hematoporphyrin (42%) and hydroxyethylvinyldeuteroporphyrin (34%) are themselves inactive in tumor PDT at the usual doses (23).

In 1984 Dougherty (8) and colleagues used gel exclusion chromatography to putatively identify the component of PDT most responsible for its photosensitizing ability as bis-1-3-(1- hydroxethyl) deuteroporphyrin-8-yl] ethyl ether plus two structural isomers. They named this substance dihematoporphyrin ether (DHE) and its structure appears in Fig. 24.1. DHE appears to exert the same biologic effect as HPD at approximately one half the dose. Recent work by Kessel has cast some doubt on the structure of the so-called 'active component', suggesting it to be an ester rather than an ether (24).

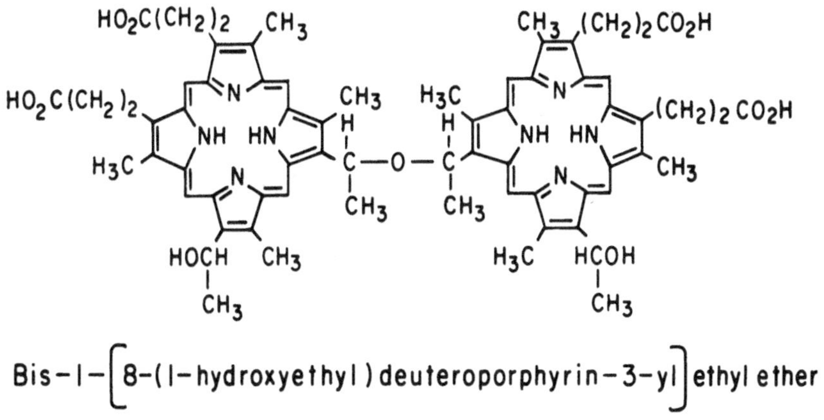

Bis−1−[8−(1−hydroxyethyl)deuteroporphyrin−3−yl]ethyl ether

Fig. 24.1. Structure of Dihematoporphyrin Ether (DHE).

Another sensitizer to receive much attention is tetraphenylporphine sulfonate (TPPS), a polar, water soluble, fairly pure, synthetic compound with tumor localizing ability as good or better than HPD (7, 25). Its clinical testing has been delayed by its apparent slow rate of serum clearance and reports of irreversible nerve toxicity detected by electron microscopy (26, 27).

The absorption spectrum of HPD appears in Fig. 24.2 along with a representation of the absorption of water and common skin pigments. Photodynamic therapy with HPD or DHE is usually performed at 630 nm. It can be appreciated that in the wavelength range of greatest tissue penetration (650-1000 nm), the strength of absorbance of HPD is quite poor. This fact has triggered the search for photosensitizing compounds with strong absorption (Soret) peaks in this range. Thus far these efforts have been concentrated in three areas: the chlorins, the phthalocyanines and the pheophorbides. The chlorins are a family of compounds related to chlorophyll. Bonellin, a naturally occurring chlorin, has shown *in vitro* activity superior to HPD at 632 nm (28). Phtalocyanines, another family of porphyrin-like compounds, have strong absorption peaks between 700 and 800 nm and likewise show *in vitro* activity in early studies (29). Finally, the pheophorbides, yet another group of photosensitizing compounds, are being studied by Nakajima and co-workers in Japan (30). Hopefully the goal of finding the 'ideal' photosensitizer will be reached over the next few years.

Mechanism of PDT

With PDT's obvious potential for clinical efficacy in mind, a review of current mechanistic concepts of PDT is in order.

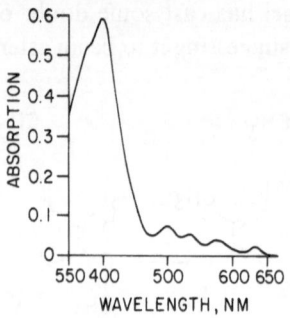

Fig. 24.2A. Absorption spectrum of HPD.

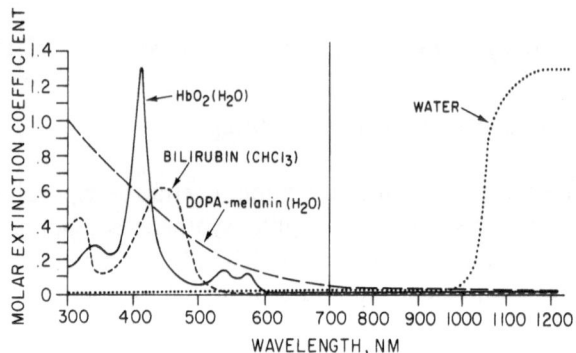

Fig. 24.2B. Absorption spectrum of skin pigments and water.

Localization in Tumor

Figure 24.3 gives the basic scheme. As noted previously, systemic administration of photosensitizer, usually a porphyrin or porphyrins, results in high sensitizer levels in tumor, inflammatory and reticuloendothelial tissue. Although early work suggested active concentration of sensitizer in tumor cells, *in vitro* studies do not give any clear cut indication that tumor cells take up or retain more porphyrin than normal cells (40, 62). Indeed the majority of tumor porphyrin is located in tumor stroma rather than in the tumor cells themselves (86).

This suggests that high tumor sensitizer levels are the result of a number of properties attributable to tumors rather than individual malignant cells. These have been outlined by Evensen (31) and include 1) increased vascular permeability to protein- porphyrin complexes when compared to normal tissue, 2) faulty lymphatic clearance with increased protein-porphyrin complex time in interstitial space, 3) increased porphyrin binding capability of collagen 4) a large population of reticuloendothelial cells (reticuloendothelial cells have been shown to readily phagocytose porphyrins), 5) increased cellular uptake at low

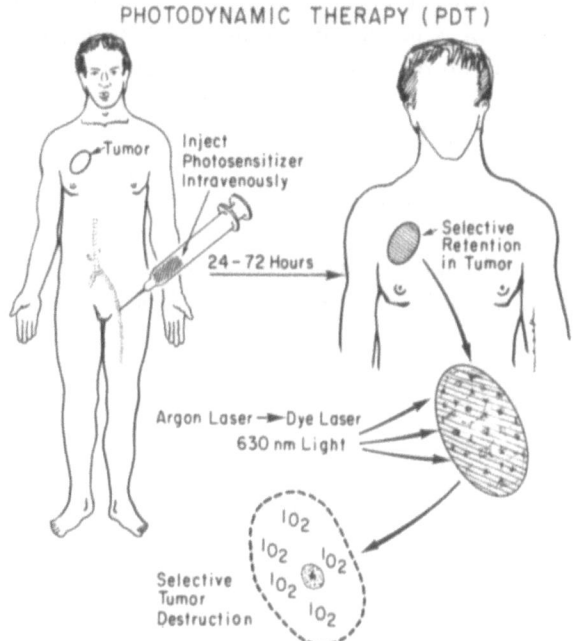

PHOTODYNAMIC THERAPY (PDT)

Tumor

Inject
Photosensitizer
Intravenously

24 - 72 Hours

Selective
Retention
in Tumor

Argon Laser → Dye Laser
630 nm Light

$^1O_2$
$^1O_2$ $^1O_2$
Selective $^1O_2$
Tumor
Destruction $^1O_2$

Fig. 24.3. Sequence of events in photodynamic therapy.

Ph (tumor cells tend to be more acidic), and 6) increased binding of porphyrins to neoplastic cell proteins and receptors.

The concentration of porphyrin, then, in any given tissue would be the result of the relative contributions of each of these factors. This could explain why certain tissues, such as liver (with a large concentration of reticuloendothelial cells and a rich, leaky vasculature) (87) have a higher porphyrin content than even most tumors.

Ultrastructural Localization

The localization of sensitizer which does actually enter the tumor cell has also been the subject of a great deal of investigation. The puzzle has been made more difficult by the fact that HPD, as noted above, is a mixture of several different porphyrins. Early research in isolated cell systems revealed high porphyrin concentration in the cell membrane and mitochondria (32-34). However, variations in chemical configuration (monomer, dimer, oligomer) as well as molecular aggregation due to hydrophobic and hydrophillic forces, can cause marked variation in fluorescence and localization behavior (35). For example, monomeric DHE fluoresces while aggregated DHE does not (36). Use of radio-labeled porphyrins plus fluorescence measurement carried out in non-polar (monomer promoting) solvents have now allowed more accurate elucidation of the ultrastructural fate of HPD (35, 37-39). Nonetheless, the intracellular environment is much more complicated than a simple aqueous system. Cells are made up of a number of micro- environments, each with variable physical and chemical properties. Therefore, intracellular localization of a sensitizer depends on the interaction of the sensitizer with intracellular components (proteins and membranes). This interaction would be expected to be different with different sensitizers (40). Since variability in polarity and solubility between different sensitizers is significant, at this point in our understanding it is difficult to predict localization behavior for specific compounds. A great deal of work remains to be done in this area.

Mechanism of Cell Killing

The actual cytotoxic species generated in the photochemical reaction is felt to be singlet oxygen, an unstable and powerful oxidizing species. Support for the role of singlet oxygen comes from experiments showing increased photodynamic damage when PDT is carried out in D_2O rather than water (43, 44). Since the lifetime of singlet oxygen in D_2O is ten times greater than its lifetime in water, this result is expected. In addition, Weishaupt et al., in 1976, showed that TA-3 mouse mammary carcinoma cells were spared photodynamic inactivation when illuminated in the presence of 1,3-diphenylisobenzofuran, a potent singlet oxygen trap (45). Indeed, beta carotene, another singlet oxygen trap, is being investigated as a means of post-treatment sensitizer 'neutralization' to avert cutaneous photosensitivity in human patients (46).

Generation of singlet oxygen is felt to occur via a type II photochemical process involving the action of a light excited sensitizer molecule with ground state molecular oxygen (Fig. 24.4) (47). This reaction produces ground state sensitizer and singlet oxygen radicals capable of oxidative reaction with proteins and nucleic acids.

Table 24.1. Mechanism of singlet oxygen generation.

^{1}Sens $\rightarrow$ ^{3}Sens (long lived excited state)
^{3} + $^3O_2$ (ground state) $\rightarrow$ ^{1}Sens (ground state) + $^1O_2$ (excited state)
$^1O_2$ (excited state) + Substrate $\rightarrow$ $^3O_2$ + Substrate (oxidized)

Sens = Sensitizer
$^1O_2$ = Singlet Oxygen

Extensive work by Christensen, Moan and other workers, has shown that PDT can cause sister chromatid exchanges and DNA single strand breaks (48-50). However, X-ray therapy results in approximately ten times more chromosomal breaks than PDT when given in clinically equivalent doses (51). This suggests that while effects on the cell nucleus can and do occur, they are not the principal means of PDT damage leading to cell death. It also suggests that PDT should not be as mutagenic as X-ray therapy (52). Membrane associated damage occurs via protein cross-linking and lipid peroxidation. This leads to inactivation of transport mechanisms and alterations in membrane permeability with subsequent cellular swelling and lysis (32, 53-57). Recently workers have shown PDT effects on mitochondria with inactivation of cytochrome C (58), uncoupling of respiration and changes in membrane calcium transport (59).

Mechanism of Tumor Destruction

Research discussed above would suggest that tumor destruction with PDT is a result of direct tumor cell death from oxidation by singlet oxygen. However, as early as 1963, Castellani (60) described *in vivo* microcirculatory changes secondary to HPD-PDT with agglutination of red blood cells and intravascular stasis. These findings were confirmed by Star et al. (61), in 1983 who demonstrated a similar phenomenon in rat mammary tumors, concluding that tumor kill following PDT was probably the result of destruction of the tumor microcirculation rather than direct tumor cell kill.

This hypothesis was elegantly tested when Henderson and co- workers (62) reported in 1984 that EMT-6 mouse tumor cells treated with standard PDT *in vivo* showed nearly normal *in vitro* colony formation when explanted into cell culture immediately after light treatment. If the cells were allowed to remain in situ after treatment, cell death occurred rapidly and progressively. This suggested that tumor cells were, in effect, 'rescued' from avascular/anoxic death by immediate explantation into the nutrient media of tissue culture. In fact, studies by Bicher (63) in 1980 had shown a precipitous drop in tumor PO_2 after PDT consistent with vascular collapse. Further studies by Henderson (62) rendering tumor cells anoxic via host death showed tumor cell death kinetics remarkably similar to the PDT treated tumor cells.

Thus it seems that, at least in several model systems, a significant if not predominant contribution to tumor destruction comes from PDT induced disruption of tumor microvasculature rather than direct cytotoxicity (41, 42). The destruction of tumor microvasculature in turn appears to be based upon singlet oxygen mediated endothelial cell damage.

Equipment for endoscopic applications

Clinically PDT is currently used for treatment of carcinoma and early detection of subclinical carcinoma. The equipment for endoscopic use of PDT is different from that of non-endoscopic applications.

Light Source

In earliest observations of what we now call PDT, the light source used was the sun. As understanding of the physical principles of PDT evolved, more sophistication in light source technology has been used. Early clinical PDT studies utilized 500 watt slide projector (tungsten) lamps with filters, or gas discharge (i.e. xenon arc) lamps with filters to transmit 630 nm light (64). The output from these sources was quite low, typically less than 50 milliwatts per square centimeter.

Lasers, invented in 1960 have been used in a number of medical applications. High intensity coherent light allows a significant increment in delivered irradiance over incandescent or gas discharge sources (65). Although the helium neon laser has an appropriate output wavelength for PDT (632 nm), its low power limits its use. Gold vapor lasers (628 nm, pulsed) are capable of high power outputs and are increasingly popular. In fact, some early studies suggest more efficient PDT with gold vapor lasers that argon dye lasers (66, 75). The most common laser used for clinical PDT, however, is the argon pumped dye laser (Fig. 24.4).

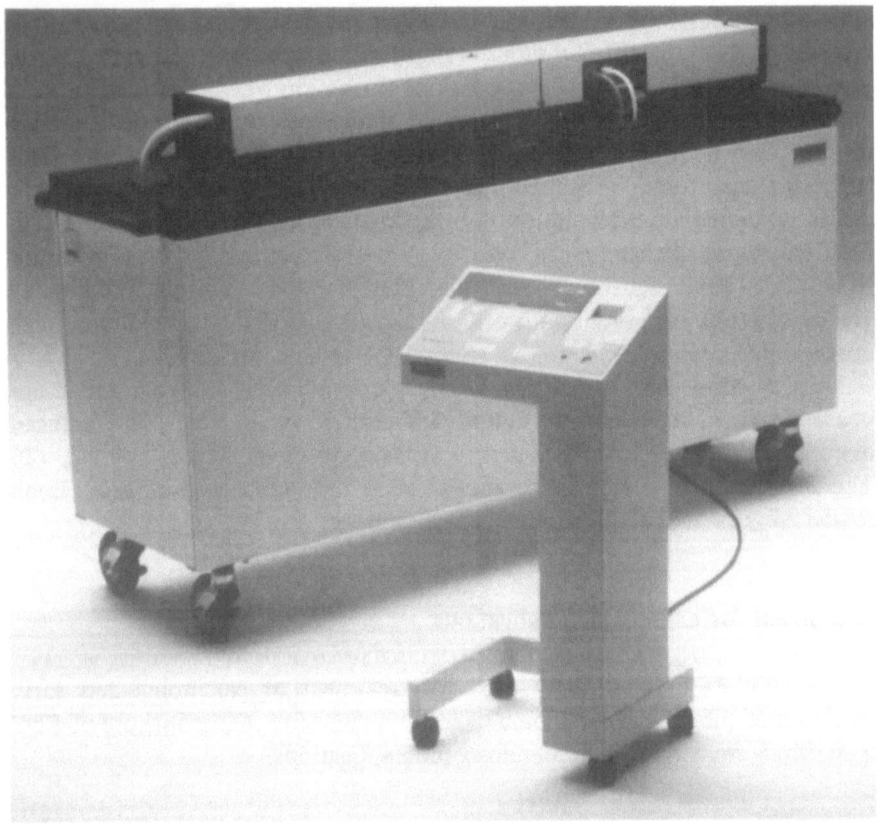

Fig. 24.4. Clinical argon dye laser.

302

This is a combination unit which uses an argon laser to activate, or pump, one of a number of dyes which emit over a wavelength range and deliver up to 3 to 4 watts. For example, an argon- rhodamine B laser can produce a tunable output over the range 594-643 nm, nicely suited to HPD-PDT. Changing the dye in an argon/dye system changes output wavelength range and therefore allows flexibility in using photosensitizers with different peak absorption wavelengths.

Delivery Systems

While focused or unfocused lamp systems may be adequate for PDT in some cutaneous tumors, laser light output is generally delivered via quartz or glass fibers which have the advantage of being small (200 to 400 microns), flexible and efficient. Major energy losses with short fibers (less than 10 meters) generally occur at input and output couplings and are 15% or less (67).

Requirements for clinical PDT have given rise to a number of distal fiber tip attachments to modify light distribution. While a straight-cut quartz fiberoptic will give a Gaussian light pattern, the use of microlenses can convert this into a more homogeneous distribution with sharp edges. Demand for interstitial treatment of tubular structures such as bronchi, or intraluminal treatment of spherical structures such as the bladder has led to the development of cylindrical and spherical diffusing tips, respectively. These are based upon scattering of light at the fiber tip by coating the tip with a material of the appropriate refractive index. The resulting illumination field can thus be cylindrical or spherical.

Fluorescence Detection Systems

As noted in the introduction, red fluorescence of porphyrins in response to incident ultraviolet irradiation was observed as early as 1923. This observation suggested that subclinical tumors could be detected by HPD administration with subsequent ultraviolet scanning and fluorescence detection. Until recently, there have been two main types of HPD fluorescence detection systems. Both of these have been predominately used in bronchoscopic applications. One, developed by Profio and Doiron (68, 69), employs a Krypton ion laser emitting at 406.7 nm (36%), 413.5 nm (60%) and 415.4 nm (4%) to deliver violet light to the bronchus via a quartz fiber passed through the operating channel of a bronchoscope. Filters then block the reflected violet light, transmitting any red fluorescence to an image intensifier with a luminous gain of 30,000 X and a green output phosphor. The low intensity red light is thus converted to bright green light. Early results in clinical use have been most impressive, as reported by Balchum to detect subclinical tumors (70).

The second system, developed by Kinsey and coworkers (71) at the Mayo

Clinic, depends upon rapid alternation of white light (for standard bronchoscopic viewing) and violet light near 405 nm from a filtered mercury arc lamp. The alternation occurs fast enough (about 30 cycles per second) such that the bronchoscopist can perform an essentially normal white light exam. Any red fluorescence emitted in response to the violet light is transmitted via a second optical fiber to a photomultiplier. The photomultiplier is in turn coupled to an audio signal generator which emits a pitch proportional to red fluorescent intensity. This allows the endoscopist to pay full visual attention to his regular exam and still detect areas suspicious by virtue of HPD fluorescence. Benson at the Mayo Clinic (72) has adapted this system for bladder carcinoma detection with encouraging results.

Aizawa et al. (73), in Japan recently added a spectroscope to these systems thus allowing separation of normal autofluorescence (less than 600 nm) from true HPD fluorescence (630 nm, 690 nm).

Most recently, Aizwa (74) has reported a new fluorescence detection system utilizing a rapidly alternating white light and eximer laser (405 nm), coupled with a spectroscope for 630 nm and 690 nm HPD emission detection.

Problems

Progress in both basic science and clinical aspects of PDT over the past ten years has been impressive. However, there are several areas where persistent problems have limited both understanding and clinical success of PDT.

Dosimetry

Extreme heterogeneity of different tumors and tissues with respect to color, density, cell size, blood flow, etc. render Maxwell's equations on the propagation of light unsolvable in these systems. Still, precise dosimetry is required for clinical PDT and depends on knowledge of the optical properties (absorbance and scattering) of each type of tissue. Extensive work in this area, notably by Svaasand (76), has revealed that a collimated beam of 635 nm (red) light passing through tissue will be reduced to 10% of its initial intensity at anywhere from 2.6 mm to 13.2 mm depending upon on the tissue chosen. Obviously dose requirements for clinical efficacy will vary to a similar degree in different tissues.

Mathematical analysis by Svaasand yields the following equation for space irradiance (power density) with interstitial PDT:

$$I = I_{os}(d/r)\, e^{-[r-d\|d]}$$

where I = space irradiance, I_{os} = space irradiance at the optical penetration depth (directly related to total power and a coupling coefficient), d = optical penetration depth (a function of scattering and absorption for that tissue), and r = distance from the fiber end. It is apparent that prediction of dosimetry will only be possible after exhaustive measurements of multiple parameters in various tissues and subsequent dose/response verification.

Instrumentation

Accurate information on dosimetry can only be utilized if technology exists for accurate delivery of the desired dose. For cutaneous and forward surface PDT, standard power meters supply the necessary data. However, interstitial treatment requires a three dimensional power meter or integrating power sphere. This technology has only recently become commercially available. Ideally, investigators should have a scanning power meter allowing measurement of output strength at various points along interstitial (Cylindrical, spherical) fiber tips. Variation in output along a cylindrical diffusing tip can lead to areas of undertreatment or over treatment if an assumption of homogeneous output is made.

Sensitizers

As discussed above the ideal photosensitizer has not been found. Research in this area hopefully will lead to the resolution of problems with current photosensitizing compounds.

Photosensitivity

Cutaneous photosensitivity in PDT patients can vary from minimal to severe (77) but nonetheless requires at least 30 days of sunlight avoidance. Solving this problem requires either a nontoxic photosensitizing compound or a means of 'quenching' systemic photosensitizer after PDT.

Mechanism

Elucidation of the cellular mechanism of PDT will certainly suggest ways of improving therapy. If the predominant mode of tumor killing with PDT is via vascular compromise, treatment strategies may be altered to deliver more energy to nutrient vessels. The impressive results seen with forward surface PDT of transplanted subcutaneous animal tumors may not be as clinically useful if these tumors are regressing due to interruption of cutaneous blood supply. That is, forward surface PDT may only be treating the vessel containing skin overlying the tumor. If the analogous tumor in man is in a deep location requiring interstitial treatment, the same results may not be attainable.

Variations in animal model, tumor model, treatment mode, and data analysis are legion among investigators in PDT. While this is not unusual in basic science research, results of PDT experiments seem especially dependent on these factors. Tumor heterogeneity, as discussed above, results in variable responses of different tumors to standard PDT. Various tumor models (i.e. human tumors growing in nude mice) may interfere or interact with PDT.

Differences in experimental results based upon the use of different lasers or sensitizers of differing purity are an ongoing problem (79). The issue of confounding hyperthermic kill during PDT must be recognized and eliminated to isolate pure PDT effects (80). Numerous experimental findings noted with PDT are different in *in vivo* versus *in vitro* systems, suggesting an important role of the tumor host (81). Lastly, different laboratory methods of treatment evaluation are in fact measuring different properties. For example, growth delay or TC 50 evaluation (*in vivo*) give different information than clonogenic assays (*in vitro*) (81).

While clinical success of PDT depends on tumor eradication only, the success of research into the basic science of heater PDT requires unraveling and control of these many intertwined variables.

The future

The future of PDT holds great promise. For certain neoplasms, i.e. superficial bladder cancer or early lung cancer, PDT may well become the treatment of choice. Certain other applications will most likely remain palliative. The technique of fluorescence detection discussed above will likely be generalized to numerous organ systems making possible early detection of malignancies currently undetectable by standard means.

Early work on the interaction of PDT with hyperthermia (Waldow et al.) (82, 83) shows an apparent synergism between PDT and hyperthermia if hyperthermia follows PDT by approximately 30 minutes. Tulip et al. (84) in Canada have early results suggesting that addition of misonidazole to tumor systems prior to PDT enhances tumor killing analogous to effects seen in radiation therapy. Mew and coworkers (85) have impressive early results with their efforts to bind photosensitizers to tumor specific monoclonal antibodies.

These novel research efforts coupled with continued work on basic cellular mechanisms should result in PDT having a significant impact on the future of cancer therapy.

References

1. Policard A. Etudes sur les aspects offerts par des tumeurs experimentales examinée à la lumière de woods. CR Soc Biol 1924;1423-1424.
2. Auler H, Banzer G. Untersuchungen über die Rolle der Prophine bei geschwulstkranken Menschen und Tieren. Z. Krebsforsche 1942;53:65-68.
3. Figge FHJ, Eeiland GS, Manganiello LOJ. Cancer detection and therapy. Affinity of neoplastic, embryonic and traumatized regenerating tissues for porphyrins and metalloporphyrins. Proc Soc Exptl Biol Med 1948;68:640-641.
4. Lipson RL. The photodynamic and fluorescent properties of a particular hematoporphyrin derivative and its use in tumor detection. Master's Thesis Univ. of Minn, 1960.
5. Lipson RL, Baldes EJ, Olsen AM. A further evaluation of the use of hematoporphyrin derivative as a new aid for endoscopic detection of malignant disease. Dis Chest 1964;46:676-679.
6. Lipson RL, Pratt JH, Baldes EJ et al. Hematoporphyrin derivative for the detection of cervical cancer. J Obstet Gyn 1964;24:78-84.
7. Winkelman J. The distribution of tetraphenylporphine- sulfonate in the tumor-bearing rat. Ca Res 1962;22:589-586.
8. Dougherty TJ, Potter WR, Weishaupt KR. The structure of the active component of hematoporphyrin derivative. In: Porphyrin Localization in Treatment of Tumors. Doiron DR and Gomer CJ (eds), Alan R. Liss, Inc. New York 1984;301- 314.
9. Rabb O. Ueber die Wirkung fluoreszierenden Stoffe auf Infusorien. A Biol 1900;39;524-546.
10. Von Tappeiner H, Jesionek A. Therapeutische Versuche mit fluoreszierenden Stoffen. Muenchen Med Wochenschr 1903;2:2042- 2044.
11. Hausmann W. Ueber die sensibilisierende Wirkung tierischer Farbstoffe und ihre physiologische Deutung. Biochem Z 1908;14:275.
12. Meyer-Betz F. Untersuchungen über die biologische (photodynamische) Wirkung des Hematoporphyrins und anderer Derivate des Blut- und Gallen-Farbstoffs. Deutsches Arch F Klin Med 1913;112:476-503.
13. Lipson RL, Gray MJ, Baldes EJ. Hematoporphyrin derivative for detection in management of cancer. In Proceedings of the 9th Int'l Congress, Harris RJC (ed), Springer-Verlag, New York 1967;393.
14. Diamond I, Granelli SG, McDonagh AF et al. Photodynamic therapy of malignant tumors. Lancet 1972;2:1175-1177.
15. Gregorie HB Jr, Horger EO, Ward JL et al. Hematoporphyrin derivative fluorescence in malignant neoplasms. Ann Surg 1968;167:820-828.
16. Dougherty TJ. Activated dyes as anti-tumor agents. J Natl Cancer Inst 1974;52:1333-36.
17. Kelly JF, Snell ME, Berenbaum MC. Photodynamic destruction of human bladder carcinoma. Br J Ca 1975;31:237-42.
18. Tomson SH, Emmett EA, Fox SH. Photodestruction of mouse epithelial tumors after oral acridine orange and argon laser. J Cancer Res 1974;34:3124-27.
19. Dougherty TJ, Grindey GB, Fiel R et al. Photoradiation therapy II. Cure of animal tumors with hematoporphyrin and light. J Natl Ca Inst 1975;55:115-21.
20. Kelly JF, Snell ME. Hematopophyrin derivative: A possible aid in the diagnosis and therapy of carcinoma of the bladder. J Urol 1976;115:150-51.
21. Regan JF, Parrish JA (eds). Much basic work on light penetration in tissue has been done by Parrish. See: The Science of Photomedicine, Plenum Press, New York/London, 1982, Chap. 6, pp. 477-625.
22. Moan J, Sandberg S, Christensen T. Hematoporphyrin derivative: Chemical composition, photochemical and photosensitizing properties. In: Porphyrin sensitization, Kessel E, Dougherty TJ (eds), Plenum Press, New York, 1981, pp. 165-179.
23. Dougherty TJ, Boyle DG, Weishaupt KR et al. Photoradiation therapy – clinical and drug advances. In: Porphyrin Sensitization, Kessel E, Dougherty TJ (eds), Plenum Press, New York, 1981, pp. 3-13.

307

24. Kessel D. Properties of the tumor localizing components of HPD. Abstract from International Meeting on Porphyrins as Phototherapeutic Agents for Tumors and Other Diseases, Sardinia, Italy, May 1985.
25. Musser A, Wagner JM, Datta-Gupta N. Distribution of tetraphynylporphinesulfonate and tetracarboxyphenylporphine in tumor bearing mice. J Natl Ca Inst 1978;61:1397-1403.
26. Sima AAF, Kennedy JC, Blakeslee D et al. Experimental porphyric neuropathy: A preliminary report. Le J Can Sci Neuro 1981;8:105-13.
27. Winkelman JW, Collins GH. Morphologic effects of tetraphenylporphinesulfonate (TPPS) upon rat peroneal nerve. Abstract from International Meeting on Porphyrins as Phototherapeutic Agents for Tumors and Other Diseases, Sardinia, Italy, May 1985.
28. Monfrecola G, Martellotta D, Galli R et al. Effect of Helium- Neon laser on human erythrocytes incubated with hematoporphyrin and bonellin: Comparative study. Abstract from International Meeting on Porphyrins as Phototherapeutic Agents for Tumors and Other Diseases, Sardinia, Italy, May 1985.
29. Ben-Hur E, Rosenthal I. Phthalocyanines: Synthetic porphyrin- like dyes with an improved potential for cancer phototherapy. Abstract from International Meeting on Porphyrins as Phototherapeutic Agents for Tumors and Other Diseases, Sardinia, Italy, May 1985.
30. Nakajima S, Hayishi H, Omote Y et al. Research for a correlation between the side chain structures of 90 different kinds of porphyrin, pheophorbide derivatives and their tumor localizing capacity. Abstract from International Meeting on Porphyrins as Phototherapeutic Agents for Tumors and Other Diseases, Sardinia, Italy, May 1985.
31. Evensen JF, Moan J, Hindar A et al. Tissue distribution of 3H-hematoporphyrin derivative and its main components, 67GA and 131I-albumin in mice bearing Lewis lung carcinoma. In: Porphyrin Localization and Treatment of Tumors, Doiron DR, Gomer CJ, (eds), Alan R. Liss New York, 1984, pp. 541-562.
32. Allison AC, Magnus IA, Young MR. Role of lysosomes and of cell membranes in photosensitization. Nature 1966;209:874- 878.
33. Docchio F, Ramponi R, Sacchi CA et al. Time-resolved fluorescence microscopy of hematoporphyrin derivative in cells. Lasers in Sur Med 1982;2:21-28.
34. Berns ME, Dahlman A, Johnson FM et al. *In vitro* cellular effects of hematoporphyrin derivative. Ca Res 1982;42:2325-2329.
35. Spikes JF. A preliminary comparison of the photosensitizing properties of porphyrins in aqueous solution in liposomal systems. In: Porphyrin Sensitization, Kessel E, Dougherty TJ (eds), Plenum Press, New York, 1981, pp. 181-92.
36. Dougherty TJ, Weishaupt KR, Boyle DG. Photodynamic therapy in cancer. In: Principles and Practices of Oncology, 2nd ed., DeVita VT, Hellman S, Rosenberg SA (eds), JB Lippincott, Philadelphia, 1985, In Press.
37. Gomer CJ, Dougherty TJ. Determination of [3H]- and [14C] hematoporphyrin derivative distribution in malignant and normal tissue. Ca Res 1979;39:146-51.
38. Kessel D. Transport and binding of hematoporphyrin derivative and related porphyrins by murine leukemia L-1210 cells. Ca Res 1981;141:1318-23.
39. Kessel D. Chemical and biochemical determinants of porphyrin localization. In: Porphyrin Localization and Treatment of Tumors, Doiron DR, Gomer CJ, (eds), Alan R. Liss, New York, 1984, pp. 405-18.
40. Spikes JD, Straight RC. Fundamental aspects of porphyrin- sensitized reactions in the photodynamic therapy of tumors. Med Biol Env 1985;13:145-54.
41 Spikes JD, Straight RC. Photodynamic behavior of porphyrins in model cell, tissue and tumor systems. In: Photodynamic Therapy of Tumors and Other Diseases, Jori G, Perria C (eds). Liberia Prodetto, (Padova, Italy), 1985.
42. Straight RC, Spikes JD. Preliminary studies with implanted polyvinyl alcohol sponges as a model for studying the role of neointerstitial and neovascular compartments of tumors in the localization, retention and photodynamic effects of photosensitizers. In: Photosensitization II, Kessel D (ed), Plenum Press, New York, 1985.
43. Sandberg S, Romslo I. Porphyrin induced photodamage at the cellular and subcellular level

as related to the solubility of the porphyrin. Clinica Chimica Acta, 1981;109:193-201.

44. Moan J, Petterson EO, Christensen P. The mechanism of photodynamic inactivation of human cells *in vitro* in the presence of hematoporphyrin. Br J Ca 1979;39:398-407.

45. Weishaupt KR, Gomer CJ, Dougherty TJ. Identification of singlet oxygen as the cytotoxic agent in photo-inactivation of a murine tumor. Ca Res 1976;36:2326-29.

46. Mathews-Roth MM. Beta carotene therapy for erythropoietic protoporphyria and other photosensitivity diseases. In: The Science of Photomedicine, Regan JD, Parrish JA, (eds), Plenum Press, New York/London, 1982, pp. 409-40.

47. Spikes JD. Porphyrins and related compounds as photodynamic sensitizers. Ann NY Acad Sci 1975;244:496-508.

48. Gomer CJ, Rucker N, Banerjee A et al. Comparison of mutagenicity and induction of sister chromatid exchange in Chinese hamster cells exposed to hematoporphyrin derivative photoradiation, ionizing radiation, or ultraviolet radiation. Ca Res 1983;43:2622.

49. Christensen T, Moan J. Photodynamic inactivation of synchronized human cells *in vitro* in the presence of hematoporphyrin. Ca Res 1979;39:3735-37.

50. Moan J, Waksvik H, Christensen T. DNA single-strand breaks and sister chromatid exchanges induced by treatment with hematoporphyrin and light or by X-rays in human NHIK 3025 cells. Ca Res 1980;40:2915-18.

51. Evensen JF, Moan J. Photodynamic action and chromosomal damage: A comparison of hematoporphyrin derivative (HPD) and light with X- irradiation. Br J Ca 1982;45:456-65.

52. Gomer CJ, Doiron DR, Rucker N et al. Examination of action spectrum, dose rate and mutagenic properties of hematoporphyrin derivative in photoradiation therapy. In: Porphyrin Localization and Treatment of Tumors, Doiron DR, Gomer CJ (eds), Alan R. Liss, Inc., New York, 1984, pp. 459-69.

53. Grossweiner LI. Membrane photosensitization by hematoporphyrin derivative. In: Porphyrin Localization and Treatment of Tumors, Doiron DR, Gomer CJ (eds), Alan R. Liss, Inc., New York, 1984, pp. 391-404.

54. Dubbelman TMAR, DeGoeij AFPM, Van Steveninck J. Protoporphyrin- induced photodynamic effects on transport processes across the membrane of human erythrocytes. Biochimica et Biophysica Acta 1980;595:133-39.

55. Kessel D. Effects of photo-activated porphyrins on cell surface properties. Biochemical Soc Transactions 1977;5:139-40.

56. Torinuki W, Miura P, Seiji M. Lysosome destruction in lipoperoxide formation due to active oxygen generated from hematoporphyrin and UV irradiation. Br J Derm 1980;102:1727.

57. Wakulckik SD, Schiltz JR, Bickers DR. Photolysis of protoporphyrin-treated human fibroblasts *in vitro*: Studies the mechanism. J Lab Clin Med 1980;96:158-67.

58. Gibson SL, Leakey PB, Crute JJ et al. Photosensitization of mitochondrial cytochrome c oxidase by hematoporphyrin derivative (HPD) *in vivo* and *in vitro*. In: Porphyrin Localization and Treatment of Tumors, Doiron DR, Gomer CJ (eds), Alan R. Liss, Inc., New York, 1984, pp. 323-34.

59. Salet C, Moreno G. Photodynamic effects of hematoporphyrin on respiration and calcium uptake in isolated mitochondria. J Rad Biol 1981;39:227-30.

60. Castellani A, Pace GP, Concioli M. Photodynamic effect of hematoporphyrin on blood microcirculation. J Path Bacteriol 1963;86:99-102.

61. Star WM, Marijnissen JPA, van den Berg-Blok AE et al. Destructive effect of photoradiation on the microcirculation of a rat mammary tumor growing in a 'sandwich' observation chamber. In: Porphyrin Localization and Treatment of Tumors, Doiron DR, Gomer CJ (eds), Alan R. Liss, Inc., New York, 1984, pp. 637-45.

62. Henderson DW, Dougherty TJ, Malone PB. Studies on the mechanism of tumor destruction by photoradiation therapy. In: Porphyrin Localization and Treatment of Tumors, Doiron DR, Gomer CJ (eds), Alan R. Liss, Inc., New York, 1984, pp. 601-12.

63. Bicher HI, Hetzel SW, Vaupel P et al. Microcirculation modifications by localized microwave hyperthermia and hematoporphyrin phototherapy. 11th European Conference on Microcirculation, Garmisch-Partenkirchen, Published in Biblthca Anat 1980;20:628-32.

64. Dougherty TJ, Kaufman JE, Goldfarb A et al. Photoradiation therapy for the treatment of malignant tumors. Ca Res 1978;38:2628- 35.

65. Surgical Application of Lasers. Dixon JA (ed), Year Book Medical Publishers, Chicago, 1984.

66. Hisazumi H, Mitao K, Misaki T et al. An experimental study of photodynamic therapy using a pulsed gold vapor laser. Abstract from International Meeting on Porphyrins as Phototherapeutic Agents for Tumors and Other Diseases, Sardinia, Italy, May 1985.

67. Steve Falk, Cooper LaserSonics, Inc., Personal communication.

68. Profio AE, Doiron DR. A feasibility study of the use of fluorescence bronchoscopy for localization of small lung tumors. Phys Med Biol 1977;22:5,949-57.

69. King EG, Man G, LeRiche J et al. Fluorescence bronchoscopy in the localization of bronchogenic carcinoma. J Ca 1982;49:777-82.

70. Balchum OJ, Doiron DR, Profio AE et al. Fluorescence bronchoscopy for localizing early bronchial cancer in carcinoma in situ. In: Recent Results in Cancer Research, Vol. 82: Springer-Verlag, Berlin and Heidelberg, 1982, pp. 97-120.

71. Kinsey JH, Cortese DA, Sanderson DR. Detection of hematoporphyrin fluorescence during fiberoptic bronchoscopy to localize early bronchogenic carcinoma, Mayo Clinic Proceedings. 1978;53:594-600.

72. Benson Jr. RC. The use of hematoporphyrin derivative (HPD) in the localization and treatment of transitional cell carcinoma (TCC) of the bladder. In: Porphyrin Localization and Treatment of Tumors, Doiron DR, Gomer CJ (eds), Alan R. Liss, Inc., New York, 1984, pp. 795-804.

73. Aizawa K, Kato H, Ono J et al. a new diagnostic system for malignant tumors using hematoporphyrin derivative, laser photoradiation and spectroscope. In: Porphyrin Localization and Treatment of Tumors, Doiron DR, Gomer CJ (eds), Alan R. Liss, Inc., New York, 1984, pp. 501-20.

74. Aizawa K, O'Hata S, Kato H et al. HPD localization using an excimer dye laser. Abstract from International Meeting on Porphyrins as Phototherapeutic Agents for Tumors and Other Diseases, Sardinia, Italy, May 1985.

75. Berns MW, Hammer-Wilson M, Walter RJ et al. Uptake and localization of HPD and 'active fraction' in tissue culture and in serially biopsied human tumors. In: Porphyrin Localization and Treatment of Tumors, Doiron DR, Gomer CJ (eds), Alan R. Liss, Inc., New York, 1984, pp. 501-20.

76. Svaasand LO. Optical dosimetry for direct and interstitial photoradiation therapy of malignant tumors. In: Porphyrin Localization and Treatment of Tumors, Doiron DR, Gomer CJ (eds), Alan R. Liss, Inc., New York, 1984, pp. 91-114.

77. Parrish JA. Photobiologic considerations in photoradiation therapy. In: Porphyrin Sensitization, Kessel E, Dougherty TJ (eds), Plenum Press, New York, 1981, pp. 91-108.

78. Dixon JA, personal communication.

79. Dougherty TJ. Variability in hematoporphyrin derivative preparations. CA Res 1982;42:118.

80. Svaasand LO, Doiron DR. Thermal distribution during photoradiation therapy. In: Porphyrin Sensitization, Kessel E, Dougherty TJ (eds), Plenum Press, New York, 1981, pp. 77- 90.

81. Berenbaum C, Bonnett R, Scourides PA. *In vivo* biological activity of the components of hematoporphyrin derivative. Br J Ca 1982;45:571-81.

82. Waldow SM, Dougherty TJ. Interaction of hyperthermia and photoradiation therapy. Lasers in Surg Med 1984;97:380-385.

83. Waldow SM, Henderson BW, Dougherty TJ. Potentiation of photodynamic therapy by heat. Effect of sequence and time interval between treatment *in vivo*. Lasers in Surg Med 1985;5:83-94.

84. Tulip J, McPhee M, Gonzales S et al. Phototherapy of the Dunning R3327 prostate cancer. Abstract for 5th Annual Mtg. of the Amer. Soc. for Laser Med. & Surg., Florida, 1985.

85. Mew D, Wat C, Towers GHN et al. Photoimmunotherapy: Treatment of animal tumors with tumor-specific monoclonal antibody-porphyrin conjugates. J Immun 1983;130(3):1473-77.

86. Bugelski PJ, Porter CW, Dougherty TJ. Autoradiographic distribution of hematopophyrin derivative in dermal and tumor tissue of the mouse. Ca Res 1979;39:96-100.

310

87. Sery TW. Photodynamic killing of retinoblastoma cells with hematoporphyrin and light. Ca Res 1979;39:96-100.

25. PHOTODYNAMIC THERAPY IN EARLY STAGE CARCINOMA

YOSHIHIRO HAYATA AND JUTARO ONO

Introduction

While attempts to employ hematoporphyrin with light in malignant disease extend for over half a century, the first studies with practical import were published in the early 1960's by Lipson, Olsen and their colleagues (1). They developed a derivative of hematoporphyrin (HPD) which reduced the side effects. Also, they showed that the material was retained at higher levels by malignant tissue than by normal tissue and that the fluorescence of the material emitted upon excitation by light could be employed for diagnostic applications. In the early 1970's, Dougherty, Weishaupt and their colleagues demonstrated that the cytocidal effect is of HPD upon stimulation by light had potential in the treatment of malignant tumors and metastatic lesions of advanced cancer (2-4). They also explored the applications of laser light in combination with HPD in advanced cases (5-8). Their studies and those of other investigators showed that this modality could obtain regression of malignant lesions (9-29).

Beginning in 1978, this modality was evaluated in an experimental canine lung cancer model previously developed in the author's institution. Initially lung cancer was induced by instillation of a carcinogen (20-methylcholanthrene, 20-MC) through a vinyl tube inserted as deeply as possible into the lower lobe bronchi of mongrel dogs and beagles. Peripheral type lung cancer was successfully induced by this method, but it was not possible to observe the development of the lesions due to their location. In order to induce central type lung cancer we began injecting 20-MC at the bifurcation of the right apical and cardiac lobe bronchi via a flexible injection catheter developed in our department for insertion via flexible endoscopes (MN-22C, Olympus Optical, Tokyo). This method successfully induced lung cancer at the injection site with a high rate of success and resulted in an experimental model that could be utilized for basic studies on lung cancer.

By means of the experimental central type lung cancer model, we evaluated the effectiveness of HPD and light systems in early stage lesions experimentally (30). Based upon these results this modality was applied in cases of cancer of the lung and other organs. We refer to this modality as photodynamic therapy (PDT) instead of photoradiation therapy (PRT) in order to prevent possible confusion with vaporization of tissue by high energy laser beams, which is a totally different approach.

D.M. Jensen and J.M. Brunetaud (eds), Medical Laser Endoscopy. 313-330.
© 1990 Kluwer Academic Publishers, Dordrecht

Equipment

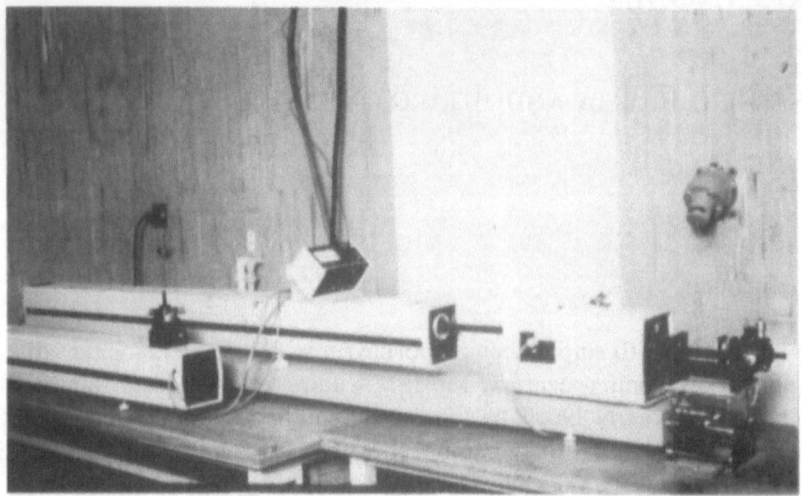

Fig. 25.1. Argon dye laser (Spectra-Physics).

Lasers

The most important point in performing PDT with HPD is to obtain sufficient penetration of the target tissue by light. Since the HPD is activated by light, areas of malignant tissue containing HPD that are not reached by light will remain unaffected, as will the malignant lesion. In cases of cancer of the respiratory, gastric and urinary tract, it is convenient to employ laser light via endoscopy, but for lesions on the body surface, a laser light source is not absolutely necessary. While a 405 nm wavelength krypton ion laser or a 514 nm wavelength argon laser are effective in exciting HPD, their tissue penetration is poor as these wavelengths are easily absorbed by hemoglobin. A 630 nm red wavelength has the best tissue penetration for PDT of lasers presently available. We therefore use argon dye laser systems (Figs. 25.1-25.3). All of these systems produce a 630 nm beam. In the system shown in Fig. 25.3, the built-in computer calculates the energy density administered.

Quartz Fibers

Single strand quartz optical fibers were employed (Quartz Products, Plainfield, NJ and Fujikura Densen, Tokyo). The laser beams are transmitted via the quartz fibers inserted into a connector at the output section of the argon dye laser. The angle of divergence of the beam from the fiber is 22°, but this can be increased by attaching microlens. For photoradiation of a circumferential lesion, such as a central type lung cancer or cancer of the

314

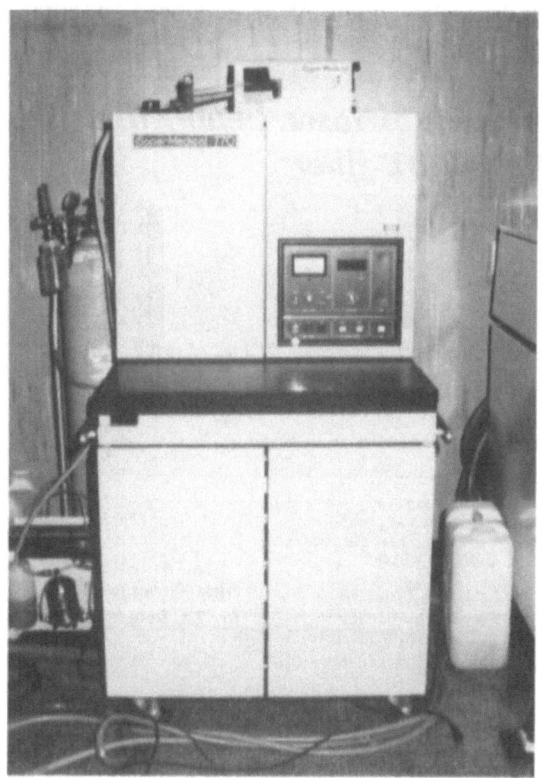

Fig. 25.2. Argon dye laser (Cooper Medical).

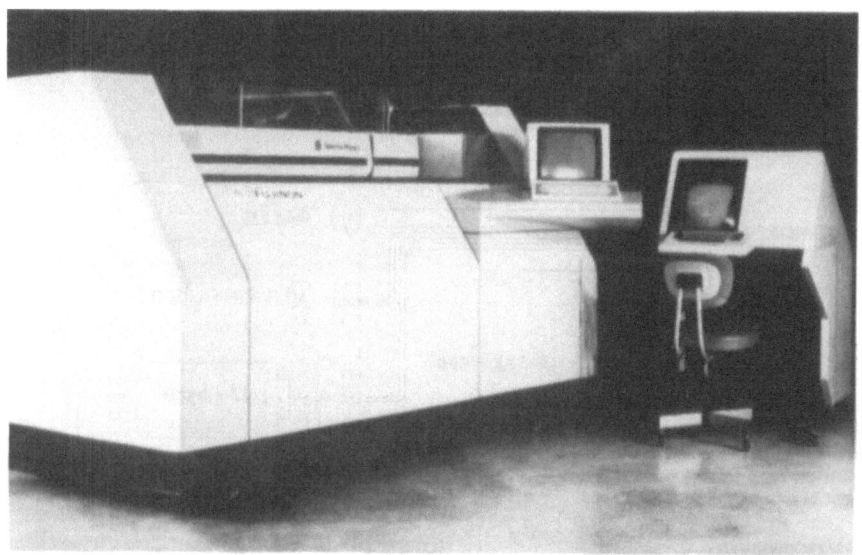

Fig. 25.3. Argon dye laser (Fujinon), the right is a computer to put out necessary energy of an argon dye laser.

esophagus, a cylindrical 360° diffusing tip developed by Potter and Dougherty is employed (Fig. 25.4).

Divergence of laser beam from the tip of the quartz fiber

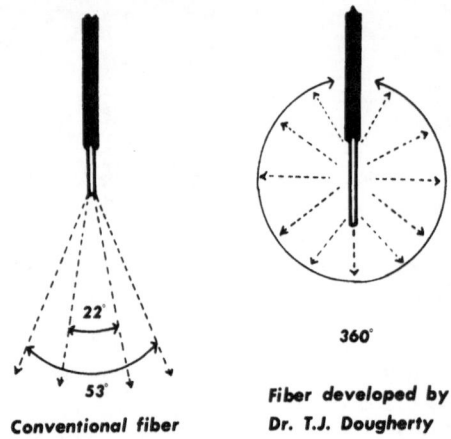

Fig. 25.4. Divergence angle of quartz fiber.

Therapeutic System

The diagram in Fig. 25.5 illustrates how the laser beam is transmitted via the quartz fiber inserted through the instrumentation channel of the fiberoptic bronchoscope. Photoradiation is performed with the tip of the fiber 1-3 cm from the lesion.

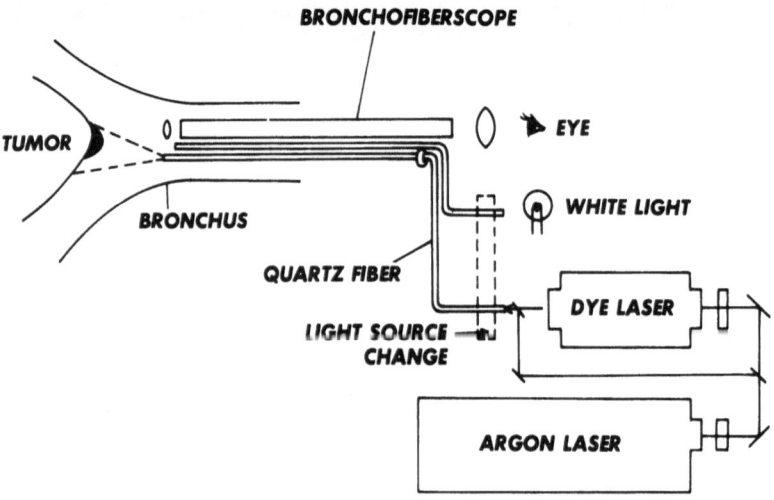

Fig. 25.5. The PDT therapeutic system.

HPD

Initially HPD was kindly provided by Dr. T.J. Dougherty of Roswell Park Memorial Institute and subsequently the same substance has been obtained commercially (Photofrin Medical, Cheektowaga, NY). Generally 2.5-5.0 mg/kg body weight is injected 72 hours before the procedure.

Technique

Insertion of the endoscope is performed under local anesthesia in all procedures. In cases of superficially proliferating lesions, care is exercised to insure that the fiber tip protrudes from the orifice of the instrumentation channel but is not in contact with tissue. When the fiber points in the correct direction and is at a distance of 1-3 cm from the lesion, the foot switch is pressed to transmit the argon dye laser beam. The power of the beam and the time of photoradiation are selected based on the individual conditions of each case, i.e. 100-600 mW for 10-30 minutes. In protruding tumors the quartz fiber is first inserted into the tumor. Because the energy density is only an approximation in cases of superficial photoradiation, we express the light density given as an estimated energy dose (e.e.d.) based on the estimation of the average distance of the tip of the quartz fiber from the lesion.

Results

PDT in Early Stage Central Type Lung Cancer

PDT was performed in 35 cases of early stage (stage Ia) central type lung cancer. These cases were diagnosed endoscopically and roentgenologically as early stage by three experts. Twenty-one of the 35 cases were treated with PDT alone because of inoperability due to poor pulmonary function in 12 and refusal of surgery in 9. The others were resected after PDT because remaining tumor was suspected after PDT. The histological type was squamous cell carcinoma in all cases except one case of adenocarcinoma. The therapeutic results of PDT are shown in Tables 25.1 and 25.2.

Complete tumor remission (no evidence of tumor endoscopically, cytologically or histologically) was obtained in all 21 non-resected cases after PDT and in 5 resected cases. Significant remission (more than 60% of the tumor volume disappeared) was obtained in the other 9 resected case.

Case No. 1 died of pneumonia 46 months after PDT, case No. 2 died of cerebral infarction 31 months after PDT, case No. 4 died of prostatic carcinoma 33 months after PDT, case no. 18 died of C.O.P.D. 23 months after PDT and case No. 21 died of liver cancer 16 months after PDT. Recurrence was the cause of deaths in cases No. 5, 8 and 10. The remaining 13 non-resected cases are

Table 25.1. Therapeutic results of PDT in inoperable early stage lung cancer cases.

Case No.	Age	Sex	Location of the tumor	Histologic type	Reasons for PDT only	Combined therapy	Survival (months)	Prognosis	
Group I									
1. JM	74	M	R.B²b	Sq. Ca.	Refused surgery		46	Dead*	
2. KO	76	M	L.B¹⁰A	,,	Poor pulm.func.	Radiation Immuno	31	Dead**	
3. TO	59	F	R.u.lobe br	,,	,,		76	Alive	
4. SK	70	M	R.u.lobe br	,,	,,		33	Dead***	
5. MC	62	M	L.B¹⁺²ab	,,	,,		16	Dead*	Rec
6. TK	70	M	R.u.lobe br	,,	,,		61	Alive	
7. YK	62	M	L.B¹⁺²	,,	Refused surgery	Chemo	61	Alive	
8. EA	71	M	L.B³	,,	,,	,,	23	Dead*	Rec
9. SH	70	M	R.u.lobe br	,,	,,	,,	27	Alive	
10. TO	75	M	L.B¹⁺²	,,	Poor pulm.func.	Radiation	26	Alive	Rec
11. MS	77	M	L.I.lobe br	Ad. ca.	Poor pulm.func.		22	Alive	
12. KT	44	M	L.u.lobe br	Sq. ca.	Refused surgery		19	Alive	
13. KT	79	M	L.B.⁶	,,	Poor pulm func.	Radiation	15	Alive	
14. CS	62	M	RB¹	,,	,,		7	Alive	
15. KY	59	M	RB³ab	,,	,,		7	Alive	
16. KC	65	M	R.u.lobe br	,,	Refused surgery		4	Alive	
Group II									
17. TU	58	M	R.B⁷	,,	Refused surgery		38	Alive	
18. YS	81	M	L.I.lobe br	,,	Poor pulm.func.		23	Dead*	
	82		R.B⁷	,,	,,		10	Dead*	
19. TK	58	M	L.B⁹	,,	Refused surgery		33	Alive	
20. TK	41	M	L.u.div.br.	,,	,,		29	Alive	
21. KM	79	M	L.I.lobe br	,,	Poor pulm.func.		16	Dead****	

N.B.: Sq.ca.: squamous cell carcinoma, u.lobe = upper lobe, pulm. func. = pulmonary function,

   * Died of pneumonia or C.O.P.D.   Group I: Biopsy (+)

  ** Died of cerebral infarction   Cytology (+)

 *** prostatic carcinoma   Group II: Biopsy (−)

**** liver carcinoma   Cytology (+)

Chemo = chemotherapy, Immuno = immunotherapy, Rec.: Recurrence

apparently disease free at 6-76 months after PDT. The 14 resected cases after PDT are apparently disease free at from 15-76 months (except for 3 fatalities).

Case No. 1 (See Atlas – Plate 75), a nodular tumor, 2.0 mm in diameter, was observed in the right B_2b of a 74 year-old male. This case was chest X-ray negative and sputum cytology positive. The case was a good indication for surgery, but the patient refused surgery adamantly. The lesion was photoradiated three times and the tumor disappeared 3 days after the first PDT. He died of pneumonia 46 months after PDT, however, autopsy revealed no tumor macroscopically or microscopically (Fig. 25.6).

Case No. 2 was a 76 year-old male with a cough. Invasive squamous cell carcinoma was detected endoscopically in left $B_{10}a$ (Fig. 25.7).

Since the case was inoperable due to poor pulmonary function, the lesion

Table 25.2. Therapeutic results of PDT in early stage lung cancer cases resected after PDT.

Case No.	Age	Sex	Location of the tumor	Histologic type	Result	Combined therapy	Survival (months)	Prognosis
Group I								
1. YA	50	M	L.u.lobe br	Sq. Ca.	SR	Chemo	76	Alive
2. TF	54	M	R.B⁸	,,	SR	,,	65	,,
3. SN	74	M	L.B¹⁺²	,,	CR	Immuno.	63	,,
4. BN	70	M	L.u.lobe br	,,	SR	Radial.	41	Dead
5. KS	62	M	L.B¹⁺² ab	,,	CR		35	Alive
6. TM	81	M	R.u.lobe br	,,	SR		32	Alive
7. KN	65	M	R.B³	,,	SR		38	Alive
8. YO	50	M	R.B¹⁰	,,	SR		26	Alive
9. KO	75	M	L.u.lobe br	,,	SR	Immuno.	23	Dead Rec*
10. SK	64	M	LB³	,,	CR		15	Alive
Group II								
11. YI	70	M	R.B²a		SR		39	Alive
12. SM	36	M	R.u.lobe br	,,	CR		36	Alive
13. NY	54	M	R.B.⁶	,,	SR		11	Dead
14. BT	62	M	L. main	,,	CR		18	Alive

N.B. = u.lobe, Sq.ca. = squamous cell carcinoma
Group I: Biopsy positive, Cytology positive
Group II: Biopsy negative, Cytology positive
*Recurrence at left main bronchus (invasion from lymph node)

was treated with PDT. He died of cerebral infarction 31 months after PDT. Clinically there was no evidence of recurrence but the patient's family did not permit an autopsy.

Case No. 3 was a 59 year-old female in whom thickening and irregularity was observed endoscopically at the orifice of the right upper lobe bronchus (Fig. 25.8). The lesion was photoradiated because of inoperability due to poor pulmonary function and slight asthma. She is apparently disease free 76 months after PDT.

Case No. 5 was a 62 year-old male. The invasive tumor on the left ($B_{1+2}ab$) was treated with PDT because of inoperability due to chronic obstructive pulmonary disease (COPD). He died of COPD 16 months after PDT, and autopsy revealed that tumor on the left $B_{1+2}ab$ had disappeared, but tumor cells were recognized in the area beyond $B_{1+2}ab$. Probably the laser beam did not reach this area sufficiently.

Case No. 8 was a 71 year-old male. The nodular tumor in left B_3 was a good indication for surgery, but was treated with PDT because he refused surgery (Fig. 25.9).

After PDT the tumor disappeared completely, and no tumor cells were observed cytologically. However, recurrence developed 20 months after PDT (Fig. 25.10). We performed lobectomy of the left upper lobe and lymph node involvement was recognized in the bronchopulmonary region. He died of pneumonia three weeks after surgery.

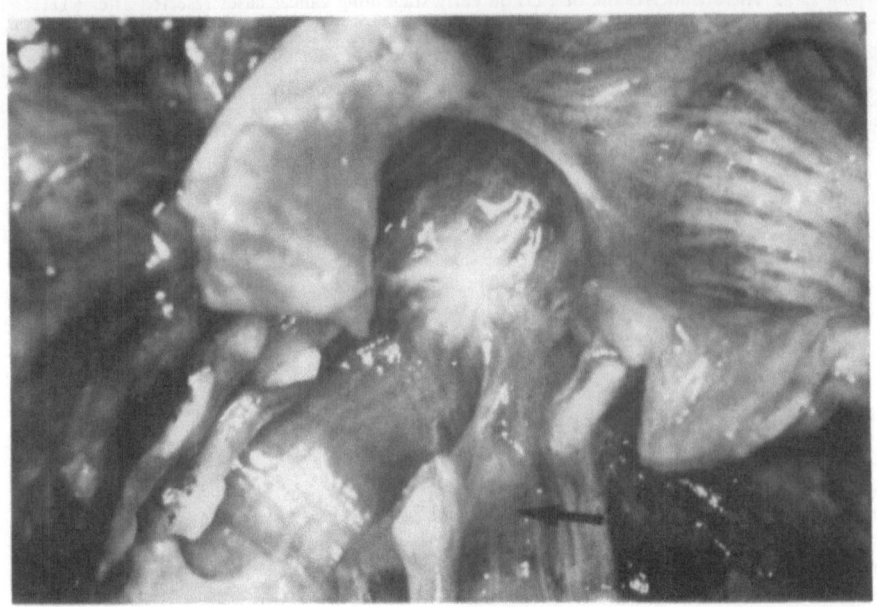

Fig. 25.6. Autopsied specimen of Case 1 (Atlas Plate 75) shows no tumor in right B_2b.

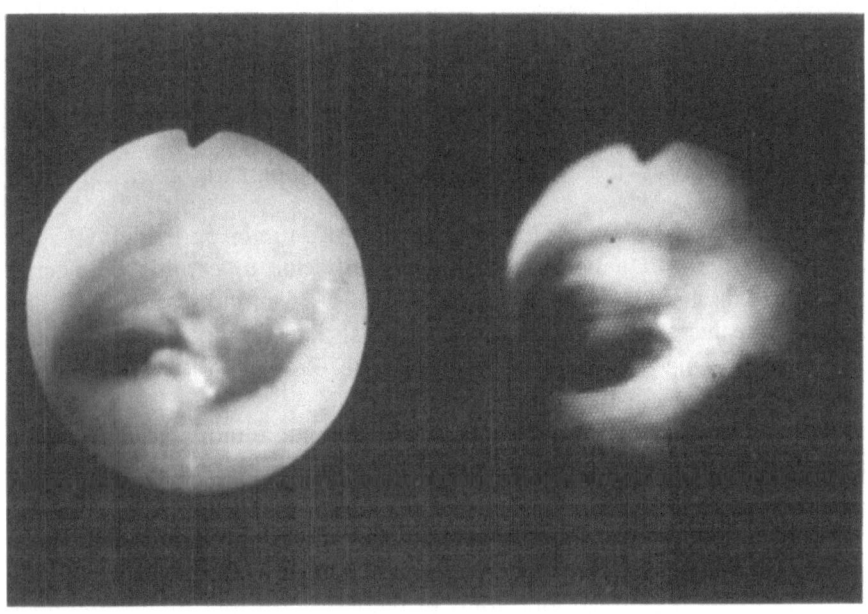

Fig. 25.7. Case No. 2. Invasive squamous cell carcinoma in left $B_{10}a$ (left). The tumor disappeared after PDT (right).

320

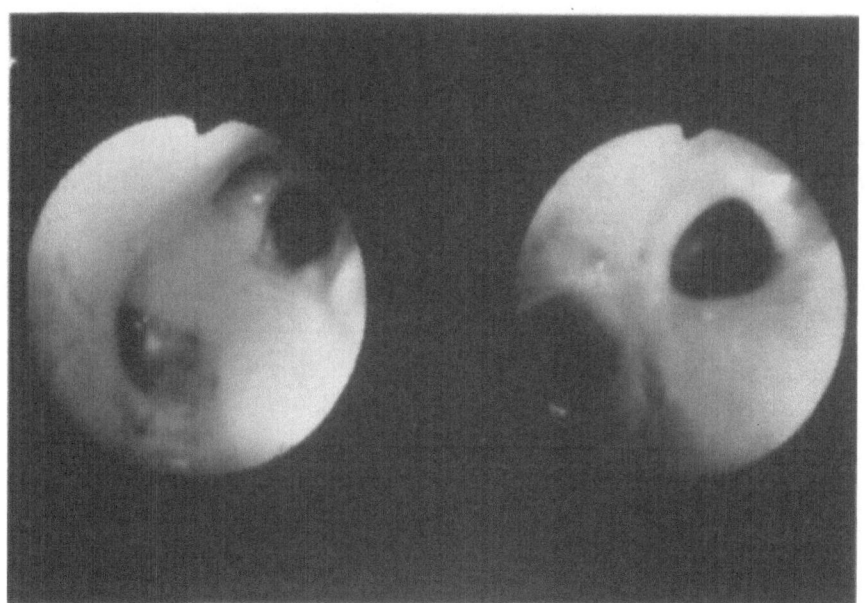

Fig. 25.8. Case No. 3, squamous cell carcinoma. Thickening and irregularity can be seen at the orifice of the right upper lobe bronchus (left). The tumor disappeared after PDT (right).

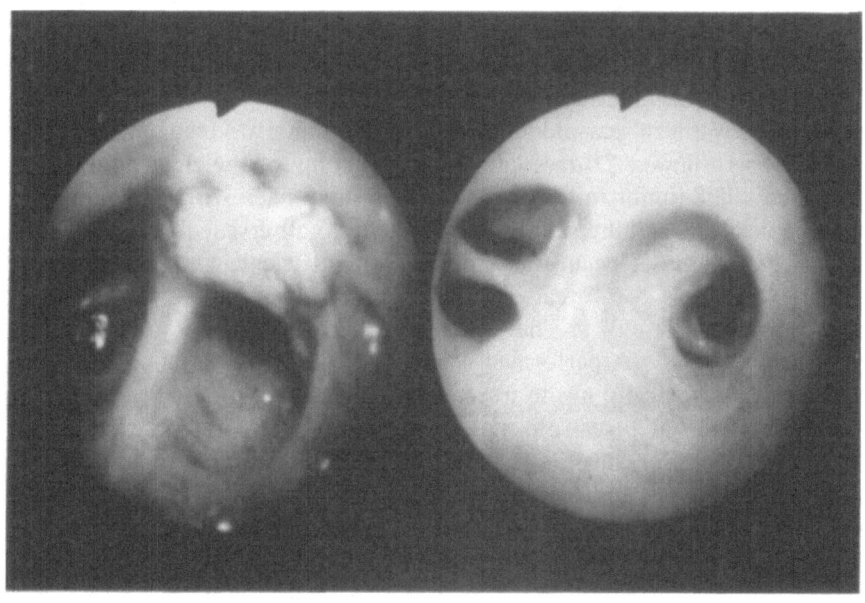

Fig. 25.9. Case No. 8 was a nodular squamous cell carcinoma tumor in left B$_3$ (left) which disappeared after PDT (right).

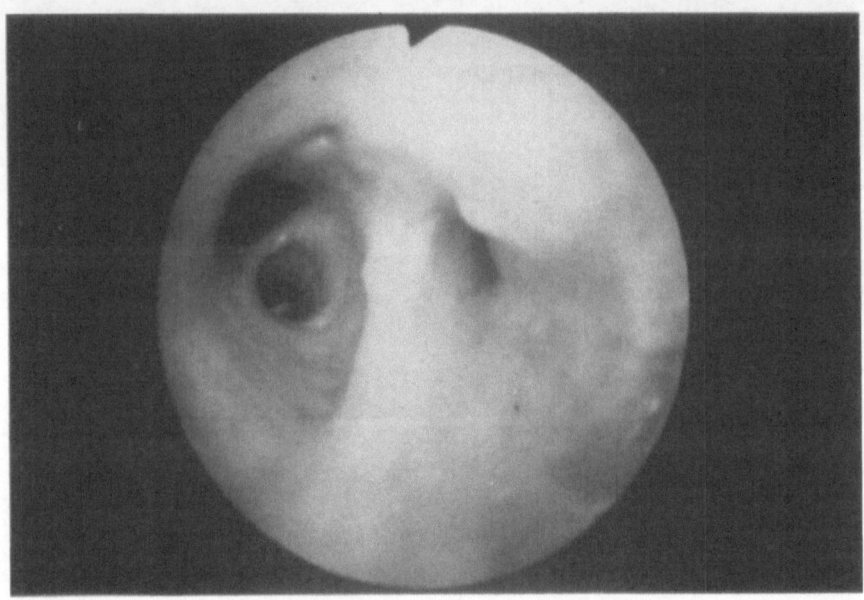

Fig. 25.10. Case No. 8, recurrence 20 months after PDT.

Case No. 1 was a 50 year-old male. An invasive tumor was recognized in the left main bronchus and the orifice of left B_{1+2} and B_3. The lesion was photoradiated superficially and pneumonectomy was performed 2 weeks after PDT because remaining tumor was suspected. In the resected specimen no tumor cells were observed in the left main bronchus. However, remaining tumor nests were observed in the orifice of left B_{1+2} and B_3. The laser beam probably did not reach these areas sufficiently (Table 25.2).

Case No. 2 was a 54 year-old male. A polypoid tumor was recognized in right B_8. PDT was followed 23 days later by bilobectomy of the right middle and lower lobes. The tumor in left B_8 had disappeared macroscopically, however, microscopically remaining small tumor nests were observed. In this case also the power of the laser beam was probably not sufficient.

Case No. 3 was a 74 year-old male. An invasive tumor was observed endoscopically in left B_{1+2}. The lesion was photoradiated and lobectomy of the left upper lobe was performed 4 weeks after PDT. No tumor cells were recognized histologically in the resected specimen.

Case No. 4 was a 70 year-old male. An invasive tumor was observed in the left upper lobe bronchus (Fig. 25.11). The lesion was photoradiated but lobectomy of the left upper lobe was performed 9 weeks after PDT because remaining tumor was suspected. The resected specimen showed that most of the tumor in the left upper lobe bronchus had disappeared, but remaining tumor nests were recognized in the orifices of B_{1+2}, B_3, B_4 and B_5. Also tumor nests remained submucosally even in the left upper lobe bronchus (Fig. 25.12).

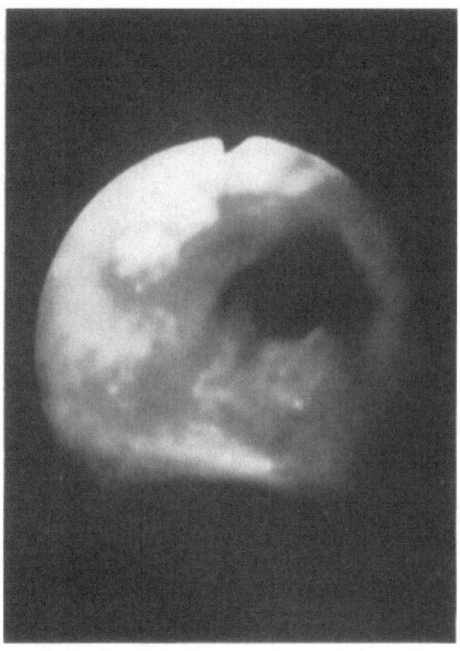

Fig. 25.11. Case No. 4, invasive tumor in the left upper lobe bronchus before PDT, squamous cell carcinoma.

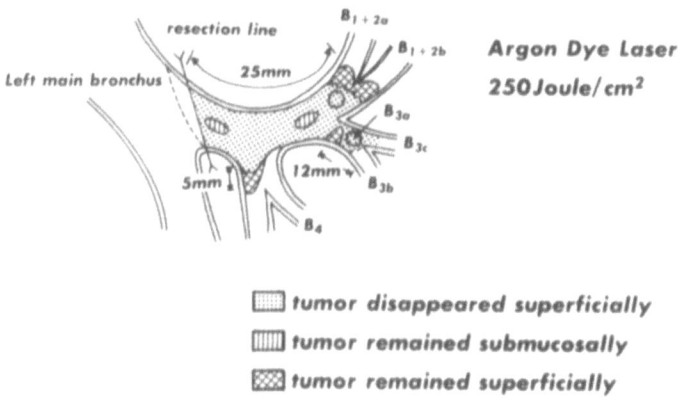

Fig. 25.12. Diagram of the histologic examination of resected specimen of case No. 12.

Case No. 5 was a 62 year-old male in whom invasive tumor was observed in left B_{1+2} (Fig. 25.13).

The lesion was treated with PDT and lobectomy of the left upper lobe was performed 6 weeks after PDT. In the resected specimen no tumor cells were recognized histologically (Fig. 25.14).

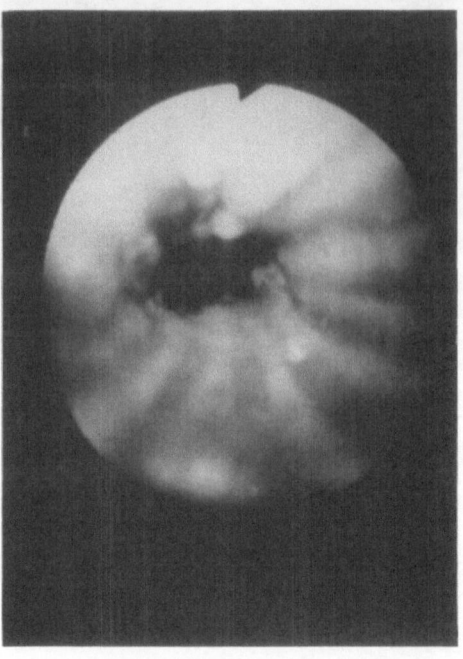

Fig. 25.13. Case No. 5, invasive tumor in left B_{1+2}ab before PDT (squamous cell carcinoma).

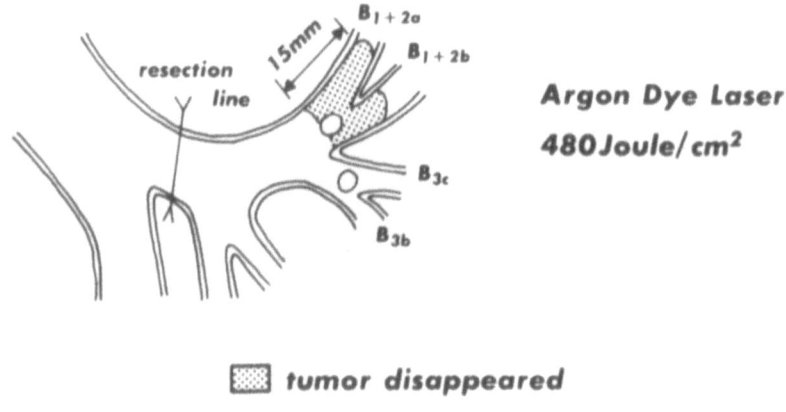

Fig. 25.14. Diagram of the resected specimen of case No. 5.

PDT in Early Stage Esophageal Cancer

PDT was performed in 7 cases of superficial esophageal cancer (early stage). Of these PDT was performed after surgical reconstruction of the esophagus in one case, in one case of refusal of surgery and in 5 cases which were inoperable due to poor pulmonary function. Complete tumor remission was obtained in all five and they are apparently disease free at from 47-79 months after PDT.

However, in the other 2 cases which were resected after PDT tumor nests were observed.

Case No. 1; a 65 year-old male, a superficial invading tumor developed in the cervical esophagus after reconstruction of the esophagus (See Plate 76 in Atlas).

The lesion was photoradiated with an energy of 480 Joules/cm². The tumor disappeared completely after PDT, and he is apparently disease free 36 months after PDT.

The reason why complete tumor remission was not obtained in two resected cases after PDT is probably that the laser beam did not reach the entire lesion in one of the cases and because the wavelength of the laser changed as a result of mechanical difficulties in the other case.

PDT in Early Stage Gastric Cancer

PDT was performed in 17 cases of early stage gastric cancer.

Five of the 17 cases were treated with PDT alone because of poor general condition in 4 and refusal of surgery in one. Complete tumor remission was obtained in all, however, recurrence developed in 2, 27 and 4 months after PDT respectively.

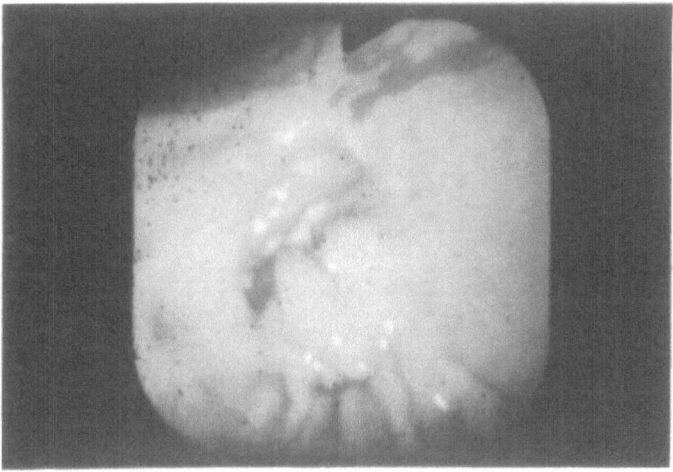

Fig. 25.15. Case No. 5 of the early stage gastric cancer. Superficial early gastric cancer in the greater curvature.

Case No. 5 was a 50 year-old male in whom superficial early stage gastric cancer was detected by a mass survey (Fig. 25.15). The case was a good indication for surgery, but he adamantly refused surgery. Therefore the lesion was photoradiated with an energy of 360 Joules/cm² and the tumor disappeared completely (Fig. 25.16). However, recurrence developed 27 months after PDT (Fig. 25.17).

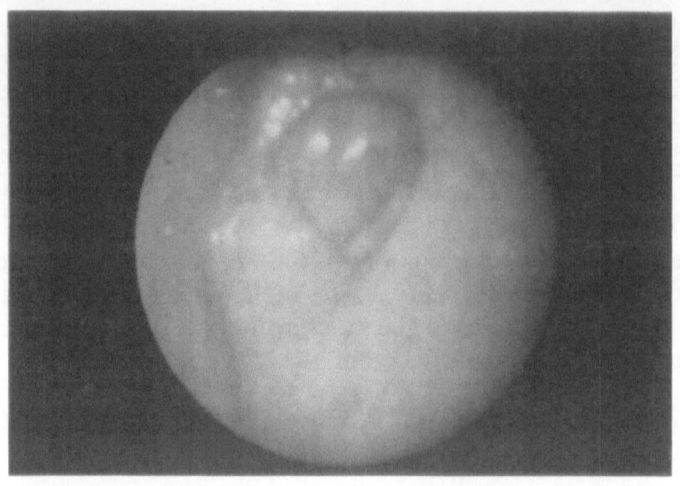

Fig. 25.16. The tumor disappeared after PDT (case No. 5, Fig. 15).

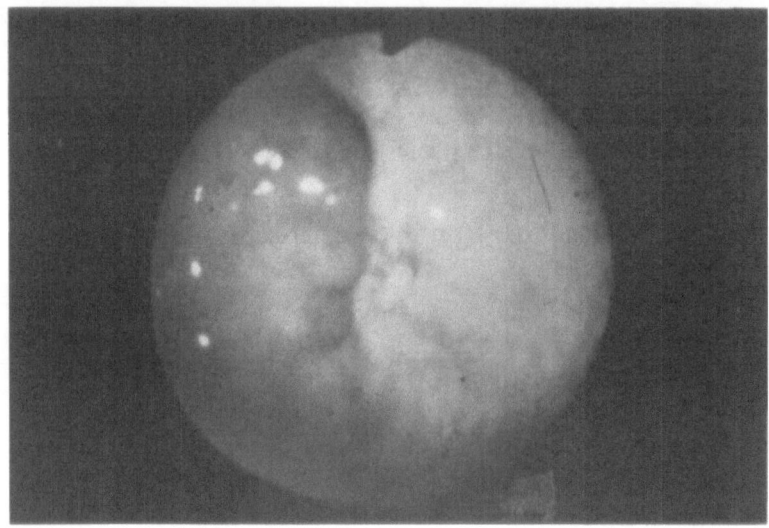

Fig. 25.17. 27 months after PDT showing recurrence (case no. 5, Fig. 15).

He again strongly refused surgery, therefore we performed PDT again recently. However, complete tumor remission was not obtained. Now we are following the case up.

Thirteen of the 17 cases were resected after PDT and complete tumor remission was verified in 6, however, remaining tumor nests were recognized histologically in the resected specimen in the other 7 cases. The reason for this is probably due to the difficult photoradiation angle due to the location of the lesion, technical failure, submucosal invasion or insufficient PDT due to peristaltic movement or gastric folds.

Discussion

Careful evaluation and selection of early stage lesions are extremely important in performing PDT in early stage cases of cancer of the lung, esophagus and stomach. In particular, endoscopic and histologic diagnosis are significant. Concerning this point, recent research has demonstrated that in central type lung cancer there are two types of intrabronchial growth. One is the primarily mucosal type, i.e. exposed in the bronchial lumen, and the other is primarily submucosal. PDT can be indicated in the former but less so in the latter. Therefore it is necessary to check endoscopic and histologic findings in meticulous detail. It may be necessary to obtain large biopsy specimens by deep bites in the bronchial wall in order to correctly assess the extent of invasion in the bronchial wall. Before treatment, this aggressive approach to staging and characterizing the cancer may lead to a better selection and better treatment results with PDT. Early stage cancers can be treated with PDT and more advanced tumors with other methods.

In early stage cancer of the lung, esophagus and stomach, complete tumor remission was achieved in some cases but not always. While complete cure by this method represents a revolutionary development, it is essential to analyze why complete cure was not achieved in some early stage cases. While correct staging is the most important factor because of the limited penetration of PDT, technical factors may preclude complete lesion treatment via endoscopy. Lesions located in sites that are difficult to view en face or circumferential lesions may require an extra effort to treat with PDT. For example, circumferential cancers in canalicular organs may require cylindrical diffusers to photoradiate the entire wall. Furthermore, in some cases the combination of non-touch and interstitial PDT technique may be necessary. Another factor accounting for differences in therapeutic results of PDT may be due to differences in histologic type. Further research will be required to delineate the role of each factor in the clinical response to endoscopic PDT. For example, squamous cell carcinoma seems more responsive to PDT than adenocarcinoma of the same stage.

Presently, PDT is indicated in cases that can be entirely visualized endoscopically. Furthermore, in submucosally invading tumors the lesion should not extend beyond the muscular layer or beyond the cartilage layer of the larger airways. The most important point is whether sufficient penetration of the lesion by light can be anticipated.

An important question is whether PDT is indicated in early stage carcinoma. Cortese et al. recently reported that it is difficult to rule out lymph node metastasis even in early stage cancer (31). Based upon these data and our own experience we feel that only certain patients should be selected for PDT: 1) those who refuse surgery or 2) those in whom PDT can reduce the extent of resection required thereby rendering them operable.

Concerning the complications of PDT and HPD slight sunburn developed in 62% of cases even though they stayed indoors for 2 weeks. Severe sunburn developed in only 3 cases. All of these patients had ignored our instructions to avoid direct sunlight. Obstructive pneumonia developed in 2 of 89 lung cancer cases. In this regard, bronchial toilet is necessary for 2 or 3 days after PDT. Bronchial fistula developed in 2 lung cancer cases and one died due to massive bleeding, but the exact relationship between PDT and these sequelae is unclear because they received radiotherapy after PDT. In esophageal cancer cases, esophageal reflux developed in some cases for 2 or 3 days after the procedure. Esophageal fistula developed in one case receiving PDT and radiotherapy. In gastric cancer epigastralgia developed in most cases after PDT but was relieved within 7 days by medical treatment.

In conclusion, we have demonstrated that complete cure can be obtained by PDT in some early stage cancer cases. However, our results also demonstrate that in some early stage cases, complete cure was not obtained by this method. While this method is clinically a powerful new weapon in the anticancer arsenal, its efficacy must be further improved.

Acknowledgement

The authors wish to express their deep gratitude to Associate Professor J.P. Barron of St. Marianna University School of Medicine for his review of the manuscript.

References

1. Lipson RL, Baldes EJ and Olsen AM. The use of hematoporphyrin in tumor detection. J Natl Cancer Inst 1961;26:1-11
2. Dougherty TJ, Grindey GB, Fiel R, Weishaupt KR and Boyle DG. Photoradiation therapy. II Cure of animal tumors with hematoporphyrin and light. J Natl Cancer Inst 1975;55:115- 121
3. Dougherty TJ, Kaufman JE, Goldfarb A, Weishaupt KR, Boyle D and Mittleman A. Photoradiation therapy for the treatment of malignant tumors. Cancer Res 1978;38:2628-2635
4. Dougherty TJ, Lawrence G, Kaufman JH, Boyle D, Weishaupt KR and Goldfarb A. Photoradiation in the treatment of recurrent breast carcinoma, Cancer Research 1979;62:231-237
5. Dougherty TJ. Hematoporphyrin derivative for detection and treatment of cancer. J Surg Oncol 1980;15:209-210
6. Dougherty TJ, Thoma RE, Boyle DG and Weishaupt DR. Interstitial photoradiation therapy for primary solid tumors in pet cats and dogs. Cancer Res 1981;41:401-404
7. Dougherty TJ. Photoradiation therapy for cutaneous and subcutaneous malignancies. J Invest Dermatol 1981;77:122- 124
8. Dougherty TJ, Boyle DG, Weishaupt DR, Henderson BA, Potter WR, Bellnier DA and Witky KE. Photoradiation therapy – Clinical and drug advances. Adv Exp Med Biol 1983:160:3-13

9. Benson RC Jr, Kinsey JH, Cortese DA, Farrow GM and Utz DC. Treatment of transitional cell carcinoma of the bladder with hematoporphyrin derivative phototherapy. J Urol 1983;130(6):1090- 1095

10. Cortese DA and Kinsey JH. Hematoporphyrin-derivative phototherapy for local treatment of cancer of the tracheobronchial tree. Ann Otol Rhinol Laryngol 1982;91:652- 655

11. Dahlman A, Wile AG, Burns RG, Mason GR, Johnson FM and Berns MW. Laser photoradiation therapy of cancer. Cancer Res 1983;43:430- 434

12. Diamond I, Granelli SG, McDonagh AG, Nielsen S, Wilson CB and Jaenicke R. Photodynamic therapy of malignant tumors. Lancet 1972;2:1175-1177

13. Doiron DR, Svaasand LO and Profio AE. Light dosimetry in tissue: Application to photoradiation therapy. Adv Exp Med Biol 1983;160:63-76

14. Douglass HO Jr, Nava HR, Weishaupt KR, Boyle D, Sugerman MG, Halpern E and Dougherty TJ. Intra-abdominal applications of hematoporphyrin photoradiation therapy. Adv Exp Med Biol 1983;160:15-21

15. Forbes IJ, Cowled PA, Leong AS, Ward AD, Black RB, Blake AJ and Jacka FJ. Phototherapy of human tumors using hematoporphyrin derivative. Med J Aust 1980;2:489-493

16. Gomer CJ, Doiron DR, Jester JV, Szirth BC and Murphree AL. Hematoporphyrin derivative photoradiation therapy for the treatment of intraocular tumors: Examination of acute normal ocular tissue toxicity. Cancer Res 1983;43:721-727

17. Hayata Y, Kato H, Konaka C, Ono J and Takizawa N. Hematoporphyrin derivative and laser photoradiation in the treatment of lung cancer. Chest 1982;81:269-277

18. Hayata Y, Kato H, Konaka C, Aida M, Ono J and Nishimiya K. Hematoporphyrin derivative and photoradiation for tumor localization and treatment of lung cancer. In: Lung Cancer 1982, Editors: S. Ishikawa, Y. Hayata, K. Suemasu, 55-72 Excerpta Medica, Amsterdam-Oxford-Princeton, 1982

19. Hayata Y, Dougherty TJ (eds). Lasers and Hematoporphyrin Derivative in Cancer. IGAKU-SHOIN Tokyo, New York 1983

20. Hayata Y, Kato H, Amemiya R et al. Indications of photoradiation therapy in early stage lung cancer on the basis of post-PRT histologic findings. Doiron D.R. ed. Clayton Foundation Symposium on Porphyrin Localization and Treatment of Tumors. 747- 758, Alan R. Liss Inc. 1984

21. Hayata Y, Kato H, Konaka C, Amemiya R, Ono J, Ogawa I, Kinoshita K, Sakai H and Takahashi H. Photoradiation therapy with hematoporphyrin derivative in early and stage I lung cancer. Chest 1984;86:169-177

22. Hisazumi H, Misaki T and Miyoshi N. Photoradiation therapy of bladder tumors. J Urol 1983;86:168-177

23. Kato H, Konaka C, Ono J, Matsushima Y, Nishimiya K, Lay J, Sawa H, Shinohara H, Saito T, Kinoshita K, Tomono T, Aida M and Hayata Y. Effectiveness of HPD and radiation therapy in lung cancer. Adv Exp Med Biol 1983;160:23-39

24. Laws ER, Cortese DA, Kinsey JH, Eagan RT and Anderson RE. Photoradiation therapy in the treatment of malignant brain tumors: A phase I (Feasibility) study. Neurosurgery 1981;9:672-678

25. Murphree AL, Gomer CJ, Doiron DR and Benedict WF. Recent developments in the genetics and treatment of retinoblastoma. Birth Defects 1982;18:681-687

26. Soma H, Akiya S, Nutahara S, Kato H and Hayata Y. Treatment of vaginal carcinoma with laser photoradiation following administration of hematoporphyrin derivative. Ann Chir Gynecol 1982;71:133-136

27. Tsuchiya A, Obara N, Niwa M et al. Hematoporphyrin derivative and laser photoradiation in the diagnosis and treatment of bladder cancer. J Urol 1983;130:79-82

28. Vincent RG, Dougherty TJ, Rao U and Doiron DR. Hematoporphyrin derivative in the diagnosis and treatment of lung cancer. Adv Ep Med Biol 1983;130:79-82

29. Vincent RG, Dougherty TJ, Rao U, Boyle DG and Potter WR. Photoradiation therapy in advanced carcinoma of the trachea and bronchus. Chest 1984;85(1):29-33

30. Hayata Y, Kato H, Konaka C, Hayashi N, Tahara M, Saito T, Ono J. Fiberoptic bronchoscopic

photoradiation in experimentally induced canine lung cancer. Cancer 1983;51:50-56

31. Cortese DA, Pairolero PC, Bergstralh EJ, Woolner LB, Uhlenhopp MA, Piehler JM, Sanderson DR, Bernatz PE, Williams DE, Taylor WF, Payne WS and Fontana RS. Roentgenographically occult lung cancer. A ten-year experience. J Thorac Cardiovasc Surg 1983;86(3):373-380.

INDEX

339

Developments in Gastroenterology

1. A. S. Peña, I.T. Weterman, C.C. Booth and W. Strober (eds.): *Recent Advances in Crohn's Disease*. Proceedings of the 2nd International Workshop on Crohn's Disease, held in Noordwijk/Leiden, The Netherlands (1980). 1981   ISBN 90–247–2475–9

2. P.M. Motta and L.J.A. Didio (eds.): *Basic and Clinical Hepatology*. 1982
   ISBN 90–247–2404–X

3. D. Rachmilewitz (ed.): *Inflammatory Bowel Diseases*. Proceedings of the 1st International Symposium, held in Jerusalem, Israel (1981). 1982   ISBN 90–247–2612–3

4. D. Fleischer, D. Jensen and P. Bright-Asare (eds.): *Therapeutic Laser Endoscopy in Gastrointestinal Disease*. 1983   ISBN 0–89838–577–6

5. S.P. Borriello (ed.): *Antibiotic Associated Diarrhoea and Colitis*. The Role of *Clostridium difficile* in Gastrointestinal Disorders. 1984   ISBN 0–89838–623–3

6. Ch.H. Gips and R.A.F. Krom (eds.): *Progress in Liver Transplantation*. 1985
   ISBN 0–89838–726–4

7. G.F. Nelis, J. Boevé and J.J. Misiewicz (eds.): *Peptic Ulcer Disease: Basic and Clinical Aspects*. Proceedings of a Symposium on Peptic Ulcer Today, held at the Sophia Zieken-huis, Zwolle, The Netherlands (1984). 1985   ISBN 0–89838–759–0

8. D. Rachmilewitz (ed.): *Inflammatory Bowel Diseases 1986*. Proceedings of the 2nd International Symposium, held in Jerusalem, Israel (1985). 1986   ISBN 0–89838–796–5

9. E.M.H. Mathus-Vliegen: *The Role of Laser in Gastroenterology*. Analysis of Eight Years' Experience. 1989   ISBN 0–7923–0425–X

10. D.M. Jensen and J.-M. Brunetaud (eds.): *Medical Laser Endoscopy*. 1990
    ISBN 0–7923–0579–5

11. D. Rachmilewitz and J. Zimmerman (eds.): *Inflammatory Bowel Diseases 1990*. Proceedings of the 3rd International Symposium, held in Jerusalem, Israel (1989). 1990
    ISBN 0–7923–0657–0

Kluwer Academic Publishers – Dordrecht / Boston / London